Alternative Remedies and Natural Products for Cancer Therapy: An Integrative Approach

Edited by

Motamarri Venkata Naga Lalitha Chaitanya
School of Pharmacy
Lovely Professional University
Phagwara, 144402
Punjab, India

Galvina Pereira
Bombay college of Pharmacy
Mumbai, India

&

Heyam Saad Ali
Pharmaceutics Department,
University of Khartoum, Khartoum
Sudan

Alternative Remedies and Natural Products for Cancer Therapy: An Integrative Approach

Editors: Motamarri Venkata Naga Lalitha Chaitanya, Galvina Pereira and Heyam Saad Ali

ISBN (Online): 978-981-5124-69-9

ISBN (Print): 978-981-5124-70-5

ISBN (Paperback): 978-981-5124-71-2

Published by Bentham Science Publishers Pte. Ltd. Singapore. All Rights Reserved.

First published in 2023.

need for a court order if at any point you breach any terms of this License Agreement. In no event will any delay or failure by Bentham Science Publishers in enforcing your compliance with this License Agreement constitute a waiver of any of its rights.

3. You acknowledge that you have read this License Agreement, and agree to be bound by its terms and conditions. To the extent that any other terms and conditions presented on any website of Bentham Science Publishers conflict with, or are inconsistent with, the terms and conditions set out in this License Agreement, you acknowledge that the terms and conditions set out in this License Agreement shall prevail.

Bentham Science Publishers Pte. Ltd.
80 Robinson Road #02-00
Singapore 068898
Singapore
Email: subscriptions@benthamscience.net

BENTHAM SCIENCE

CONTENTS

FOREWORD

Cancer is the second leading cause of mortality worldwide. Integrative therapies and botanicals are sought for their ability to exhibit anti-carcinogenic activity *via* interfering with the onset and progression of cancer at various stages such as cellular proliferation, differentiation, apoptosis, angiogenesis, and metastasis. Nature offers a vast untapped repository of biomolecules possessing structural diversity that could be mined for their potential application in cancer therapy. Integrative medicine is now acknowledged worldwide, and efforts are going on to understand these systems through the lenses of modern science. The authors of the book "Alternative Remedies and Natural products for Cancer: An Integrative Approach" have brought an excellent compilation of recent findings in this domain and present an elaborate discussion on the mechanisms, efficacy, and utility of complementary systems approach to alleviation, mitigation and techniques for addressing varied types of cancers. Through this book, the authors emphasize, educate and appreciate the importance of the translational role of botanical and integrative approaches such as acupuncture, yoga, alternative therapies, the role of phytochemicals, dietary supplements, *etc*. This book provides a holistic view of all the translational approaches and botanicals used in cancer treatment and acquaints us with modern techniques in anticancer drug discovery from a botanical perspective which will be very useful especially to researchers, medical practioners, P.G. students, PhD scholars and society including the common man in order to understand the reality of translational approaches in addressing cancer, its treatment and prevention

Monica Gulati
School of Pharmacy
Lovely Professional University
Phagwara, 144402
Punjab, India

PREFACE

The purpose of the book is to understand, emphasize, and appreciate the role of complementary and alternative medicine systems like Ayurveda, Acupuncture, Yoga, Mudras, Aromatherapy, and Homeopathy in the management of cancer. One of the vital factors that affect the development and spread of this disease is the lack of immunity and resistance. Through this book, we intend to offer our readers an amalgamation of interesting topics like natural immune-boosting foods, recipes, and herbs that fight against cancer coupled with modern drug discovery techniques such as in silico methods, High-throughput screening, and methods to convert these herbs into leads with suitable illustrations. This book emphasizes the role of spirulina, super green foods, weeds, African herbs, mushrooms, multi-targeting anticancer phytochemicals, and terpenoids as modern anticancer botanicals in the 21st century and botanicals acting on important targets like human topoisomerases I & II, and caspases in addressing cancer through translational approaches. The contents of the proposed books cater to a diverse audience from domains of food and nutrition, pharmaceuticals, medicine, and practitioners of CAMS and help them in understanding the ethnopharmacological, nutraceutical, phytochemical, and systems approach to cancer therapy.

Motamarri Venkata Naga Lalitha Chaitanya
School of Pharmacy
Lovely Professional University
Phagwara, 144402
Punjab, India

Galvina Pereira
Bombay college of Pharmacy
Mumbai, India

&

Heyam Saad Ali
Pharmaceutics Department
University of Khartoum
Khartoum, Sudan

List of Contributors

Akey Krishna Swaroop	Department of Pharmaceutical Chemistry, JSS College of Pharmacy, JSS Academy of Higher Education & Research, Ooty, The Nilgiris, Tamil Nadu, India
Awotunde Oluwasegun Samson	Department of Biochemistry, Habib Medical School IUIU, Kampala, Uganda
Aditya Kulkarni	Research Scientist, Atenporus lifesciences, Bangalore, India
Bijesh Kumar Biswal	Cancer Drug Resistance Laboratory, Department of Life Science, National Institute of Technology Rourkela, Odisha-769008, India
Charu Kamal Yerneni	Flamma USA, Pennsylvania, USA
Gnana Ruba Priya Muthaiah	Department of pharmaceutical chemistry, College of Pharmaceutical Sciences, Dayananda Sagar University, Bangalore, Karnataka, India
Galvina Pereira	Bombay College of Pharmacy, Kalina, Mumbai, India
Gana Manjusha Kondepudi	Vignan Institute of Pharmaceutical Technology, Visakhapatnam, Andhra Pradesh, India
Heyam Saad Ali	Pharmaceutics Department, University of Khartoum, Khartoum, Sudan
Jubie Selvaraj	Department of Pharmaceutical Chemistry, JSS College of Pharmacy, Ooty-643001, Tamil Nadu, India
Kuppuswamy Uma	PSG College of Pharmac, Coimbatore, Tamil Nadu, India
Madhavi Patel	Parul Institute of Pharmacy, Parul University, Limda, Vadodara, Gujarat, India
Maida Engels S.E.	PSG College of Pharamacy, Coimbatore, Tamil Nadu, India
Motamarri Venkata Naga Lalitha Chaitanya	School of Pharmacy, Lovely Professional University Phagwara, 144402 Punjab, India
Malakapogu Ravindra Babu	Department of Pharmacognosy, School of Pharmaceutical Sciences, Lovely Professional University, Phagwara, India
Mugambwa Joseph Yusuf	Department of Biochemistry, Habib Medical School IUIU, Kampala, Uganda
Munmun Panda	Cancer Drug Resistance Laboratory, Department of Life Science, National Institute of Technology Rourkela, Odisha-769008, India
Mandar Mulik	Principal. K.M. Kundnani College of Pharmacy, Mumbai, Maharashtra, India
Mukesh Gangar	Aten Porus Life sciences, Bangalore, India
Nandhakumar Sathyamoorthy	Department of Pharmaceutic, Faculty of Pharmacy, Dr. M.G.R. Educational and Research Institute, Chennai, Tamil Nadu, India
Omogbadegun Olu Richard	Department of Biochemistry, Habib Medical School IUIU, Kampala, Uganda
Pavan Kumar Chintamaneni	Department of Pharmaceutics, School of Pharmacy, GITAM Deemed to be University, Hyderabad, India

Poonam Agrawal	Natucare Herbessence Pvt. Ltd, Thane, Maharashtra, India
Prabha Thangavelu	Department of Pharmaceutical Chemistry, Nandha College of Pharmacy, Affiliated to The Tamil Nadu Dr. MGR Medical University-Chennai, Erode-638052, Tamil Nadu, India
Rashmi Saxena Pal	Department of Pharmacognosy, School of Pharmaceutical Sciences, Lovely Professional University, Phagwara, India
Rokeya Sultana	Department of Pharmacognosy, Yenepoya Pharmacy College and Research Centre, Under Yenepoya Deemed to be University, Mangalore, Karnataka, India
Seema Sajjan Singh Rathore	Department of pharmaceutical chemistry, College of Pharmaceutical Sciences, Dayananda Sagar University, Bangalore, Karnataka, India
Surya Kant Tripathi	Cancer Drug Resistance Laboratory, Department of Life Science, National Institute of Technology Rourkela, Odisha-769008, India
Stuti Biswal	Cancer Drug Resistance Laboratory, Department of Life Science, National Institute of Technology Rourkela, Odisha-769008, India
Swati Patil	Principal. K.M. Kundnani College of Pharmacy, Mumbai, Maharashtra, India
Sai Kiran S.S. Pindiprolu	Department of Pharmacology, Aditya Pharmacy College, Surampalem, Andhra Pradesh, India
Sakshi Sharma	Department of Botany, DAV College, Amritsar-143001, Punjab, India
Sandeep Goyal	Aten Porus Lifesciences, Bangalore, India
Varsha Jayakar	Department of Studies and Research in Biochemistry, Mangalore University, Jnana Kaveri Post Graduate Centre, ChikkaAluvara, Kodagu, Karnataka, India
Vikas Jhawat	School of Medical and Allied Sciences, GD Goenka University, Gurugram-122103, India
Vishnu Nayak Badavath	Department of Pharmaceutical Chemistry, College of Pharmacy, Chitkara University, Chitkara, Panjab, India
Vishal Patel	Vasu Research Centre, A Div. of Vasu Healthcare Pvt. Ltd, Vadodara, Gujarat, India

CHAPTER 1

Clinical Role of Modern Ayurveda in Treating Cancer

Galvina Pereira[1,*], **Motamarri Venkata Naga Lalitha Chaitanya**[2] and **Rashmi Saxena Pal**[3]

[1] *Bombay College of Pharmacy, Kalina, Mumbai, India*

[2] *School of Pharmacy, Lovely Professional University Phagwara, 144402 Punjab, India*

[3] *School of Pharmaceutical Sciences, Lovely Professional University, Phagwara, India*

Abstract: "Ayurveda", an ancient Indian science of living which originated about 5000 thousand years ago, establishes ways of living a healthy life by establishing harmony between body, mind, and spirit. Ayurveda suggests lifestyle and dietary changes for the management of cancer and cancer like symptoms. Though the occurrence of this disease about five thousand years ago was sparce, yet the ayurvedic texts do mention some symptoms that can be aliased to cancer. These are often treated by different Ayurvedic procedures and formulations. Majority of these formulations balance the elements in our body referred to as "*Tridoshas*" which are *vatta, pitta* and *kapha*. It has been reported that the herbs, lifestyle and dietary changes that act by balancing "*Tridoshas*" show beneficial effects on cancer at various stages of the disease. Medicinal plants that possess a set of defined attributes such as bitter, pungent, astringent biopotency, act as excellent candidates for prevention, mitigation and treatment of cancers. Moreover, using systems pharmacology and bioactivity-guided fractionation, it is now possible to decipher the molecular mechanism of action of these potent anti-cancer herbs. An amalgamation of Ayurvedic systems and modern medicine put together as "Modern Ayurveda" is proving efficient in cancer therapy.

Keywords: Ayurveda ayush, Cancer treatment, *Grandhi* and *Arbuda*, Herbs, Neoplasm, Tridosha.

INTRODUCTION

Ayurveda meaning "Science of Life" is an ancient Indian system of medicine which dates to more than 5000 years ago. Ayurveda focuses on the holistic healing *viz.* well-being of body, mind and soul for elimination of disease conditions. Ayurveda is still practiced worldwide in the 21st century with more

* **Corresponding author Galvina Pereira:** Bombay College of Pharmacy, Kalina, Mumbai, India; E-mail: galvinaferr@gmail.com

Motamarri Venkata Naga Lalitha Chaitanya, Galvina Pereira, & Heyam Saad Ali (Eds.)

than 7 lakh practitioners currently registered in India itself. The ayurvedic practitioners called *vaidyas*, use patient-centric method of treatment, after a personalized diagnosis [1, 2]. This system is well documented in the ancient scripts and focusses on curing the root cause of diseases rather than being a mere symptomatic treatment.

The interest in traditional medicine has recently resurged owing to an increase in incidences of chronic diseases, cases of antibiotic resistance amongst micro-organisms, multi-drug resistant cancers and the emergence of newer disease conditions such as COVID-19. Ayurvedic therapies have been proven beneficial in the management of various disease conditions which are thought to be incurable by allopathic system of medicine, *e.g.*, diabetes, arthritis, and most importantly cancer [3 - 5].

Ayurveda describes the health condition of individual as a combination of *Tridoshas* (body humor) *viz vata* (air), *pita* (fire) and *kapha* (water) based on motion, digestion and cumulation, which remain constant throughout one's life [6]. The imbalance or inequilibrium of these doshas is referred to as "*vikruti*" and leads a disease condition [7]. The physical or mental condition of an individual can cause this imbalance, eventually affecting the body.

Ayurveda uses varied approaches which aid in the mitigation and treatment of disease conditions. These include massage, meditation, yoga, diet, medicine and surgery. It also uses techniques such as panchakarma for detoxification of body [8, 9]. The ayurvedic practitioners prescribe consumption of certain drugs to cure a person of disease conditions. Many Ayurvedic medicines, referred to as "*rasayanas*" are based on herbal products. Medicinal plants (*dravyas*) have been consumed traditionally for their healing properties. The usage and preparations of medicinal plants have also been listed in Ayurvedic scriptures. These Ayurvedic drugs include some of the most commonly found flora in the Asian subcontinent [10]. Ayurvedic drugs are formulated into different dosage forms for enhancing their palatability, potency, and shelf-life. Ayurvedic scriptures mention various formulations such as *arka, taila, ghrita, vati, asava, arista, lepa etc.* to obtain the best properties of single herb, polyherbal or herbo-mineral preparations [11].

CANCER: AYURVEDIC PERSPECTIVE

The incidences of disease conditions such as cancer in the time of development of Traditional Medicinal systems were minimal, as a result, very few texts describe this condition. With the onset of the 21st century, the incidences of cancer are on the rise owing to changes in diet, lifestyle, stress, environment, *etc.* The vital books of Ayurvedic medicine *viz.*, *Charaka Samhita* and *Sushruta Samahita* describe methods of cancer detection, mitigation, management, and cure [7].

Pathophysiology of Cancer as per Ayurveda

Cancer is a condition manifested when cells in the human body undergo uncontrolled division and inflammation. The different factors that lead to precipitation or build-up of tumours in the body have been postulated in ancient texts. Mostly abnormal interactions between *prakriti* (genotype) and environmental factors vitiate the *doshas* (body humour) and impair immunity, which can lead to aberrant cell growth and sometimes cancer. Table **1** summarizes the effect of different food and other factors on *doshas*. Moreover, the interaction between vitiated *doshas* (body humour) and weak *dhatus* (body tissues) manifests as cancers of a specific organ [12].

Table 1. Types of doshas and their corresponding aggravating factors [12]

Dosha (Body Humor) Involved	Aggravating Factors
Vata	Excessive consumption of bitter, pungent, astringent, dry foodstuff and stress.
Pitta	Excessive consumption of sour, salty, fried food and excessive anger.
Kapha	Excessive consumption of sweet, oily food and sedentary lifestyle.

Another theory about the cause of cancers in a body, obtained from the traditional texts, as described by Rao (1994) states that cancers can arise out of metabolic imbalances in body, involving proteins and enzymes. The body fire (*dhatwagni*) regulates the metabolic processes in the body. This body fire can be classified into four categories: low (*mand*), medium (*sama*), high (*tikshna*) and nil (*vishama*) depending upon intensity and is responsible for all enzymatic processes in the body. When the body fire decreases to nil condition (*vishama*), the cell losses its characteristic pattern of protein synthesis, leading to the production of altered proteins and metabolism of amphibolic substances. The presence of these substances is characteristic of a tumour cell [13].

An additional theory from *Sushruta Samhita* states that the consumption of Kapha aggravating substances decreases the intensity of body fire which in turn slows down the digestive and metabolic processes resulting in the formation and accumulation of toxins (*ama*) in our body. The toxins then interact with different body tissues (*dhatus*) and alter its functioning, slowly leading to systemic blockade and stagnation thus initiating various pathological processes [14]. When this overrides the limit, there is a diversion of flow in these channels and alteration in the functions of body tissues. This leads to the formation of neoplasms into various organs and tissues. The decrease in the body fire, is inversely proportional to the related tissue size. Consequently, the tissue size increases resulting from cell proliferation and tissue growth. If these events further continue, this might lead to the formation of neoplasm (*arbudas*) [15]. Generally, *vata* is correlated to anabolic phase whereas *kapha* is correlated to the catabolic phase of growth. Cancer originates out of metabolic imbalances viz. aggravation of *vata* and suppression of *kapha*. Cancerous growth in one particular organ is managed by the body by compensation from other body parts leading to weight loss. In benign neoplasm (*Vataja, Pittaja* or *Kaphaja*), one or two of the three bodily systems (humors) are out of control, but this condition is not considered to be too harmful because the body is still able to coordinate among these systems. Malignant tumours (*Tridosaja*) are very harmful because in these, all the three major bodily systems lose mutual co-ordination and thus cannot prevent tissue damage, resulting in a deadly morbid condition [16]. The pathogenesis of disease has been described by Shatkriyakala (meaning six stages of progress of a disease), which helps the practitioner in the assessment of different stages of spread of these diseases, mentioned in Table **2**.

Table 2. The six stages of pathogenesis of disease

No.	Stage	Ayurvedic term	State of the pathogenesis
1.	**Dosha accumulation at one's own location**	***Sanchaya***	Pre-clinical observations
2.	**Vitiation at own site**	***Prakopa***	Pre-clinical observations, generally curable
3.	**Stage of Spread**	***Prasara***	The spread of disease to other organs can be controlled by treating the root cause. Without any intervention, the vitiated doshas start to affect other organs. Generally vata is dosha responsible for the spread.
4	**Stage of localisation**	***Sthanasamshraya***	The vitiated doshas settle at site outside the affected organ depending upon the affinity of other organs.
5	**Stage of manifestation**	***Vyaktha***	At this stage, all the clinical symptoms of the disease appear due to interaction of Dosha with dhatu (body tissue).
6	**Stage of chronicity**	***Bheda***	Clinical symptoms aggravate and the progression of the disease is almost complete and the complications arising out of the disease reach to a maximum often leading to high chances of mortality.

The vital books in Ayurveda describe ways to achieve good health by synchronising ones' lifestyle with nature and universal clock, viz., the solar, lunar, and seasonal calendars. Few examples of this include:

a. *Dincharya* meaning following optimum daytime routine viz. waking up between 3 am- 6 am (*Brahma mahurta*) to improvise normal peristaltic movements.
b. *Ratricharya* meaning following optimum nighttime routine such as the consumption of light and easily digestible food at night and sleeping by 10 pm.
c. *Ritucharya* meaning following optimum seasonal routine (which mentions the consumption of cooling food substances and avoiding hot and spicy food during summer and *vice versa*.

Ayurveda also recommends health-promoting foods and methods of consuming them, ways of social and personal behaviour (*sadvritta*), and management of mental stress (*manasa tivra*) using techniques such as meditation and yoga. Ayurveda believes that mental fluctuations are caused by an overload of incoming information perceived by our senses, which influences gene expression. The mind-body connection can lead to physical disorders [17]. Ayurveda also states that one must avoid etiological factors that aggravate *Vata* and *Kapha*. Many body purification techniques are available in Ayurveda that eliminate accumulated toxins. One such technique is *Panchakarma* in which the accumulated toxins in the body are removed by five treatments viz *Virechan* (superficial cleansing using herbal pastes or powders), *Vaman* (inducing vomiting or purging by consumption of herbal preparations), *Basti* (faecal clearance by utilizing enemas, warm oils *etc*), *Rakta moksha* (Bloodletting) and *Nasya* (clearing of nasal passages by inhalation of steam, medicinal oils and herbal preparations). These treatments may vary from person to person depending upon their health condition and the doshas involved.

Ayurveda in Cancer Treatment

To improve their disease condition, Ayurvedic practitioners recommend specific diet modifications, such as limiting proteinaceous foods like meat, which aid in the growth and proliferation of cancer cells, avoiding cold biopotency substances because they suppress the digestive fire, and consuming food substances that rejuvenate the body's healing potential. A meta-analysis study of 85 herbs used in cancer, carried out by Singh *et al*, 2002 reports that herbs with bitter (*Katu*), pungent (*Tikta*) and astringent (*Kasaya rasa*) taste, hot biopotency (*Usna virya*) and catabolic active metabolites (*Katu vipaka*) herbs with dry, coarse, light, and sharp biophysical properties have significantly greater possibilities of producing anticancer effects [14].

Katu rasa (a pungent taste or substance that produces a burning sensation and psychological irritation) stimulates the body fire (*agni*), thereby activating the digestive and antioxidant enzymes, decreasing inflammation, and decongesting all the body channels and accumulative growths like tumours. Ayurveda reports the usage of numerous herbal ingredients for the mitigation and cure of tumours and cancer-like symptoms commonly addressed as *"Apachi," "Gulma," "Granthi,"* and *"Arbuda,"* which mean minor and major forms of neoplasm, respectively. Surgery, therapeutic heat burn (*agni karma*), and caustic therapy (*kshara karma*) were all traditional *arbuda* treatment methods.

Surgical management of neoplasms includes the principles of fomentation by external application, cleansing by internal medication, treatment for evacuation of the tumor's contents, cauterization with acids or alkalis to avoid recurrence, and post-operative care for healing the wound. Consumption of immunoboosting drugs, *gaumudra* (cow urine) therapy, and rasayan (herbal or herbo-mineral preparations) therapy have also been indicated for cancer management. Body purification and detoxification processes are carried out through the consumption of certain internal and external applications that eliminate vitiated doshas and have primarily been used for cancer medical management. According to Ayurvedic concepts, all cancer therapies treat the affected tissues indirectly by eliminating vitiated *doshas*, rejuvenating *doshas*, and restoring immunity in cancer patients [12]. Ayurveda also prescribes consumption of purified cannabis for the treatment of chronic pain associated with this disease [18].

Ayurveda in Post Cancer Therapy

Major limitations of allopathic therapy are the adverse effects on the body owing to chemotherapy, radiation therapy which affect the growth and replication process of healthy cells especially in the tissues surrounding the affected area. In Ayurveda they are thought to be manifestations of aggravated pitta mostly affecting the vasculature leading to haemorrhage and vascular inflammation. Ayurvedic herbs act as Adjuvant to chemo-radiotherapy thereby improving their quality-of-life Panchakarma treatment post cancer therapy is reported to reduce the adverse effects of chemo-radiotherapy as well [19]. The post cancer therapies also work on establishment of a diet, exercise and lifestyle regimen to prevent recurrence of this disease.

CLINICAL ROLE OF MODERN AYURVEDA

With the era of evidence-based medicine, some of the molecular targets of Ayurvedic medicine have been identified and validated. The rich knowledge of phytochemistry further aids in understanding the molecular mechanism of action of different herbs or herbal preparations. Both Ayurvedic as well as allopathic practitioners around the world are open to prescribing standardized herbal formulations containing drugs mentioned in ancient Ayurvedic text. There is surge in number of scientific articles documenting the clinical benefits of administering traditional formulations for treatment of cancer [20] With the development of modern analytical techniques sensitive to even picogram level of a biomarker and with OMICS studies, understanding the underlying mechanisms of ayurvedic medicines is much simpler [21].

"Ayurnutrigenomics" is an emerging branch of nutrigenomics which recommends personalized nutrition based on one's genomic constitution often referred in Ayurveda as "*prakriti*" [22].

The effects of various Ayurvedic formulation processes on phytochemical composition are now being studied [23]. Several clinical trials are now being carried out to validate the efficacy of this system of medicine [24].

Meditation and sticking to a daily routine are said to benefit our bodies by lowering the amount of free radicals produced, which causes oxidative damage to the cells. Maintaining a sleep cycle as per the circadian rhythm is vital for maintaining homeostasis in the body, which in turn regulates metabolic processes and prevents the accumulation of toxins [25].

Some of the anti-cancer herbs prescribed in Ayurveda act by improving tissue metabolism, body health, and immunomodulation [26]. There are several reports documenting the effects of different Ayurvedic approaches and formulations. With the recent surge in cases of drug-resistant cancers, many of these are also prescribed as adjuvants to cancer therapy. *Triphala rasayana,* a combination of *Phyllanthus emblica* L., *Terminalia chebula* Retz., and *Terminalia bellerica* Roxb. fruit powders, has been shown in clinical studies to have anti-cancer and radioprotective effects due to its higher content of astringent principle tannins that act as antioxidants [27, 8]. Withanolides present in Ashwagandha (*Withania somnifera*) root exhibit an anti-cancer effect by activating tumour suppressor cells, inhibiting angiogenesis, and restricting proliferation of cancer cells [28]. Manikay Bhasma, an Ayurvedic nanomedicine made up of purified gemstones such as ruby, orpiment, and arsenic sulfide, was proven to show anticancer activity by inducing oxidative stress in cancer cells, which causes the release of Cyt C, loss of mitochondrial membrane potential, activation of caspases, and DNA degradation, eventually leading to a cytotoxic effect [29]. The bioactive flavonoids from holy basil (*Ocimum sanctum*), viz., orientin and vicenin, have shown radioprotective effects on human lymphocytes [30]. A summary of a few herbs and their effects in the treatment and mitigation of cancer and cancer-like symptoms is summarised in Table **3**.

Table 3. Modern Mechanism of actions of Ayurvedic herb / Formulation used in treatment of Cancer

Ayurvedic Herb / Formulation used	Modern mechanism of action	Chemical constituents	Reference
Triphala (*Terminalia chebula, Phyllanthus emblica, Terminalia bellerica*)	Radioprotective effect when exposed to 10 Gy of gamma radiation.	Gallic acid, ellagic acid, chebulic acid.	[13]
Tinospora cordifolia	Triggers autophagy and apoptosis in HCT-116 Colon cancer cells.	Glycosides, steroids sesquiterpenoid, phenolics, polysaccharides, diterpenoid lactones.	[32, 33]
Drakchasava (*Vitis vinefera*)	Antioxidant.	Resveratrol, pterostilbene.	[34]
Ocimum sanctum	Inhibits matrix metalloproteinase, free radical scavenging and radioprotective.	Ursolic acid, eugenol and apigenin.	[35]
Aegle marmelos	Inhibits cell proliferation.	Lupeol, marmelin	[36]
Allium sativum	Induces CYP450 3A4.	Alliin, allicin, Sulphur containing compounds	[37]
Bacopa monnieri	Inhibits cell proliferation and shows apoptosis in Ehrlish ascites tumor cell lines, activates Caspase -3 and downregulates Bcl-2 gene.	Bacosides and dammarane triterpenoids	[38]
Withania somnifera	Anti-apoptotic, anti-inflammatory, immunomodulatory.	Withaferin, tannins	[39]
Andrographis paniculata, Annona atemoya, Phyllanthus niruri, Piper longum, Podophyllum hexandrum, Tinospora cordifolia, Semecarpus anacardium, Vitis vinifera, Baliospermum montanum, Madhuca indica	Reduce side effects of cancer associated complications.	Complex mixture of phytoconstituents	[40]
Curcuma longa	Chemoprotective, anti-inflammatory and interferes with cell signalling pathways.	Curcuminoids	[41]
Zingiber officinale	Inhibition of NFκB activation	Gingerols, resins	[42]
Datura stramonium	Causes oxidative damage and damages mitochondrial membrane potential, stimulates the proliferation of human peripheral blood mononuclear cells.	Neophytadiene, β-damascenone and β-eudesmol	[43]

(Table 3) cont.....

Ayurvedic Herb / Formulation used	Modern mechanism of action	Chemical constituents	Reference
Vinca rosea	Interaction with tubulin and microtubules in mitotic spindle.	Vincristine, Vinblastine, vinorelbine, vincristine and vindesine	[44]
Colchicum autumnale	Inhibition of microtubule formation.	Colchicoside, thiocolchicoside	[45]
Andrographis paniculate	Inhibits cell proliferation and metastasis.	Andrographolide, andrographoside	[46]
Podophyllum hexandrum	Arrests cell mitosis	Podophyllin	[47]
Picrorhiza kurroa	Induction of signal transducers inhibiting apoptosis.	Picrosides	[48]
Phyllanthus niruri	Anti-oxidant and cytotoxic.	Gallic acid and flavonoids	[49]
Calotropis gigantea	Inhibits Wnt signalling.	Calatropin	[50]

Challenges in Practicing Modern Ayurveda

When one tries to integrate the ancient Ayurvedic practices, techniques, and formulation into mainstream medicine, they often encounter several hurdles which need to be addressed and thoroughly investigated. First, the method of diagnosis in Ayurveda are different when compared to allopathic or any other form of medicine [20]. Next the ayurvedic medications are formulated based on ones "*Prakruti*" and involves treatment of "*dosha*" rather than symptoms so there is a personalized approach, and the medications may vary even if two individuals present a common problem. With increasing urbanization, it is difficult to procure fresh herbs for preparation of Ayurvedic formulations, as a result, the formulation quality and potency may differ [51]. It is very difficult to mimic the Ayurvedic manufacturing practices on an industrial scale which require process alterations and thereby needs standardization prior and determination of toxic metals or components to their usage [52, 53].

The spiritual and the cleansing approaches used in Ayurveda are very difficult to administer and validate in modern clinical trial setting [54]. An attempt is made by the Central Council for Research in Ayurvedic Sciences (CCRAS), Ministry of AYUSH to lay down guidelines for evaluation of Ayurvedic interventions and their evaluation using both modern as well as ayurvedic techniques [55]. The prescription of these medicines in clinical setting now depends on the evidence and reports of clinical trials. More solid the evidence, stronger is the recommendation [24]

CONCLUSION

With the validation of ayurvedic concepts of *"tridosha"*, *"prakruti"*, *"jatharagni"*, we correlate them with the genetic composition and metabolic process. The mechanism of action of more and more Ayurvedic formulations can now be predicted. The phytochemical knowledge of herbal drug now makes it possible to study these interactions at molecular level. With the onset of computational techniques like network pharmacology, molecular docking it is now possible to predict the molecular mechanism of action and the bioactive fraction [56]. With an increasing number of clinical trials on Ayurvedic herbs, many bioactive molecules such as curcumin, buccatin, withaferin, andrographolide, *etc.* have already been marketed and integrated in allopathic as well as modern ayurvedic cancer therapies. Several formulation approaches such as microspheres, nano particles, nanoemulsions, *etc.* help in enhancing the efficacy and targeting these bioactives at the desired site of action. Once, standardized and validated for their efficacy, and safety, Ayurvedic formulations can readily be assimilated into the mainstream therapy.

REFERENCES

[1] Narayana DBA, Durg S. Ayurveda: (W)here is the evidence. J Ayurveda Integr Med 2021; 12(2): 408-11.https://www.sciencedirect.com/science/article/pii/S0975947620300590 [http://dx.doi.org/10.1016/j.jaim.2020.07.001] [PMID: 32951967]

[2] Mukherjee PK, Nema NK, Venkatesh P, Debnath PK. Changing scenario for promotion and development of Ayurveda – way forward. J Ethnopharmacol 2012; 143(2): 424-34. https://www.sciencedirect.com/science/article/pii/S0378874112005053 [http://dx.doi.org/10.1016/j.jep.2012.07.036] [PMID: 22885133]

[3] Semwal DK, Chauhan A, Mishra S, Semwal R. Ayurvedic research and methodology: Present status and future strategies. Ayu 2015; 36(4): 364-9. https://pubmed.ncbi.nlm.nih.gov/27833362 [http://dx.doi.org/10.4103/0974-8520.190699] [PMID: 27833362]

[4] Gundeti M, Dedge A, Reddy G, Srikanth N. 278. Integrative (Ayurveda) oncology: Where we are and Way ahead. J Ayurveda Integr Med 2018; 9(2) (Suppl. 1): S11. https://www.sciencedirect.com/science/article/pii/S0975947618301578 [http://dx.doi.org/10.1016/j.jaim.2018.02.047]

[5] Gundeti MS, Rammanohar P, Bhat SG, Narayanam S. Ayurveda in Cancer Care in India: Scope, Challenges, and Suggested Approaches. J Altern Complement Med 2018; 24(9-10): 1023-4. [http://dx.doi.org/10.1089/acm.2018.0161] [PMID: 30247971]

[6] Govindaraj P, Nizamuddin S, Sharath A, *et al.* Genome-wide analysis correlates Ayurveda Prakriti. Sci Rep 2015; 5(1): 15786. [http://dx.doi.org/10.1038/srep15786] [PMID: 26511157]

[7] Dhruva A, Hecht FM, Miaskowski C, Kaptchuk TJ, Bodeker G, Abrams D. Correlating traditional Ayurvedic and modern medical perspectives on cancer: results of a qualitative study. J Altern Complement Med 2014; 20(5): 364-70.

[8] Ahmed S, Ding X, Sharma A. Exploring scientific validation of Triphala Rasayana in ayurveda as a source of rejuvenation for contemporary healthcare: An update. J Ethnopharmacol 2021; 273: 113829.https://www.sciencedirect.com/science/article/pii/S0378874121000556 [http://dx.doi.org/10.1016/j.jep.2021.113829] [PMID: 33465446]

[9] Sharma H, Chandola HM, Singh G, Basisht G. Utilization of Ayurveda in health care: an approach for prevention, health promotion, and treatment of disease. Part 2--Ayurveda in primary health care. J Altern Complement Med 2007; 13(10): 1135-50.
[http://dx.doi.org/10.1089/acm.2007.7017-B] [PMID: 18166127]

[10] Sun C, Nirmalananda S, Jenkins C, *et al.* First ayurvedic approach towards green drugs: anti cervical cancer-cell properties of Clerodendrum viscosum root extract. Anticancer Agents Med Chem 2013; 13(10): 1469-76.
[http://dx.doi.org/10.2174/18715206113139990138] [PMID: 23387970]

[11] Mukherjee PK, Harwansh RK, Bahadur S, *et al.* Development of Ayurveda – Tradition to trend. J Ethnopharmacol 2017; 197: 10-24. https://www.sciencedirect.com/science/article/pii/S0378874116307826
[http://dx.doi.org/10.1016/j.jep.2016.09.024] [PMID: 27633405]

[12] Chauhan A, Semwal DK, Mishra SP, Semwal RB. Ayurvedic concept of Shatkriyakala : a traditional knowledge of cancer pathogenesis and therapy. J Integr Med 2017; 15(2): 88-94. https://www.sciencedirect.com/science/article/pii/S209549641760311X
[http://dx.doi.org/10.1016/S2095-4964(17)60311-X] [PMID: 28285613]

[13] Rao SD. Dhatwagni vyapara in carcinogenesis. Anc Sci Life 1994; 14(1-2): 61-7.
[PMID: 22556677]

[14] Tripathi JS Sr, Singh RH. Possible Correlates of Free Radicals and Free Radical Mediated Disorders in Ayurveda with Special Referance to Bhutagni Vyapara and Ama at molecular Level. Anc Sci Life 1999; 19(1-2): 17-20.
[PMID: 22556911]

[15] Balachandran P, Govindarajan R. Cancer—an ayurvedic perspective. Pharmacol Res 2005; 51(1): 19-30.https://www.sciencedirect.com/science/article/pii/S1043661804001094
[http://dx.doi.org/10.1016/j.phrs.2004.04.010] [PMID: 15519531]

[16] Charaka, Charaka Samhita of Agnivesa Text with Englishtranslation and critical exposition based on Cakrapani Datta'sAyurved Dipika by Dr. Ram Karan Sharma and vaidyaBhagwan Dash (Volume III) Chaukhambha Sanskrit SeriesOffice Varanasi, India p. 341-342 2005.

[17] Sharma P KD. Role of Kalpa Chikitsa in the management of Lynch syndrome- A case report. J Fam Med Prim Care 9(5): 2487-91.

[18] Tavhare S, Acharya R, Reddy RG, Dhiman K. Management of chronic pain with *Jalaprakshalana* (water-wash) *Shodhita* (processed) *Bhanga* (*Cannabis sativa* L.) in cancer patients with deprived quality of life: An open-label single arm clinical trial. Ayu 2019; 40(1): 34-43.
[http://dx.doi.org/10.4103/ayu.AYU_43_19] [PMID: 31831967]

[19] Metri K, Bhargav H, Chowdhury P, Koka PS. Ayurveda for chemo-radiotherapy induced side effects in cancer patients. J Stem Cells 2013; 8(2): 115-29.
[PMID: 24698988]

[20] Edavalath M, Bharathan BP. Methodology for developing and evaluating diagnostic tools in Ayurveda – A review. J Ayurveda Integr Med 2021; 12(2): 389-97.https://www.sciencedirect.com/science/article/pii/S0975947621000103
[http://dx.doi.org/10.1016/j.jaim.2021.01.009] [PMID: 33678559]

[21] Mukherjee PK, Venkatesh M, Gantait A. 3.14 - Ayurveda in Modern Medicine: Development and Modification of Bioactivity. Chemistry, Molecular Sciences and Chemical Engineering. Oxford: Elsevier 2010.

[22] Banerjee S, Debnath P, Debnath PK. Ayurnutrigenomics: Ayurveda-inspired personalized nutrition from inception to evidence. J Tradit Complement Med 2015; 5(4): 228-33.https://www.sciencedirect.com/science/article/pii/S222541101500019X
[http://dx.doi.org/10.1016/j.jtcme.2014.12.009] [PMID: 26587393]

[23] Sekar S, Vinothkanna A. Polyherbal and submerge fermented medicines of Ayurveda: Convergence of tradition with scientific trends and needs. S Afr J Bot 2019; 121: 410-7.https://www.sciencedirect.com/science/article/pii/S0254629918312249 [http://dx.doi.org/10.1016/j.sajb.2018.12.009]

[24] Sridharan K, Sivaramakrishnan G. Clinical trials in Ayurveda: Analysis of clinical trial registry of India. J Ayurveda Integr Med 2016; 7(3): 141-3.https://www.sciencedirect.com/science/article/pii/S0975947616300407 [http://dx.doi.org/10.1016/j.jaim.2016.08.009] [PMID: 27658912]

[25] Nair LP. Lekshmy, ML, Chandran,H. Haroon I. Ayurvedic perspective of Circadian Rhythm. J Ayurveda Integr Med Sci 2021; 6(2): 187-94.

[26] Dash MK, Joshi N, Gautam DNS, Jayakumar R, Tripathi YB. Ayurvedic supportive therapy in the management of breast cancer. J Herb Med 2021; 29: 100490.https://www.sciencedirect.com/science/article/pii/S2210803321000701 [http://dx.doi.org/10.1016/j.hermed.2021.100490]

[27] Baliga MS. Triphala, Ayurvedic formulation for treating and preventing cancer: a review. J Altern Complement Med 2010; 16(12): 1301-8. [http://dx.doi.org/10.1089/acm.2009.0633] [PMID: 21138390]

[28] Saggam A, Tillu G, Dixit S, *et al. Withania somnifera* (L.) Dunal: A potential therapeutic adjuvant in cancer. J Ethnopharmacol 2020; 255: 112759.https://www.sciencedirect.com/science/article/pii/S0378874119347646 [http://dx.doi.org/10.1016/j.jep.2020.112759] [PMID: 32173425]

[29] Jha S, Trivedi V. Manikya Bhasma is a nanomedicine to affect cancer cell viability through induction of apoptosis. J Ayurveda Integr Med 2021; 12(2): 302-11. [http://dx.doi.org/10.1016/j.jaim.2020.11.001] [PMID: 33358658]

[30] Pandey G. Anticancer herbal drugs of India with special reference to ayurveda. 1-153.2002;

[31] Jagetia GC, Baliga MS, Malagi KJ, Sethukumar Kamath M. The evaluation of the radioprotective effect of Triphala (an ayurvedic rejuvenating drug) in the mice exposed to γ-radiation. Phytomedicine 2002; 9(2): 99-108.https://www.sciencedirect.com/science/article/pii/S0944711304700884 [http://dx.doi.org/10.1078/0944-7113-00095] [PMID: 11995956]

[32] Sharma N, Kumar A, Sharma PR, *et al.* A new clerodane furano diterpene glycoside from Tinospora cordifolia triggers autophagy and apoptosis in HCT-116 colon cancer cells. J Ethnopharmacol 2018; 211: 295-310.https://www.sciencedirect.com/science/article/pii/S0378874117325278 [http://dx.doi.org/10.1016/j.jep.2017.09.034] [PMID: 28962889]

[33] Patil S, Ashi H, Hosmani J, *et al. Tinospora cordifolia* (Thunb.) Miers (Giloy) inhibits oral cancer cells in a dose-dependent manner by inducing apoptosis and attenuating epithelial-mesenchymal transition. Saudi J Biol Sci 2021; 28(8): 4553-9.https://www.sciencedirect.com/science/article/pii/S1319562X21003065 [http://dx.doi.org/10.1016/j.sjbs.2021.04.056] [PMID: 34354441]

[34] Paul B, Masih I, Deopujari J, Charpentier C. Occurrence of resveratrol and pterostilbene in age-old darakchasava, an ayurvedic medicine from India. J Ethnopharmacol 1999; 68(1-3): 71-6. [http://dx.doi.org/10.1016/S0378-8741(99)00044-6] [PMID: 10624864]

[35] Singh V, Kumar K, Purohit D, *et al.* Exploration of therapeutic applicability and different signaling mechanism of various phytopharmacological agents for treatment of breast cancer. Biomed Pharmacother 2021; 139: 111584. [http://dx.doi.org/10.1016/j.biopha.2021.111584] [PMID: 34243623]

[36] Lampronti I, Martello D, Bianchi N, *et al.* In vitro antiproliferative effects on human tumor cell lines of extracts from the Bangladeshi medicinal plant Aegle marmelos Correa. Phytomedicine 2003; 10(4): 300-8.https://www.sciencedirect.com/science/article/pii/S0944711304702263

[http://dx.doi.org/10.1078/094471103322004794] [PMID: 12809360]

[37] Li G, Qiao CH, Lin RI, Pinto J, Osborne MP, Tiwari RK. Antiproliferative effects of garlic constituents in cultured human breast-cancer cells. Oncol Rep 1995; 2(5): 787-91. [http://dx.doi.org/10.3892/or.2.5.787] [PMID: 21597817]

[38] Kalyani MI, Lingaraju SM, Salimath BP. A pro-apoptotic 15-kDa protein from *Bacopa monnieri* activates caspase-3 and downregulates Bcl-2 gene expression in mouse mammary carcinoma cells. J Nat Med 2013; 67(1): 123-36. [http://dx.doi.org/10.1007/s11418-012-0661-z] [PMID: 22467255]

[39] Vashi R, Patel BM, Goyal RK. Keeping abreast about ashwagandha in breast cancer. J Ethnopharmacol 2021; 269: 113759. [http://dx.doi.org/10.1016/j.jep.2020.113759] [PMID: 33359916]

[40] Kosta S, Tiwari A, Jain R. Ayurveda and cancer. Pharmacognosy Res 2010; 2(6): 393-4. [http://dx.doi.org/10.4103/0974-8490.75463] [PMID: 21713145]

[41] Giordano A, Tommonaro G. Curcumin and Cancer. Nutrients 2019; 11(10): 2376. [http://dx.doi.org/10.3390/nu11102376]

[42] Habib SHM, Makpol S, Hamid NAA, Das S, Ngah WZW, Yusof YAM. Ginger extract (Zingiber officinale) has anti-cancer and anti-inflammatory effects on ethionine-induced hepatoma rats. Clinics (São Paulo) 2008; 63(6): 807-13.https://pubmed.ncbi.nlm.nih.gov/19061005 [http://dx.doi.org/10.1590/S1807-59322008000600017] [PMID: 19061005]

[43] Chandan G, Kumar C, Verma MK, Satti NK, Saini AK Sr, Saini RV. *Datura stramonium* essential oil composition and it's immunostimulatory potential against colon cancer cells. 3 Biotech 2020; 10(10): 451. [http://dx.doi.org/10.1007/s13205-020-02438-4] [PMID: 33062579]

[44] Moudi M, Go R, Yien CYS, Nazre M. Vinca alkaloids. Int J Prev Med 2013; 4(11): 1231-5.https://pubmed.ncbi.nlm.nih.gov/24404355 [PMID: 24404355]

[45] Kumar A, Sharma PR, Mondhe DM. Potential anticancer role of colchicine-based derivatives. Anticancer Drugs 2017; 28(3): 250-62. [http://dx.doi.org/10.1097/CAD.0000000000000464] [PMID: 28030380]

[46] Dai L, Wang G, Pan W. Andrographolide Inhibits Proliferation and Metastasis of SGC7901 Gastric Cancer Cells. BioMed Res Int 2017; 2017: 1-10. [http://dx.doi.org/10.1155/2017/6242103] [PMID: 28194420]

[47] Zhao S, Baik OD. Application of ultrasound as pretreatment for extraction of podophyllotoxin from rhizomes of *Podophyllum peltatum*. Ultrason Sonochem 2012; 19(1): 22-31.https://www.sciencedirect.com/science/article/pii/S1350417711001052 [http://dx.doi.org/10.1016/j.ultsonch.2011.05.012] [PMID: 21664168]

[48] Soni D, Grover A. Picrosides from *Picrorhiza kurroa* as potential anti-carcinogenic agents. Biomed Pharmacother 2019; 109: 1680-7.https://www. sciencedirect .com/science /article /pii/S0753332218351965 [http://dx.doi.org/10.1016/j. biopha.2018 .11.048] [PMID: 30551422]

[49] Araújo Jr, Soares LAL. Growth inhibitory effects of Phyllanthus niruri extracts in combination with cisplatin on cancer cell lines. World J Gastroenterol 2012; 18(31): 4162-6168.

[50] Park HY, Toume K, Arai MA, Sadhu SK, Ahmed F, Ishibashi M. Calotropin: A Cardenolide from Calotropis gigantea that Inhibits Wnt Signaling by Increasing Casein Kinase 1α in Colon Cancer Cells. Chem Bio 2014; 15(6): 872-8. [http://dx.doi.org/10.1002/cbic.201300786]

[51] Katiyar CK. Ayurvedic pharmaceutics, manufacturing processes and novel drug delivery systems in ayurveda. Springer Singapore 2019; c: 33-52.

[http://dx.doi.org/10.1007/978-981-13-2062-0_4]

[52] Vaidya VN, Tatiya AU, Elango A, Kukkupuni SK, Vishnuprasad CN. Need for comprehensive standardization strategies for marketed Ayurveda formulations. J Ayurveda Integr Med 2018; 9(4): 312-5.

[53] Rammanohar P. Chapter 31 - Toxicity of Ayurvedic Medicines and Safety Concerns: Ancient and Modern Perspectives.History of Toxicology and Environmental Health. 2019; pp. 441-58.

[54] Warrier M. Seekership, Spirituality and Self-Discovery: Ayurveda Trainees in Britain. Asian Med (Lieden) 2008; 4(2): 423-51.
[http://dx.doi.org/10.1163/157342009X12526658783691] [PMID: 20617123]

[55] CCRAS. General guidelines for clinical evaluation of ayurvedic interventions. 1-123.2018;

[56] Bender A, Fauzi FM, Koutsoukas A, *et al.* Linking Ayurveda and Western medicine by integrative analysis. J Ayurveda Integr Med 2013; 4(2): 117-9.
[http://dx.doi.org/10.4103/0975-9476.113882] [PMID: 23930045]

CHAPTER 2

Aromatherapy: An Adjuvant Treatment in Cancer

Poonam Agrawal[1,*]

[1] *Natucare Herbessence Pvt. Ltd., Thane, Maharashtra, India*

Abstract: Aromatherapy is a complementary healing therapy that uses aromatic essential oils to improve the health of the body and mind. Essential oils with healing properties, like geranium oil, rosemary oil, lavender oil, patchouli oil, and others, have been used to treat cancer. Cancer is often treated using chemotherapy and/or radiation therapy. Nausea and vomiting are often side effects of chemotherapy and radiotherapy. Subsequently, these cancer therapies lead to various psychological disorders, such as stress, anxiety, and depression, in cancer patients. Hence, the a need to assist cancer patients in overcoming these disorders. Aromatherapy, which is a blend of essential oils, has been reported to improve disorders that arise during complicated cancer therapies such as chemotherapy and radiation. Research on cancer populations has revealed that patients exposed to essential oils *via* inhaler devices had reduced anxiety, stress, nausea, and poor sleep. The effects of aromatherapy are reported to be due to the binding of chemical components in the essential oil to receptors in the olfactory bulb, impacting the brain's emotional center, the limbic system. Aromatherapy has also been reported to relieve pain, muscular tension, and fatigue. Aromatherapy practitioners treat specific conditions using various combinations of oils and different modes of application. Aromatherapy can thus be used as a potential supplement treatment to improve complications in cancer; however, further studies are needed to estimate the protocol and standard dosage. Given the difficulties of cancer treatment, aromatherapy can play an important role in treating patients' psychological aspects.

Keywords: Aromatherapy, Aromatherapy practitioners, Brain's emotional center, Cancer therapies, Cancer, Chemotherapy, Essential oil, Geranium oil, Lavender oil, Psychological aspects, Patchouli oil, Radiation, Rosemary oil.

INTRODUCTION

Cancer is one of the greatest health challenges in the world. GLOBOCAN 2020 estimated about 19.3 million new cancer cases and 10.0 million cancer deaths in 2020 [1]. Although various advanced treatment and therapies are available, patients suffer from various complications such as such as loss of appetite, malnutrition, loss of hair, vomiting, dryness of mouth, fatigue, nausea, pain, wea-

* **Corresponding author Poonam Agrawal:** Natucare Herbessence Pvt. Ltd., Thane, Maharashtra, India; E-mail: galvinaferr@gmail.com

kness, and psychological disorders like anxiety, depression and stress [2]. Thus, the need arises for developing complementary and alternative methods which are not only effective in relieving cancer complications, but also having less side-effects. Alternative therapies have been commonly used in reducing the discomfort of the patients with cancer [3].

Aromatherapy has varied applications as complementary treatment in different diseases [4, 5]. This treatment is considered to be one of the natural ways of healing person's mind, body and soul. Aromatherapy comprises of the use of essential oils extracted from natural resources such as plants to treat various disorders [6]. Essential oils are known to be highly concentrated extracts with characteristic odor.

Literature survey reveals that aromatherapy can be used to improve complications arising in cancer patients such as fatigue, nausea, vomiting, loss of appetite, psychological disorders, *etc* [7 - 10].

Classification of Aromatherapy

Aromatherapy can be applied or administered in three ways, namely [11]: Medical aromatherapy is where essential oils are administered internally *via* oral, rectal, or vaginal routes. Only steam-distilled and expeller-pressed essential oils are used internally. Subtle aromatherapy is the inhalation of essential oils for psychological treatment. It is also called aromacology. In this therapy, essential oils are absorbed through the nasal membrane, which reaches the olfactory nerves and stimulates impulses. This impulse travels to the limbic system of the brain, where it has a relaxing and psychological effect [12]. Traditional aromatherapy uses essential oils applied topically by massage. It can be used in two forms: for therapeutic use or for cosmetic use. Therapeutically, essential oils can have physical as well as psychological effects.

Essential Oil Aromatherapy mainly comprises the controlled use of essential oils obtained from plants and administering them internally or externally based on individual needs to promote good health or treat any disorder. Essential oils are volatile oils extracted from various parts of aromatic plants. Essential oils are stored in secretory parts of the plant such as oil cells, resin sacs, epidermis, trichomes, *etc*. Essential oils are extracted from plants using various processes such as steam distillation, expression, enfleurage, solvent extraction, maceration, and supercritical fluid extraction [11]. Essential oils chemically consist of monoterpenes, aldehydes, ketones, esters, alcohols, *etc* [13]. They are volatile in nature and have a characteristic odour. Every individual plant produces varied types of essential oil that differ in chemical composition [14]. Due to variations in chemical composition, clinical effects can be distinctly different.

Essential Oil Chemical Composition

On the basis of the chemical structure, essential oils are broadly categorized into oxygenated compounds and hydrocarbon compounds [15]. Oxygenated compounds comprise esters, alcohols, phenols, aldehydes, ketones, oxides, *etc.* Hydrocarbons consist of mainly terpenes which have the basic isoprene (C_5) unit. Terpenes are further classified as monoterpenes (C_{10}), sesqueterpene (C_{15}), and diterpene (C_{20}). Terpenes can also be acyclic, monocyclic, or bicyclic.

Plants are used in Aromatherapy. Some well-known essential oils occur in Thymus vulgaris, Rosmarinus officinalis, Ocimum, Salvia officinalis, Lavender, Chamomile, and Melissa officinalis [11]. The most commonly used essential oils or aromas in cancer treatment are lavender, peppermint, orange, and chamomile [11]. Lavender is known to improve sleep quality and relieve psychological disorders. Peppermint is reported to be used for nausea and vomiting. Orange finds application in reducing anxiety, depression, *etc* [11]. Some of the essential oils derived from plants that can be used in aromatherapy for cancer patients are listed in Table **1**. Essential oils are typically dispersed in carriers, which are obtained by cold pressing or fixing vegetable oils such as sweet almond, grape seed, and so on. Many fixed vegetable oils such as calendula (Calendula officinalis) and St. John's wort (Hypericum perforatum) are known for their therapeutic activity. Other carriers include honey, Aloe vera and specially formulated gel and wax.

Table 1. Essential oil from plants for aromatherapy in cancer patients

Essential oil	Constituent	Possible mechanism	Ref
Eucalyptus oil	major- 1,8- cineol	Reduces the production of inflammatory cytokines that stimulate cancer cell growth.	[27]
Thymus fallax	Carvacrol, thymol	Cytotoxicity by anti-oxidant mechanism	[28]
Boswellia sacra	α-pinene, myrcene, boswellic acid	Antiproliferative	[29]
Lippia alba	Geranial, geraniol	Citral dependent cytotoxicity.	[30]
Zanthoxylum rhoifolum	β-caryophyllene, α-pinene, myrcene	Cytotoxicity.	[31]
Peppermint oil	Menthol	Reduces chemotherapy induced nausea and vomiting.	[32]
Cymbopogon flexuosus	Citral	Induces apoptosis.	[33]
Patchouli oil	α-guaiene, seychellene, α-patchoulene	Induces apoptosis and decreases cell growth.	[34]
Rosewood oil	Linalool	Cytotoxicity.	[35]

(Table 1) cont.....

Essential oil	Constituent	Possible mechanism	Ref
Commiphora gileadensis	Sabinene, ß-caryophyllene, α-pinene	Anti-proliferative.	[36]

Anti-Cancer Mechanism of Action of Essential Oil

Essential oils have been shown to have anticancer properties *via* a variety of mechanisms, including cancer prevention and tumour cell action (Fig. **1**). Their mechanism includes an antimutagenic property. In this mechanism, essential oils prevent mutagens from entering the cell [16]. Other antimutagenic mechanisms include the inhibition of drug-metabolizing enzymes such as the phase I cytochrome P450 enzyme [17]. Vegetables containing essential oils such as garlic and onion have been reported to increase phase II enzymes such as glutathione S-transferase (GST), uridine 5'-diphospho-glucuronosyltransferase (UGT), quinone reductase (QR), and epoxide hydrolase (EH) [18 - 20]. Recently, citral was reported to inhibit cell proliferation and tumour growth by inducing oxidative stress [21]. Camphene isolated from Piper cernuum was reported to induce apoptosis by the caspase-3 pathway activation as well as activating the endoplasmic reticulum stress signal [22]. In another work, it was reported that carvacrol induced apoptosis in a metastatic breast cancer cell line by permeation through the mitochondrial membrane, resulting in cytochrome C release, induction of caspases through poly ADP ribose polymerase (PARP) cleavage, and DNA fragmentation [23, 26]. PKB (Protein Kinase B) is a vital molecule for cellular metabolism, transcription, cell cycle progression, and survival [24]. The vapour of essential oil obtained from Litsea cubeba seed induced cell cycle arrest and apoptosis in lung carcinoma cells [25]. Terpineol has been shown to inhibit cell proliferation in a lung cell line by decreasing NF-B transcription in tumour cells [25]. Another mechanism consists of the antioxidant property of essential oils, which results in the prevention of cancer. Eugenol extracted from clove oil is known to induce antioxidant properties by reacting with reactive oxygen species (ROS) and preventing DNA or protein damage [26, 27].

Aromatherapy And Cancer Clinical Trials

Patients with different types of cancer were studied using blends of essential oil in various forms. The studies are summarized in Table **2**. A total of 16 clinical trials are reported from 2017 to 2019. The age range of participants was between 28 to 72 years. Massage and inhalation aromatherapy were majorly used in the study. The aromas were used either in pure or in combination form. The most common aromas include lavender, ginger and chamomile. Complications such as anxiety, nausea, vomiting, pain, sleep quality, and oral mucositis were studied.

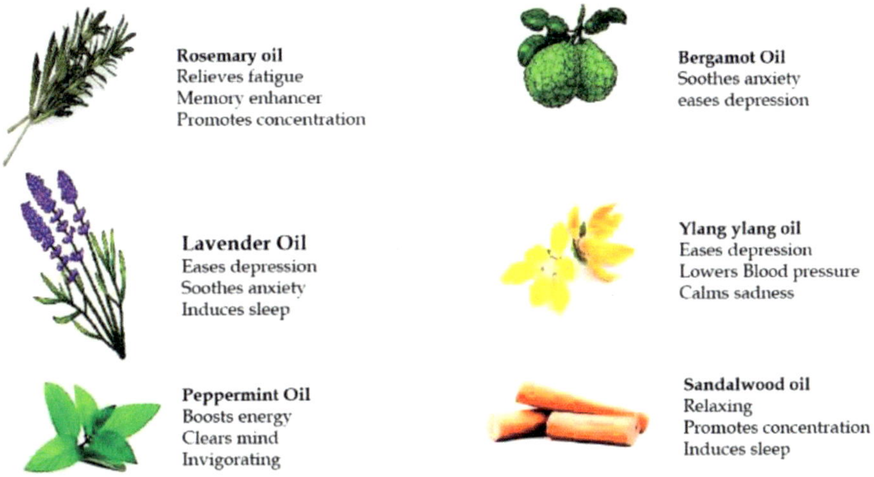

Fig. (1). Essential oils or aroma used in mood management.

Table 2. Role of Araomatherapy in treatment of cancer

Type of cancer	Number of participants	Gender (Male/ Female)	Country	Outcomes	Type of Aromatherapy	Dose, Frequency	Result	Ref
Multiple	123	39/84	Turkey	Pain and anxiety	Inhalation aromatherapy using Lavender and Eucalyptus,, once	3 drops once, 3 min duration, Once	Effective on pain but not on anxiety.	[38]
Multiple	60	29/31	Turkey	Pain	Inhalation aromatherapy using orange, chamomile, and lavender.	3 drops, Every night	Positive effect on pain.	[39]
Multiple	45	17/28	Iran	Sleep quality	Inhalation aromatherapy using Rosa damascene.	5 drops, Every night for 2 weeks	Positive effect on sleep. quality	[40]
Gastrointestinal	46	27/19	Turkey	Painful paresthesia, Neuropathic Pain and Fatigue	Massage aromatherapy using peppermint, chamomile, and rosemary.	50 ml, 40 min three times a week for 6 week; 18 session	Positive effect on pain and fatigue.	[41]

(Table 2) cont.....

Type of cancer	Number of participants	Gender (Male/ Female)	Country	Outcomes	Type of Aromatherapy	Dose, Frequency	Result	Ref
Colorectal cancer	80	44/36	Turkey	Anxiety, Sleep quality	Massage aromatherapy using Lavender	5 ml twice a day, 10 min duration, 2 session	Positive effect on both.	[42]
Breast Cancer	100	0-100	China	Anxiety, Pain	1. Massage aromatherapy 2. Inhalation aromatherapy using Bergamot, Geranium, lavender.	1. Weekly, 3.1 hour for 4 weeks 2. 3 drops 15 min, 15 min 1 day	Positive effect on anxiety, depression.	[43]
Breast Cancer	75	0-75	Turkey	Nausea, Vomiting	Inhalation/Massage aromatherapy using peppermint, bergamot, and cardamom.	2 ml for inhalation once every 21 days; 3 min inhalation, 20 min massage	Effect on Nausea and Vomiting.	[44]
Multiple Type	49	30/19	USA	Nausea, Vomiting	Inhalation aromatherapy using essential oil of ginger.	4 drops, three session	No effect	[45]
Acute Myeloid Leukemia (AML)	50	28/22	USA	Insomnia, Symptom burden	1. Inhalation aromatherapy using wheatgerm with lavender, peppermint, or chamomile. 2. Inhalation Aromatherapy	one drop of each aromas, daily. Every Night, 14 sessions	Positive effect on insomnia, Symptom burden.	[46]
Breast	153	0/153	Japan	Vital signs, Quality of Life	Inhalation aromatherapy using ylang–ylang, orange, and lavende	1 day, 3.19 h	No effect.	[47]
Head and neck	19	15/5	Australia	Oral mucositis, pain, nutrition status	Gargle using manuka, kanuka oils.	2 drops in 15 ml warm water, 3-5 times daily; 24-40 session, 8 days	Positive effect on oral mucositis, Pain, nutrition status.	[48]

(Table 2) cont.....

Type of cancer	Number of participants	Gender (Male/ Female)	Country	Outcomes	Type of Aromatherapy	Dose, Frequency	Result	Ref
Thyroid	71	16/55	Japan	Salivary Gland Damage	Inhalation aromatherapy using Citrus lemon, Zingiber.	0.5-1 ml three times daily, 10 min, 2 weeks	Positive effect on Salivary Gland Damage.	[49]
Breast cancer	60	0/60	Malaysia	Nutritional status	Inhalation aromatherapy using ginger Oil.	2 drops, three times a day. 2 min, 42 session, two weeks.	Positive effect on nutritional status.	[50]
Multiple	60	22/38	India	Anxiety	Massage and Inhalation aromatherapy using lavender Oil.	6 drops, every hour. 3.10 min	Positive effect on anxiety.	[51]
Haematological	39	16/23	United Kingdom	Cortisol and prolactin; Quality of Life	Massage aromatherapy	0.5 hourly for 2 h and at 24 h.	Positive effects.	[52]
Cervical	60	0/60	Indonesia	Nausea, Vomiting	Inhalation aromatherapy using ginger.	5 drops, once time, 10 min	Positive effects.	[53]

Anxiety and Aromatherapy

From Table **2**, it was observed that massage aromatherapy improved anxiety symptoms. The most effective aromas reported were lavender, chamomile and bergamot. In case of inhalation aromatherapy, lavender can be used.

Quality of Life and Aromatherapy

From Table **2**, it was observed that massage aromatherapy improved quality of life. Lavender was most commonly used.

Pain and Aromatherapy

Massage or inhalation aromatherapy both showed significant decrease in pain. Most commonly used aroma was lavender for pain relief. Gargle using aroma also decreased significant amount of pain in one study.

Nausea and Vomiting and Aromatherapy

Inhalation aromatherapy showed significant relief in nausea and vomiting in cancer patients. Most commonly used aromas are peppermint, ginger and cardamom.

Sleep Quality and Aromatherapy

Both massage and inhalation approach in aromatherapy showed improvement in sleep quality. Lavender was most commonly used aroma

Fatigue

Massage aromatherapy showed improvement in fatigue. The most commonly used aroma was chamomile.

Essential Oil Safety

Essential oils may decrease or increase the effectiveness of certain drugs, depending on the quantity of oil used, the concentration of oil, and the method of aromatherapy used. During cancer therapy, changes in skin may occur. Therefore, testing an essential oil on skin becomes vital, to observe rash or redness specially in case of topical application [11].

CONCLUSION

Aromatherapy can be effectively used for reducing physical and psychological disorders. Essential oil has reportedly showed improvement in various complications arising in the treatment of cancer patients. However it must be used as alternative or as an adjuvant treatment after consulting with aromatherapists. The most commonly used aromas are lavender, peppermint, chamomile, and orange. The reports generally indicate aromatherapy to be safe. Additionally, cost associated with aromatherapy is less. Hence the need arises that more research is carried out in aromatherapy, for reducing the various complications arising in cancer treatment.

Bax: B-cell lymphoma 2-associated X protein; Bcl-2: B-cell lymphoma 2; CAT: catalase; CDK: cyclin-dependant kinase; CytC: cytochrome C; CytP450: cytochrome P450; EH: epoxide hydrolase; EO: essential oil; ER: endoplasmic reticulum; ETC: electron transport chain; GPx: glutathione peroxidase; GSH: glutathione; GST: glutathione *S*-transferase; mdm2: murine double minute 2; mTOR: mechanistic target of rapamycin; MITO: mitochondria; NFκB: nuclear factor-κB; PARP: poly ADP ribose polymerase; pPDK1: protein pyruvate dehydrogenase kinase 1; PKB: protein kinase B; QT: quinone reductase; ROS:

reactive oxygen species; SOD: superoxide dismutase; UGT: uridine 5'-diphospho-glucuronosyltransferase.

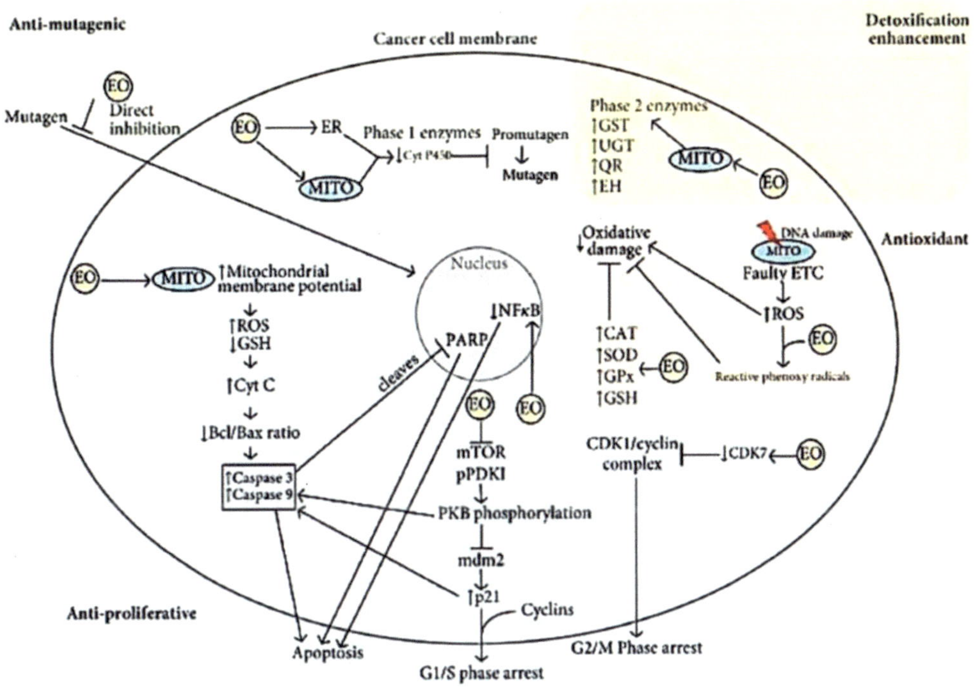

Fig. (3). Mechanism of action of essential oil as anticancer agents [16]

REFERENCES

[1] Sung H, Ferlay J, Siegel RL, *et al.* Global cancer statistics 2020: GLOBOCAN estimates of incidence and mortality worldwide for 36 cancers in 185 countries. CA Cancer J Clin 2021; 71(3): 209-49. [http://dx.doi.org/10.3322/caac.21660] [PMID: 33538338]

[2] Madmoli M. Evaluation of chemotherapy complications in patients with Cancer: A systematic review. Int J Res Stud Sci Eng Technol 2018; 5(12): 59-64.

[3] Varker KA, Ansel A, Aukerman G, Carson WE III. Review of complementary and alternative medicine and selected nutraceuticals: background for a pilot study on nutrigenomic intervention in patients with advanced cancer. Altern Ther Health Med 2012; 18(2): 26-34. [PMID: 22516882]

[4] Balouchi A, Rahnama M, Hastings-Tolsma M, Shoja MM, Bolaydehyi E. Knowledge, attitude and use of complementary and integrative health strategies: a preliminary survey of Iranian nurses. J Integr Med 2016; 14(2): 121-7. [http://dx.doi.org/10.1016/S2095-4964(16)60245-5] [PMID: 26988433]

[5] Rezaie-Keikhaie K, Hastings-Tolsma M, Bouya S, *et al.* Effect of aromatherapy on post-partum complications: A systematic review. Complement Ther Clin Pract 2019; 35: 290-5. [http://dx.doi.org/10.1016/j.ctcp.2019.03.010] [PMID: 31003672]

[6] Ali B, Al-Wabel NA, Shams S, Ahamad A, Khan SA, Anwar F. Essential oils used in aromatherapy: A systemic review. Asian Pac J Trop Biomed 2015; 5(8): 601-11.

[http://dx.doi.org/10.1016/j.apjtb.2015.05.007]

[7] Babashahi Kohanestani F, Ahmadi F, Memarian R. The effect of Lavender aromatherapy program on the pain intensity of patients with AML undergoing chemotherapy. J Urmia Nurs Midwifery Faculty 2013; 11(3)

[8] Heydarirad G, Keyhanmehr AS, Mofid B, Nikfarjad H, Mosavat SH. Efficacy of aromatherapy with Rosa damascena in the improvement of sleep quality of cancer patients: A randomized controlled clinical trial. Complement Ther Clin Pract 2019; 35: 57-61. [http://dx.doi.org/10.1016/j.ctcp.2019.01.017] [PMID: 31003687]

[9] Louis M, Kowalski SD. Use of aromatherapy with hospice patients to decrease pain, anxiety, and depression and to promote an increased sense of well-being. Am J Hosp Palliat Care 2002; 19(6): 381-6. [http://dx.doi.org/10.1177/104990910201900607] [PMID: 12442972]

[10] Lua PL, Salihah N, Mazlan N. Effects of inhaled ginger aromatherapy on chemotherapy-induced nausea and vomiting and health-related quality of life in women with breast cancer. Complement Ther Med 2015; 23(3): 396-404. [http://dx.doi.org/10.1016/j.ctim.2015.03.009] [PMID: 26051575]

[11] Dunning T. Aromatherapy: Overview, safety and quality issues. OA Alternative Medicine 2013; 1(1): 1-6. [http://dx.doi.org/10.13172/2052-7845-1-1-518]

[12] Lee M, Lee H, Khalil M, Lim H, Lim HJ. Aromatherapy for managing pain in primary dysmenorrhea: A systematic review of randomized placebo-controlled trials. J Clin Med 2018; 7(11): 434. [http://dx.doi.org/10.3390/jcm7110434] [PMID: 30423839]

[13] Wildwood C. The Encyclopedia of Aromatherapy. Healing Arts Press 1996.

[14] Bakkali F, Averbeck S, Averbeck D, Idaomar M. Biological effects of essential oils – A review. Food Chem Toxicol 2008; 46(2): 446-75. [http://dx.doi.org/10.1016/j.fct.2007.09.106] [PMID: 17996351]

[15] Blowman K, Magalhães M, Lemos MFL, Cabral C, Pires IM. Anticancer properties of essential oils and natural products. Evid Based Complement Alternat Med 2018; 2018: 1-12. [http://dx.doi.org/10.1155/2018/3149362] [PMID: 29765461]

[16] De Flora S, Ramel C. Mechanisms of inhibitors of mutagenesis and carcinogenesis. Classification and overview. Mutat Res 1988; 202(2): 285-306. [http://dx.doi.org/10.1016/0027-5107(88)90193-5] [PMID: 3057362]

[17] Gudi VA, Singh SV. Effect of diallyl sulfide, a naturally occurring anti-carcinogen, on glutathione-dependent detoxification enzymes of female CD-1 mouse tissues. Biochem Pharmacol 1991; 42(6): 1261-5. [http://dx.doi.org/10.1016/0006-2952(91)90263-5] [PMID: 1888335]

[18] Haber D, Siess M-H, De Waziers I, Beaune P, Suschetet M. Modification of hepatic drug-metabolizing enzymes in rat fed naturally occurring allyl sulphides. Xenobiotica 1994; 24(2): 169-82. [http://dx.doi.org/10.3109/00498259409043230] [PMID: 8017091]

[19] Sparnins VL, Barany G, Wattenberg LW. Effects of organosulfur compounds from garlic and onions on benzo[*a*]pyrene-induced neoplasia and glutathione S-transferase activity in the mouse. Carcinogenesis 1988; 9(1): 131-4. [http://dx.doi.org/10.1093/carcin/9.1.131] [PMID: 3335037]

[20] Sanches LJ, Marinello PC, Panis C, *et al.* Cytotoxicity of citral against melanoma cells: The involvement of oxidative stress generation and cell growth protein reduction. Tumour Biol 2017; 39(3) [http://dx.doi.org/10.1177/1010428317695914] [PMID: 28351318]

[21] Girola N, Figueiredo CR, Farias CF, *et al.* Camphene isolated from essential oil of *Piper cernuum* (Piperaceae) induces intrinsic apoptosis in melanoma cells and displays antitumor activity *in vivo.*

Biochem Biophys Res Commun 2015; 467(4): 928-34.
[http://dx.doi.org/10.1016/j.bbrc.2015.10.041] [PMID: 26471302]

[22] Arunasree KM. Anti-proliferative effects of carvacrol on a human metastatic breast cancer cell line, MDA-MB 231. Phytomed 2010; 17(8-9): 581-8.

[23] Fayard E, Tintignac LA, Baudry A, Hemmings BA. Protein kinase B/Akt at a glance. J Cell Sci 2005; 118(24): 5675-8.
[http://dx.doi.org/10.1242/jcs.02724] [PMID: 16339964]

[24] Seal S, Chatterjee P, Bhattacharya S, *et al.* Vapor of volatile oils from litsea cubeba seed induces apoptosis and causes cell cycle arrest in lung cancer cells. PLoS ONE 2012.

[25] Hassan SB, Gali-Muhtasib H, Göransson H, Larsson R. Alpha terpineol: a potential anticancer agent which acts through suppressing NF-kappaB signalling. Anticancer Res 2010; 30(6): 1911-9.
[PMID: 20651334]

[26] Sharifi-Rad J, Sureda A, Tenore G, *et al.* Biological Activities of Essential Oils: From Plant Chemoecology to Traditional Healing Systems. Molecules 2017; 22(1): 70.
[http://dx.doi.org/10.3390/molecules22010070] [PMID: 28045446]

[27] Merchán Arenas DR, Acevedo AM, Vargas Méndez LY, Kouznetsov VV. Scavenger activity evaluation of the clove bud essential oil (Eugenia caryophyllus) and eugenol derivatives employing ABTS +· decolorization. Sci Pharm 2011; 79(4): 779-91.
[http://dx.doi.org/10.3797/scipharm.1109-11] [PMID: 22145105]

[28] Schor J. Eucalyptus Oil: A Possible Aid for Cancer Patients. Botanical Medicine, Oncology, Pain Medicine 2010.

[29] Çetinus E, Temiz T, Ergül M, Altun A, Çetinus Ş, Kaya T. Thyme essential oil inhibits proliferation of DLD-1 colorectal cancer cells through antioxidant effect. Cumhuriyet Medical Journal 2013; 35(1): 14-24.
[http://dx.doi.org/10.7197/1305-0028.1757]

[30] Suhail MM, Wu W, Cao A, *et al. Boswellia sacra* essential oil induces tumor cell-specific apoptosis and suppresses tumor aggressiveness in cultured human breast cancer cells. BMC Complement Altern Med 2011; 11(1): 129.
[http://dx.doi.org/10.1186/1472-6882-11-129] [PMID: 22171782]

[31] Mesa-Arango AC, Montiel-Ramos J, Zapata B, Durán C, Betancur-Galvis L, Stashenko E. Citral and carvone chemotypes from the essential oils of Colombian *Lippia alba* (Mill.) N.E. Brown: composition, cytotoxicity and antifungal activity. Mem Inst Oswaldo Cruz 2009; 104(6): 878-84.
[http://dx.doi.org/10.1590/S0074-02762009000600010] [PMID: 19876560]

[32] Silva SL, Figueiredo PM, Yano T. Cytotoxic evaluation of essential oil from *Zanthoxylum rhoifolium* Lam. leaves. Acta Amazon 2007; 37(2): 281-6.
[http://dx.doi.org/10.1590/S0044-59672007000200015]

[33] Tayarani-Najaran Z, Talasaz-Firoozi E, Nasiri R, Jalali N, Hassanzadeh M. Antiemetic activity of volatile oil from Mentha spicata and Mentha × piperita in chemotherapy-induced nausea and vomiting. Ecancermedicalscience 2013; 7: 290.
[PMID: 23390455]

[34] Kumar A, Malik F, Bhushan S, *et al.* An essential oil and its major constituent isointermedeol induce apoptosis by increased expression of mitochondrial cytochrome c and apical death receptors in human leukaemia HL-60 cells. Chem Biol Interact 2008; 171(3): 332-47.
[http://dx.doi.org/10.1016/j.cbi.2007.10.003] [PMID: 18070620]

[35] Jeong JB, Choi J, Lou Z, Jiang X, Lee SH. Patchouli alcohol, an essential oil of *Pogostemon cablin*, exhibits anti-tumorigenic activity in human colorectal cancer cells. Int Immunopharmacol 2013; 16(2): 184-90.
[http://dx.doi.org/10.1016/j.intimp.2013.04.006] [PMID: 23602914]

[36] Sœur J, Marrot L, Perez P, *et al.* Selective cytotoxicity of *Aniba rosaeodora* essential oil towards epidermoid cancer cells through induction of apoptosis. Mutat Res Genet Toxicol Environ Mutagen 2011; 718(1-2): 24-32.
[http://dx.doi.org/10.1016/j.mrgentox.2010.10.009] [PMID: 21070863]

[37] Amiel E, Ofir R, Dudai N, Soloway E, Rabinsky T, Rachmilevitch S. β-Caryophyllene, a compound isolated from the biblical balm of gilead (*Commiphora gileadensis*), is a selective apoptosis inducer for tumor cell lines. Evid Based Complement Alternat Med 2012; 2012: 1-8.
[http://dx.doi.org/10.1155/2012/872394] [PMID: 22567036]

[38] Yayla EM, Ozdemir L. Effect of inhalation aromatherapy on procedural pain and anxiety after needle insertion into an implantable central venous port catheter: A quasi-randomized controlled pilot study. Cancer Nurs 2019; 42(1): 35-41.
[http://dx.doi.org/10.1097/NCC.0000000000000551] [PMID: 29199999]

[39] İlter SM, Ovayolu Ö, Ovayolu N. The Effect of Inhaler Aromatherapy on Invasive Pain, Procedure Adherence, Vital Signs, and Saturation During Port Catheterization in Oncology Patients. Holist Nurs Pract 2019; 33(3): 146-54.
[http://dx.doi.org/10.1097/HNP.0000000000000322] [PMID: 30973434]

[40] Heydarirad G, Keyhanmehr AS, Mofid B, Nikfarjad H, Mosavat SH. Efficacy of aromatherapy with Rosa damascena in the improvement of sleep quality of cancer patients: A randomized controlled clinical trial. Complement Ther Clin Pract 2019; 35: 57-61.
[http://dx.doi.org/10.1016/j.ctcp.2019.01.017] [PMID: 31003687]

[41] Izgu N, Ozdemir L, Bugdayci Basal F. Effect of aromatherapy massage on chemotherapy- induced peripheral neuropathic pain and fatigue in patients receiving oxaliplatin: An open label quasi-randomized controlled pilot study. Cancer Nurs 2019; 42(2): 139-47.
[http://dx.doi.org/10.1097/NCC.0000000000000577] [PMID: 29200001]

[42] Ayik C, Özden D. The effects of preoperative aromatherapy massage on anxiety and sleep quality of colorectal surgery patients: A randomized controlled study. Complement Ther Med 2018; 36: 93-9.
[http://dx.doi.org/10.1016/j.ctim.2017.12.002] [PMID: 29458940]

[43] Xiao Y, Li L, Xie Y, Xu J, Liu Y. [Effects of aroma therapy and music intervention on pain and anxious for breast cancer patients in the perioperative period]. Zhong Nan Da Xue Xue Bao Yi Xue Ban 2018; 43(6): 656-61. [Effects of aroma therapy and music intervention on pain and anxious for breast cancer patients in the perioperative period].
[PMID: 30110009]

[44] Zorba P, Ozdemir L. The preliminary effects of massage and inhalation aromatherapy on chemotherapy-induced acute nausea and vomiting: A quasi-randomized controlled pilot trial. Cancer Nurs 2018; 41(5): 359-66.
[http://dx.doi.org/10.1097/NCC.0000000000000496] [PMID: 28426542]

[45] Evans A, Malvar J, Garretson C, Pedroja Kolovos E, Baron Nelson M. The use of aromatherapy to reduce chemotherapy-induced nausea in children with Cancer: A randomized, double-blind, placebo-controlled trial. J Pediatr Oncol Nurs 2018; 35(6): 392-8.
[http://dx.doi.org/10.1177/1043454218782133] [PMID: 29947285]

[46] Blackburn L, Achor S, Allen B, *et al.* The effect of aromatherapy on insomnia and other common symptoms among patients with acute leukemia. Oncol Nurs Forum 2017; 44(4): E185-E193 .
[http://dx.doi.org/10.1188/17.ONF.E185-E193] [PMID: 28640576]

[47] Tamaki K, Fukuyama AK, Terukina S, *et al.* Randomized trial of aromatherapy *versus* conventional care for breast cancer patients during perioperative periods. Breast Cancer Res Treat 2017; 162(3): 523-31.
[http://dx.doi.org/10.1007/s10549-017-4134-7] [PMID: 28181131]

[48] Maddocks-Jennings W, Wilkinson JM, Cavanagh HM, Shillington D. Evaluating the effects of the essential oils Leptospermum scoparium (manuka) and Kunzea ericoides (kanuka) on radiotherapy

induced mucositis: A randomized, placebo controlled feasibility study. Eur J Oncol Nurs 2009; 13(2): 87-93.
[http://dx.doi.org/10.1016/j.ejon.2009.01.002] [PMID: 19297246]

[49] Nakayama M, Okizaki A, Takahashi K. A randomized controlled trial for the effectiveness of aromatherapy in decreasing salivary gland damage following radioactive iodine therapy for differentiated thyroid Cancer. BioMed Res Int 2016; 2016: 1-6.
[http://dx.doi.org/10.1155/2016/9509810] [PMID: 28042578]

[50] Salihah N, Mazlan N, Lua PL. The effectiveness of inhaled ginger essential oil in improving dietary intake in breast-cancer patients experiencing chemotherapy-induced nausea and vomiting. Focus Altern Complement Ther 2016; 21(1): 8-16.
[http://dx.doi.org/10.1111/fct.12236]

[51] Santosh D, Joseph S, Jose A, *et al.* Anxiolytic and antiemetic effects of aromatherapy in cancer patients on anticancer chemotherapy. Pharmacologyonline 2011; 3: 736-44.

[52] Stringer J, Swindell R, Dennis M. Massage in patients undergoing intensive chemotherapy reduces serum cortisol and prolactin. Psychooncology 2008; 17(10): 1024-31.
[http://dx.doi.org/10.1002/pon.1331] [PMID: 18300336]

[53] Sriningsih I, Elisa E, Lestari KP. Aromatherapy ginger use in patients with nausea & vomiting on post cervical Cancer chemotherapy. Jurnal Kesehatan Masyarakat 2017; 13(1): 59-68.
[http://dx.doi.org/10.15294/kemas.v13i1.5367]

CHAPTER 3

The Traditional Immune Boosting Recipes

Rokeya Sultana[1,*]

[1] *Department of Pharmacognosy, Yenepoya Pharmacy College and Research Centre, Under Yenepoya Deemed to be University, Mangalore, Karnataka, India.*

Abstract: The immune system is amazingly complicated and vital for our survival. Several different systems and cell types of our body work effortlessly in ideal synchrony throughout the body to fight off pathogens and clear up dead cells. Our immune systems perform an implausible job by putting up a wall that can safeguard the disease-causing microorganisms. Our immune system requires equilibrium to function smoothly, so a person must eat and drink healthy balanced foods for getting energy and nutrients. The immunity related diseases may occur due to several factors such as seasonal change, environment factors, virus attacks, and simple stress. To combat these, we need to consume immunity-boosting foods and nutrients rich in antioxidants like *Alium sativum, Alium cepa, Citrus limon, Withania somnifera,Moringa oleifera, Curcuma longa, etc.*, which can build up the immunity. The traditional system of medicine like Ayurveda and Siddha system of medicine quoted several traditional immune-boosting recipes like Maha- sudharshnachoornam, Talisadichoornam, Dhanavantam, Gulika-churnam, sitophaladichoornam, *etc.* Several times it is proven that lifestyle and dietary changes can result in a better immune system. A healthy lifestyle includes consuming foods which help in boosting immunity. In addition to keeping a balanced diet in our daily life, there is a necessity for traditional immunity-boosting agents simultaneously. Traditional immunity-boosting agents are usually rich in vitamins, antioxidants, and other minerals and the requisite nutrients for maintaining equilibrium in the immune system. In this chapter, detailed information about Traditional immunity-boosting agents will be discussed.

Keywords: *Alium sativum*, *Alium cepa*, Antioxidants, *Citrus limon*, *Curcuma longa*, Disease-causing, Dhanavantam, Environment factors, Gulika-churnam, Healthy lifestyle, Immune system, Immunity, Immunity-boosting agents, Microorganisms, *Moringa oleifera*, Maha- sudharshnachoornam, Pathogens, Seasonal change, Safeguard, Simple stress, Sitophaladichoornam, Traditional, Talisadichoornam, Vitamins, Virus attacks, *Withania somnifera*.

[*] **Corresponding author Rokeya Sultana:** Department of Pharmacognosy, Yenepoya Pharmacy College and Research Centre, Under Yenepoya Deemed to be University, Mangalore, Karnataka, India; E-mail: rokeya009ster@gmail.com & drrokeyasultana@yenepoya.edu.in

Motamarri Venkata Naga Lalitha Chaitanya, Galvina Pereira, & Heyam Saad Ali (Eds.)

INTRODUCTION

***Immunity*:** Immunity can be defined as a very complex biological system which is endowed with the capacity to recognize and withstand anything that belongs to the body itself, and to distinguish and decline what is foreign. The immune system protects us from various invading pathogenic microorganisms and other immunosuppressive diseases like cancer. Immune system is a complex network of different specialized cells, tissues and chemical mediators (Fig. **1**) [1]. The immune system always plays a vital role in the defence system against any infection [2].

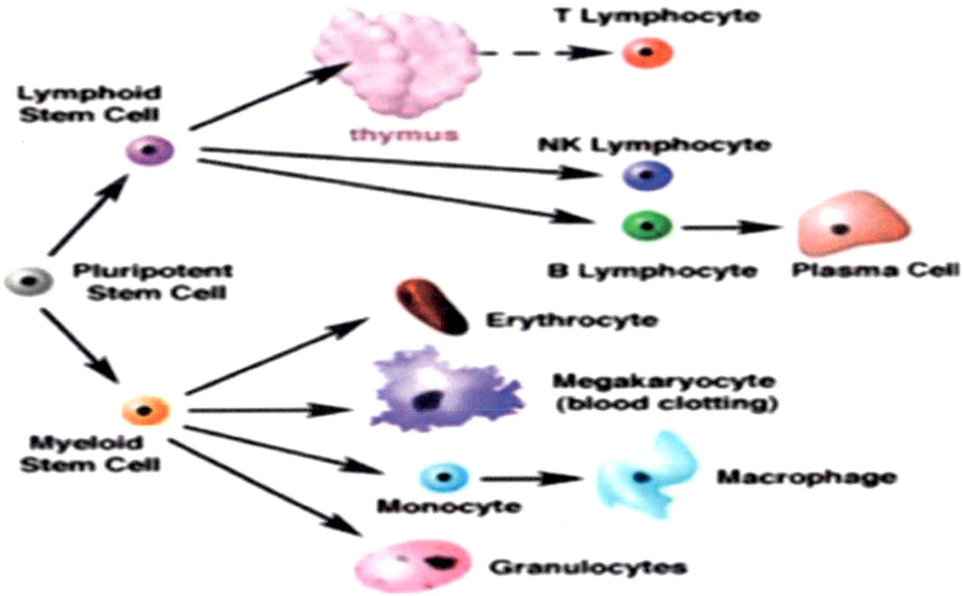

Fig. (1). Complex network of immune system [1].

Types of immunity: There are two types of immunity. Natural or innate immunity and adaptive immunity. All animals possess an ancient system of defence against the pathogens in which they are susceptible, which is called as innate, or natural, immunity and this includes two parts. The first part is called humoral innate immunity which involves a variety of substances found in the humors or body fluids. They interfere with the growth of pathogens or clump with them together to eliminate them from the body. The second part is called cellular innate immunity which is carried out by different cells called as phagocytes, which ingest as well as degrade pathogens. Innate immunity is nonspecific that is, it is not directed against specific invaders of the body but against any pathogens which enter into the body. Vertebrates have additional and more sophisticated defence mechanisms system, called adaptive immunity, which can recognize and destroy specific substances.

***Immune Response*:** The defensive reaction of the adaptive immune system is called the immune response. Any substance capable of generating such a response is called an antigen, or immunogen. Antigens are not foreign microorganisms and tissues; they are toxins or enzymes in the microorganisms or tissues that the immune system considers foreign. When an antigen enters the body, it may be partly neutralized by components of the innate immune system. It may be attacked by phagocytes or by preformed antibodies that act together with the complement system. For a strong immune system, the body requires energy and nutrients. This depends on what an individual consumes regularly. Moreover, it is important to understand that strong immunity is not built overnight, but by religiously consuming healthy food that has high nutritional value. The immune system protects the body from any kind of bacterial or viral infections by preventing them from invading our bodies (Fig. **2**) [3]. Thus a stronger immune system is an essential means of fighting bacterial or any other viral infections [4].

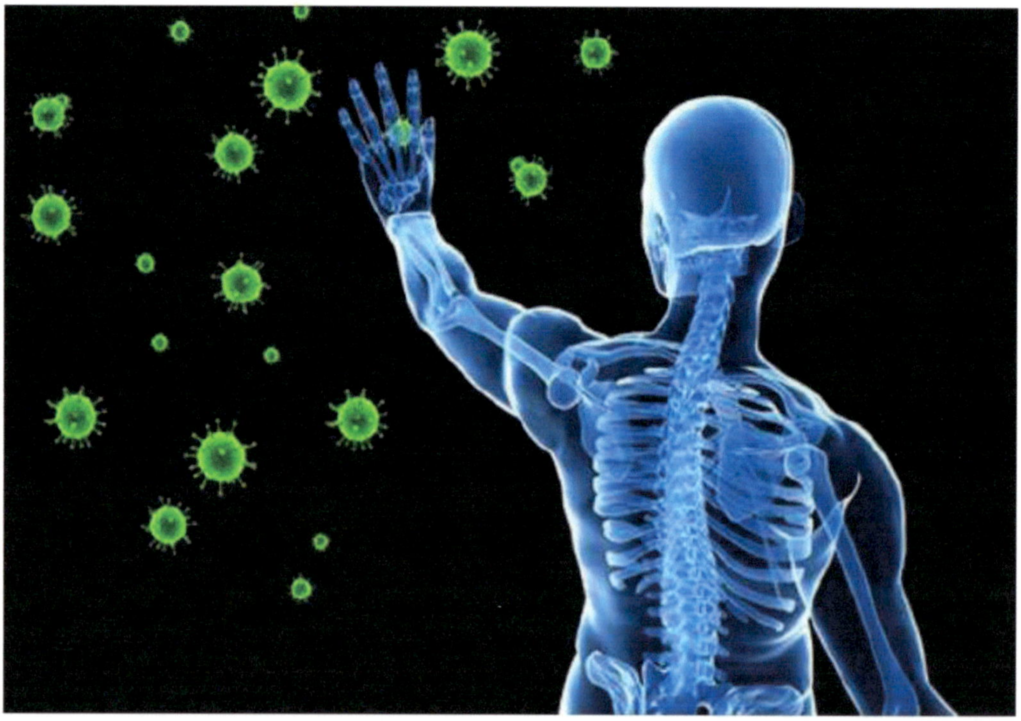

Fig. (2). The immune system depicting to protect the body from any kind of bacterial or viral infections [3].

***Immunostimulants*:** Substances (drugs and nutrients) that stimulate the immune system by inducing activation or increasing the activity of any of its components are called Immunostimulants, also known as immunostimulators. One of the most important sources of an immunostimulator that are being explored extensively currently comes from plant derived substances [5]. A large population of India uses plants for its healing, preventive, curative and much therapeutic property together with immunostimulatory property [6].

Certain medicinal plants promote positive health and maintain organic resistance against infection by re-establishing body equilibrium. Many polysaccharides isolated from higher plants are considered to be biological response modifiers and enhance various immune responses, like complement activation, proliferation of lymphocytes and stimulation of macrophages.

Plant flavonoids are also used as immunostimulators, which is important for growth, development and immunity [7]. Various synthetic agents are used as immunostimulative agents such as levamisole, thalidomide, but there are various side effects of these agents such as nephrotoxicity, hepatotoxicity, bone marrow depression, gastrointestinal disturbance and so on. Because of the side effects associated with synthetic agents and as plants are safer, much more effective and cheaper, conventional immunomodulator plants can be explored [8]. Many Plant drugs are rejuvenators, and nutritional supplements as well as possess strong antioxidant activities and act as potent immunomodulators by exerting antagonistic action on oxidative stressors, giving rise to the formation of different free radicals. They are used mainly to combat the effects of ageing, atherosclerosis, cancer, diabetes, rheumatoid arthritis, autoimmune disease and Parkinson's disease.

Traditional System of Medicine and its Role in Immunity Boosting

India is known for its traditional or alternative medicinal systems such as Ayurveda, Siddha, and Unani. Medical systems are found mentioned even in the ancient Vedas and other scriptures. The Ayurvedic concept appeared and developed between 2500 and 500 BC in India. More than 80 percent of people in developing countries cannot afford the most basic medical procedures, drugs, and vaccines. Among wealthier populations in both developed and developing countries thus, alternative practices are adjuncts or alternatives to Western medical approaches. Alternative practices are popular although proof of their safety and effectiveness is modest. Evidence-based research in Ayurveda is receiving larger acceptance in India and abroad. India has an ancient heritage of traditional herbal medicines. With the emerging interest in the world to adopt study of the traditional system and to exploit their potentials based on different healthcare systems [9], the World Health Organization estimates that about 80% of the populations living in the developing countries rely almost exclusively on traditional medicine for their primary health care needs [10]. India is the largest producer of medicinal plants. There are currently about 250,000 registered medical practitioners of the Ayurvedic system, as compared to about 700,000 of the modern medicine. In India, around 20,000 medicinal plants have been recorded; however, traditional practitioners use only 7,000–7,500 plants for curing different diseases. In India, around 25,000 effective plant-based formulations are used in traditional and folk medicine.

The use of herbal drugs for treating various diseases predates human history that forms the origin of much of the modern medicine. Herbs are traditionally used in many therapeutic practices, if not as the main, then as the accompanying therapy in combination with medications, aimed at boosting immunity for prevention. Traditional medicines are being used by those people who do not use or cannot be helped by conventional medicinal system [11]. Some common medicinal plants having nutraceutical potential and their primary use in traditional medicine are being given in Table **1**.

Table 1. Common medicinal plants having nutraceutical potential and their primary use in traditional medicine.

Plant name	Common name	Uses
Asparagus racemosus **[12]**	Shatavari	A potent Ayurvedic rejuvenative. It supplies many female hormones and mostly recommended for those women who have hysterectomies. It also helps to maintain urinary tract and strengthens the immune system and also purifies the blood.
Commiphora mukul **[13]**	Guggul	A major ingredient in joint and immunocare and regarded as a remedy in Ayurvedic medicine; it increases white blood cell count to provide strong immuno-modulating properties. It also protects against the common cold as well as used in various other conditions like lower cholesterol and triglycerides, while maintaining the HDL to LDL ratio.
Cyperus scariosus **[14]**	Nagarmusta	Useful in supporting healthy genitourinary system and has hepatoprotective properties.
Garcinia cambogia **[15]**	Garcinia	Fruits contain biologically active compounds (−) hydroxycitric acid, which is known to inhibit the synthesis of lipids and fatty acids. HCA inhibits the enzyme ATP-citrate lyase that leads to reduce production of acetyl CoA, which is a key substance in fat and carbohydrate metabolism. Therefore, formation of LDL and triglycerides is very low. It also suppresses appetite by promoting synthesis of glycogen. That way the brain gets signals of fullness and satisfaction sooner. Garcinia contains significant amounts of vitamin C and is used as a heart tonic.

(Table 1) cont.....

Plant name	Common name	Uses
Glycyrrhiza glabra **[16]**	Yashtimadhu, Licorice	It is a versatile medicine in India and China, for gastrointestinal health. It is a mild laxative, soothes and tones the mucous membranes, and relieves muscle spasms. It is an antioxidant, cancer protecting, botanical boosting, and helps in certain immune functions such as interferon production. Its mode of action is as an antimutagen, preventing damage to genetic material that can eventually result in cancer.
Gymnema sylvestre **[17]**	Gurmarar	Its Sanskrit name means literally "sugar destroyer," has a glycolytic action, and reduces the strength of a glucose solution. It has been used in Ayurveda to regulate sugar metabolism for several centuries. It increases insulin production, regeneration of pancreas cells, and the site of insulin production. Another property is abolishing the taste of sugar, so that Gurmarar has been effective to suppress and neutralize the craving for sweets.
Melia azadirachta **[18]**	Nimba, Neem	It has strong disease alleviating activity, used as a tonic and astringent that promotes healing. The extract has antispasmodic action. Its usage in Ayurvedic medicine for thousands of years has proved its detoxifying properties. It has shown most beneficial effects for the circulatory, digestive, respiratory, and urinary systems.
Momordica charantia **[19]**	Karela, Bitter melon	Karela has been widely used in Ayurvedic medicine. It contains Gurmarin, a polypeptide considered to be similar to bovine insulin, and has a strong sugar regulating effect by suppressing the neural responses to sweet taste stimuli.
Moringa pterygosperma **[20]**	Shigru, Horseradish tree	Shigru contains physiologically active principles that is effective in a broad range of health needs. It contains "Pterygospermin," an antibiotic-like substance.
Mucuna pruriens **[21]**	Kiwanch, Kapikachchhu, Cow-itch plant	It is a good natural source of *L. dopa*. In the Ayurvedic system it is reported as an effective tonic for nervous system. Studies have demonstrated its usefulness maintaining optimum performance of the nervous system.
Nardostachys jatamansi **[22]**	Jatamansi, Musk root	Jatamansi is a relaxing plant, effective for mental health. It is used in various Ayurvedic formulations as a potent ingredient. It has been shown effective in maintaining a restful sleep and with many menopausal symptoms.
Piper longum **[23]**	Pippali, Indian Long Pepper	Pippali is a powerful stimulant for both the digestive and the respiratory systems and has a rejuvenating effect on lungs. It plays an important role in the release of metabolic heat energy. This effect is the result of increased thyroid hormone level in the body. Pippali a typical Ayurvedic complementary component whose benefit is to increase the bioavailability and enhance absorption of the other active ingredients.
Piper nigrum **[24]**	Maricha, Black pepper	The black pepper is one of the most important spices which is widely used to amplify the body's ability to absorb nutrients contained in the food and aid the digestive process.

(Table 1) cont.....

Plant name	Common name	Uses
Bergenia ligulata **[25]**	Pasanavheda	It has the unique property like diuretic action with optimum urinary tract health. This important drug supports bladder by acting on the crystalloid-colloid balance and keeping calcium salts in solution.
Terminalia chebula **[26]**	Haritaki	Haritaki is a safe and effective purgative, expectorant, and tonic. It is an important ingredient of the classical Ayurvedic formulation "Triphala" which has a combination of three fruits. Tiphalpha is an important Ayurvedic medicine, which promotes health through successive steps of purification and detoxification. It is known to have strong antimutagenic activity, because of its very rich content vitamin C.
Tinospora cordifolia **[27]**	Guduchi	Guduchi is a rich source of natural vitamin C and effective in inhibiting the growth of bacteria and in building up the immune resistance and has immune-boosting ability. The use of this plant increases white blood cells the killing ability of macrophages, the immune cells responsible for fighting invaders.
Withania somnifera **[28]**	Ashwagandha	In Ayurvedic medicines Ashwagandha holds a place similar to Ginseng in traditional Chinese medicinal therapies. It is also called the "Indian Ginseng." It has been used for thousands of years as a popular remedy in Ayurvedic systems for many conditions. It is one of the best health tonics and restorative agents that have been used to treat general debility.
Zingiber officinale **[29]**	Sunthi, Ginger	Ginger is considered an adjuvant in many Ayurvedic formulas in which it enhances absorption and prevents gastrointestinal side effects. It is a very common spice which is used in Ayurvedic medicine to improve digestion and to prevent nausea. These properties help bowel movements and relax the muscles which control the digestive system.

Medicinal Plants Used in Alternative/Traditional Medicines

Traditional treatments with herbal drugs using different parts such as plant's seeds, berries, roots, leaves, bark and flowers are increasing due to therapeutic reasons. Drugs with herbal origin have a prolonged history of use, outside the conventional medicine. The use of herbal supplements has increased dramatically over the past 30 years. Traditional medicine has been a productive resource for revealing novel lead molecules for modern drug discovery. The Ayurvedic and Siddha system of medicines not only provides that alternative, but also scores over the side effects and cost factor of allopathic medicine Immunomodulators are becoming very popular. Ayurvedic drugs have promising profile as far as drug development from natural source is concerned. The Rasayana herbs seem to operate through immunostimulant, immunoadjuvant, and immunosuppressant activities or by affecting the effector arm of the immune response. Several medicinal plants used in the Indian traditional system known as Rasayana (devoted to enhancement of the body's resistance) have attracted the attention of scientists world-wide [30] and are listed in Table **2** along with their chemical constitutes and therapeutic activities.

Table 2. Medicinal Plants used in Rasayana Therapy

Sl no	Herb name	Chemical constituents	Therapeutic activities
1.	*Withania somnifera* [31]	Withanolides I-VII, Withaferine A	Immuno modulator, Strength promoting, Adaptogenic.
2.	*Emblica officianlis* [32]	Ascorbic acid, Gallic acid, Chebulinic acid, Chebulagic acid	Jaundice, bleeding disorders, gastritis, antidiabetic activity.
3.	*Terminalia bellerica* [33]	Tannin	Purgative
4.	*Bacopa monnieri* [34]	Bacoside A	Anti laprotic, antipyretic, anti-diabetic, antiinflammatory, anxiolytic, memory enhancer
5.	*Sida cordifolia* [35]	Ephedrine, Sitoindoside X, Vasicine, Vasicinone	Filariasis and bleeding piles
6.	*Eclipta alba / Eclipta prostrata* [36]	Wedelolactone, dimethylwedelolactone	Hepatoprotective, dermetosis and dyspnoea
7.	*Celatrus paniculatus* [37]	Alkaloids piperine, piperilongumine (piplartine) piperlonguminine, methyl - 3,4,5 -trimethoxycinnamate	Memory enhancing, Skin affections
8.	*Piper longum* [38]	Alkaloids piperine, piperilongumine (piplartine) piperlonguminine, methyl - 3,4,5 -trimethoxycinnamate	Bioavailability enhancer, Anti-bacterial, antifungal, anti helmenthic activities
9.	*Mucuna prurita/ Mucuna pruriens* [39]	L- 3,4 dihydroxy phenylalanine (L–dopa)	Anti Parkinsonian and aphrodisiac
10.	*Asparagus recemosa* [40]	Steroidal glycosides shatavarine I- IV, Polycyclic alkaloid 9,10-dihydrophenanthrene derivate racemosol	Anti Parkinsonian and aphrodisiac
11.	*Gmelina arborea* [41]	Linoleic acid	Haemorrhagic disorders, cardiac diseases, disurea
12.	*Tinospora cordifolia* [42]	Sesquiterpene tinocordifolin, sesquiterpene glucoside, tinocordifolioside, arabino galactane	Immuno modulatory, hepato protective
13.	*Plambagozeylanica* [43]	Plumbagine, 3- chloroplumbagine, 3,3-biplumbagine	In colic and appetizer
14.	*Embilica ribes* [44]	Embilin	Contraceptive and anthelminthic

(Table 2) cont.....

Sl no	Herb name	Chemical constituents	Therapeutic activities
15.	*Commiphorawightii* [45]	Resin, gum, volatile oil consist of myrcene, dimyrcene, poly myrcene, Resin- Z gulggulsterone, Eguggulstcronc, Z- guggulstcrol, guggulsterol l-V	Anti-inflammatory, anti hyperlipidemic, cervical adenitis
16.	*Curcuma longa* [46]	Curcumin (curcumin 1)	Anti-inflammatory, antipluritis antidiabetic, anti dermetosis, antihelmenthic, wound healing
17.	*Allium sativum* [47]	Hypocholesterolaemic	Allyl alcohol, sulphur compounds like Allicine, Allin diallyl sulphide
18.	*Rubia cordifolia* [48]	Rubiadin (1, 3-dihydroxy-2-methyl anthraquinone) Alizarin, Purpurin	Anti tumor, blood dysentery
19.	*Hygrocarpus laurifolia* [49]	Hypnocarpic acid, Chalmoorgic acid, oleic acid and palmitic acid	Skin disorders, itching, non-healing wound, sinuses and abscess.
20.	*Convolvulus pluricaulis* [50]	Convoline, convolidine, convolvine, confoline, convosine, palmitic acid, linoleic acid β sitosterol, tropane	Reduce gastric ulcers, stress, control neurotoxic, levels, improves memory, analgesic property, cure hyperthyroid

Common Plants Used as Immunity Boosters Recipies

Some well-known plants used in traditional system of medicines are *Alium sativum, Alium cepa, Citrus limon, Withaniasomnifera,Moringa oleifera* and *Curcuma longa* that are briefly *discussed* here.

Alium sativum: *Allium sativum* L. (Fig. **3**), which is a species of the onion family, Alliaceae, is one of the most used plants, both medically and as an ingredient. Historically, garlic originated in central Asia over 6,000 years ago [52]. The beneficial effects of *Allium sativum* (garlic) on health have been emphasised for centuries. Garlic is still used in folk medicine all over the world to treat a variety of diseases. It has been extensively used throughout history for its prophylactic and therapeutic effects. Garlic's biological activity includes cardiovascular benefits, free radical scavenging, immune stimulating, anti-cancer, and anti-infectious properties. Garlic contains numerous compounds, including allicin, ajoene, and alliin, which have the potential to influence immunity. A literature survey reported that garlic and its complex constituents have been investigated as promising candidates for improving the immune system. Several immunological parameters, including serum total immunoglobulin concentration and T-cell subtype CD4+, were normalised in Wistar rats in an *in vivo* study by treating them with garlic oil 30 minutes before administering diazinon. In addition, combining garlic oil with levamisole significantly restores the T-helper 1/T-helper 2 balance in Wistar rats. In addition, the immune-enhancing activity of garlic polysaccharides can be greatly improved through selenylation modification; in 14-day-old chickens, selenizing garlic polysaccharides promotes lymphocyte proliferation, enhances interferon and IL-2, and raises the serum antibody titre. Consumption of aged garlic extract was also found to lessen the duration and severity of cold and flu symptoms, as well as boost immune system performance.Garlic contains several immune-modulating compounds, but polysaccharides stand out as the most significant [53].

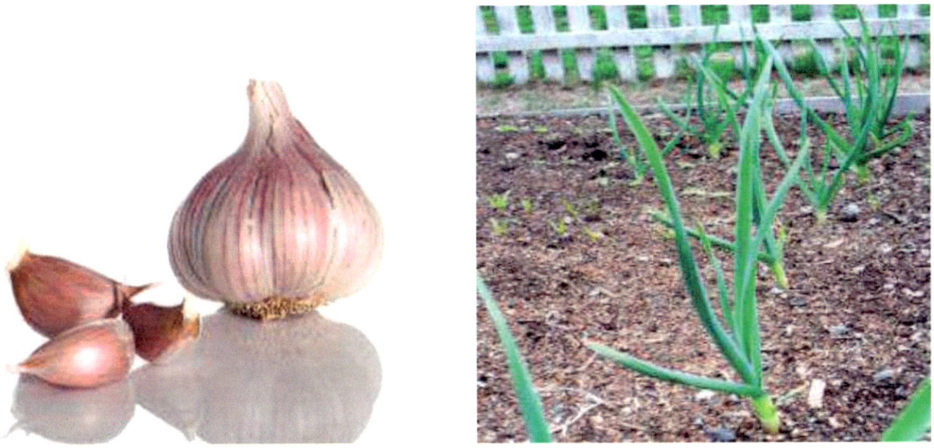

Fig. (3). Garlic and its plants [51].

***Alium cepa*:** Commonly called as onion (Fig. **4**) [54] is one of the oldest cultivated plants, utilized worldwide as both vegetable and flavouring agent. It is a biennial plant with adventitious and fibrous roots and 3–8, distichous, glaucous leaves. The bulb is made of concentric, enlarged fleshy leaf bases. The outer leaf base dries and becomes thin and variously coloured, forming the protective coat, while the inner leaf bases thicken when the bulb develops. The mature bulb can be globose, ovoid or elongate and its size varies depending on the cultivar. Onion is rich in several phytonutrients that are recognized as important elements of the Mediterranean diet but it has received attention also for its biological properties and potential application in the treatment and prevention of a number of diseases [55]. *Onion* is known to contain many vitamins and minerals and is rich in sulphur amino acids. Moreover, a variety of secondary metabolites has been identified in this species, such as flavonoids (Particularly flavonols and anthocyanin), phytosterols and saponins. Reducing Th2 cytokines (IL-4, IL-5, and IL-13) and increasing CD4 cells, IFN-c level, and IFN-c/IL4 ratio (Th1/Th2 balance) were all indicators of the plant's and quercetin's immunomodulatory effects [56].

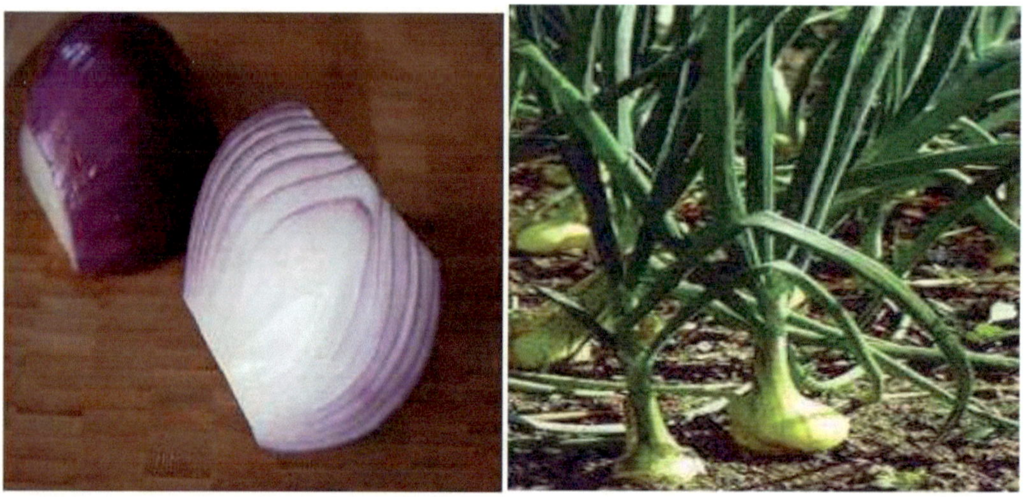

Fig. (4). Onion and its plants [54].

Citrus limon: Citrus limon (L.) Burm. f. (Fig. **5**) [57] is a tree with evergreen leaves and green and yellow edible fruits from the family *Rutaceae*. The lemon tree is a small, thorny tree that grows well throughout the tropical and subtropical regions of the world. Lemons are cultivated in modest amounts for home use almost everywhere that citrus trees can survive, but large-scale commercial production is limited to the subtropical regions since more humid tropical environments enhance pest and disease problems for both fruit and tree. The main raw material of Citrus limon is the fruit, particularly the essential oil and juice obtained from it. The Citrus limon fruit stands out as having well-known nutritional properties, but it is worth remarking that its valuable biological activities are underestimated in modern phytotherapy. Lemon contains high levels of flavonoids, especially flavanones and flavone glycosides. Flavonols, flavone aglycones, and polymethoxyflavones are also present but at lower concentrations than those of flavanones and flavones [58]. The main constituents present reported are flavanones and flavones such as eriocitrin, Quercetin, hesperidin, C-glycosides of diosmetin and apigenin, and diosmetin 7-O-rutinoside (diosmin). Reducing Th2 cytokines such as IL-4, IL-5, and IL-13 and increasing CD4 cells, IFN-c level, and IFN-c/IL4 ratio (Th1/Th2 balance) are all indicators of the plant's and quercetin's immunomodulatory effects [59].

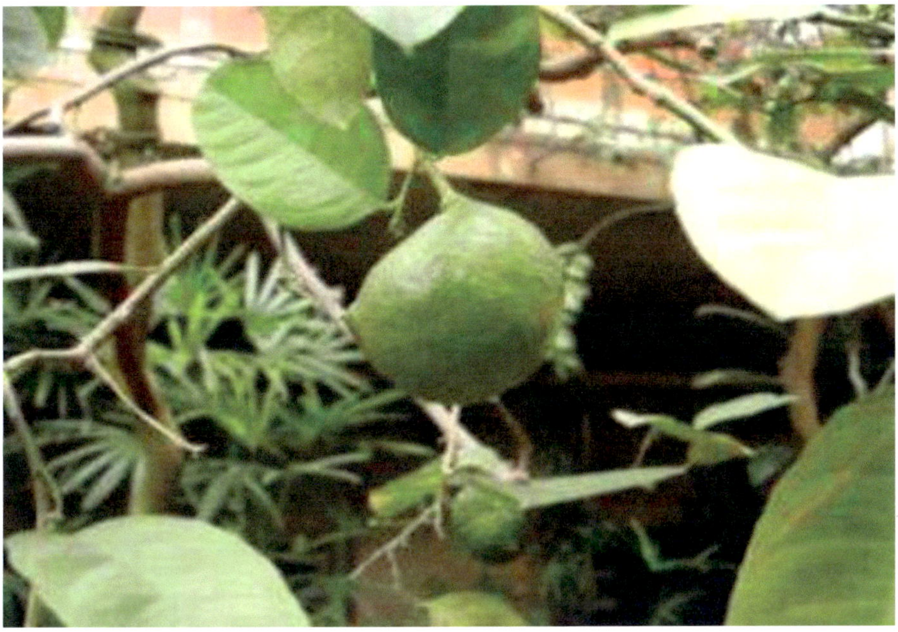

Fig. (5). Lemon and its plants [57].

Withania somnifera: Ashwagandha (Withania somnifera, fam. Solanaceae) is commonly known as "Indian Winter cherry" or "Indian Ginseng" (Fig. **6**) [60]. Ashwagandha, the magical herb, is considered to be nature's gift to mankind. The Sanskrit term Ashwagandha translates to "smell of horse", and rightly so. Traditionally, it is believed that a person who consumes this herbal medicine will gain horse-like strength and vitality. It is a small shrub with yellow flowers and a red fruit, native to India, North Africa, and the Middle East. For centuries, Ayurvedic medicine has used it to treat people for their day-to-day woes such as stress, anxiety, exhaustion, lack of sleep. It is one of the most important herb of Ayurveda (the traditional system of medicine in India) used for millennia as a Rasayana for its wide ranging health benefits. Ashwagandha is used as a household remedy by Indians, who consider it as the best tonic for old people and children, and as aphrodisiac by young people. It is one of the best nervine tonics of Ayurveda, the most ancient system of Medical Sciences. The biologically active chemical constituents of Withania somnifera (WS) include alkaloids (isopelletierine, anaferine, cuseohygrine, anahygrine, *etc.*), steroidal lactones (withanolides, withaferins) and saponin, Sitoindosides and acylsterylglucosides in Ashwagandha are anti-stress agents. Active principles of Ashwagandha, for instance the sitoindosides VII-X and Withaferin-A, have been shown to have significant anti-stress activity against acute models of experimental stress [61].

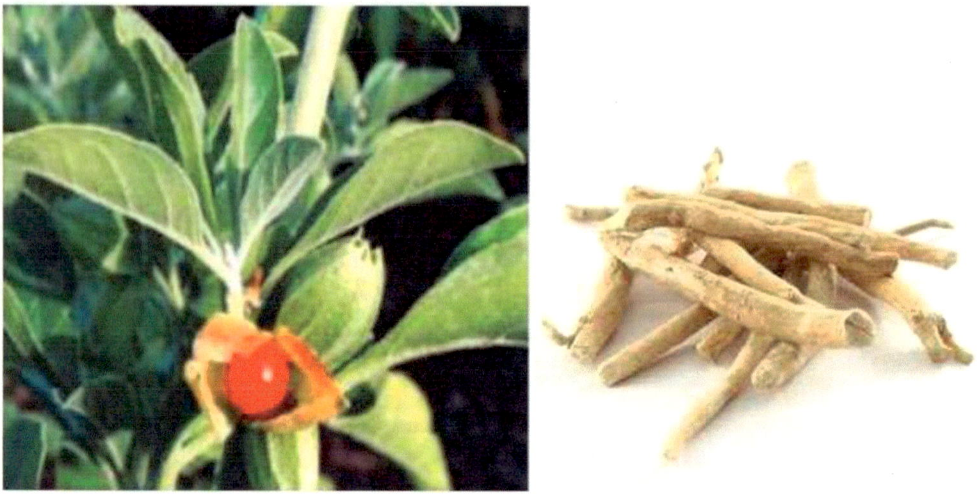

Fig. (6). Ashwagandha plants and roots [60].

Many of its constituents support immunomodulatory actions [62]. The aerial parts of Withania somnifera contain 5-dehydroxy withanolide-R and withasomniferin-A and several naturally occurring withanolides, including chantriolide A, physalins A, B, C, and O, viscosalactone B, WA, withanolides D, E, F, and withaferin A 4,27-diacetate, a diacetyl derivative of WA, are known to alter NF-B regulation [63].

Ashwagandha is popularly used for boosting immunity, anti-ageing, joint pain and insomnia. Due to its active ingredient called withanolides, Ashwagandha is also used as an "adaptogen" to help the body cope with daily stress, as a general tonic and for improving thinking ability. It also improves the brain's memory functions like attention and concentration, hence helping with the symptoms of Parkinson's, Alzheimer's and other neurodegenerative diseases. It enables the body to reserve and sustain vital energy throughout the day while promoting sound, peaceful sleep at night." These varied benefits are what make Ashwagandha a go-to choice in Indian herbal medicine [64].

Moringa oleifera: *Moringa oleifera* belong to family Moringaceae, small deciduous tree native to tropical Asia but also naturalized in Africa and tropical America, called as horseradish tree or drumstick tree (Fig. **7**) [65]. The fruit physically resembles a stick, therefore a similar name given as drum stick. It is known for high nutritional and medicinal value. It is widely used as a nutritive herb and possesses valuable pharmacological activities. Dietary consumption of its part is therein promoted as a strategy of personal health preservation and self-medication in various diseases. It is widely used in folkloric medicine of Africa and Asia. Dietary consumption of its part is therein promoted as a strategy of personal health preservation and self-medication in various diseases [66]. The different traditional uses are shown in Fig. (**8**) [67]. The different parts of this plant are reported to possess anticancer, antihyperlipidemic, antidiabetic, antiulcer, analgesic, antifertility, anticonvulsant, hepatoprotective, *etc. Moringa oleifera* have been used for decades to combat malnutrition. In M. oleifera the phytoconstituents such as sterols, flavonoids, β-sitosterol, glycosides, anthocyanins, proanthocyanidin *etc* present in adequate amount; and this make the plant medicinally important and/or nutritionally valuable [68].

Curcuma longa: *Curcuma longa* L. (turmeric) of ginger family (Zingiberaceae) belongs to the group of oldest cultivated spice plants in the south-east Asian countries (Fig. **9**) [69]. For many years rhizome of this plant has been used also as a safe and active drug for the treatment of various chronic diseases. The active substance of turmeric - curcumin (diferuloylmethane), possesses multiple therapeutic properties. Important Biological activities are anti-inflammatory, antioxidant and cancer preventive properties. Multiple *in vitro* studies employing a wide variety of immune cells have shown that curcumin has immunomodulatory properties. In IFN- or TNF—activated macrophages and NK cells, curcumin has been shown to suppress COX-2 and NO, NF-B, iNOS, and lipoxygenase, thereby inhibiting inflammatory responses [70].

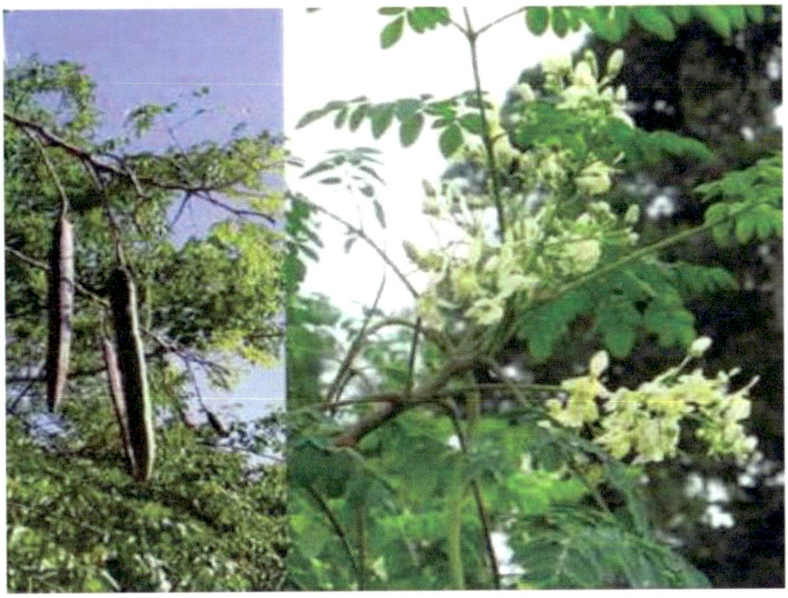

Fig. (7). *Moringa oleifera* plants and fruits [65].

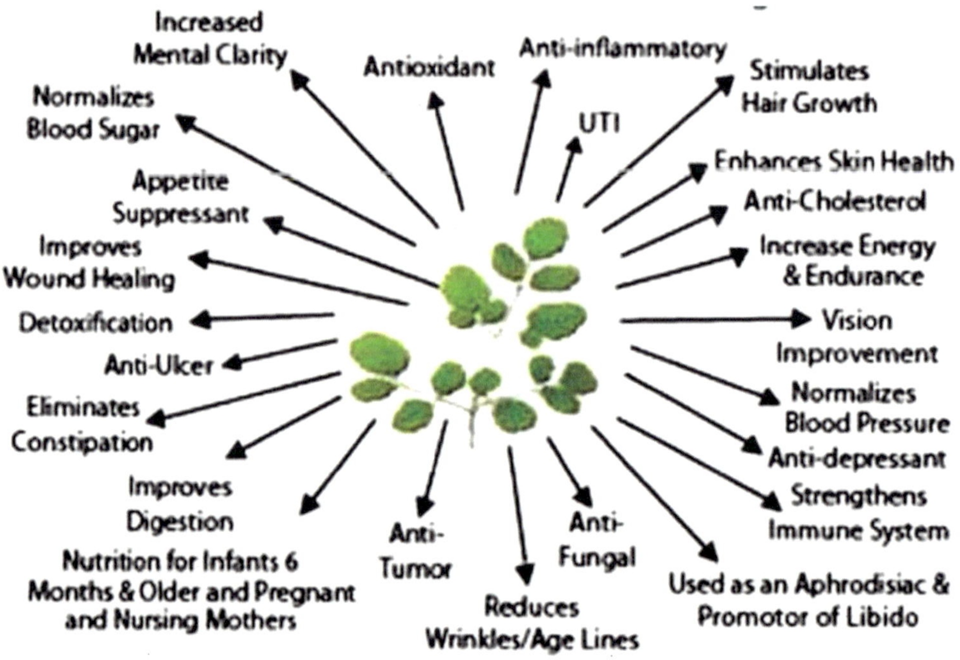

Fig. (8). Traditional medicinal uses of Moringa [67].

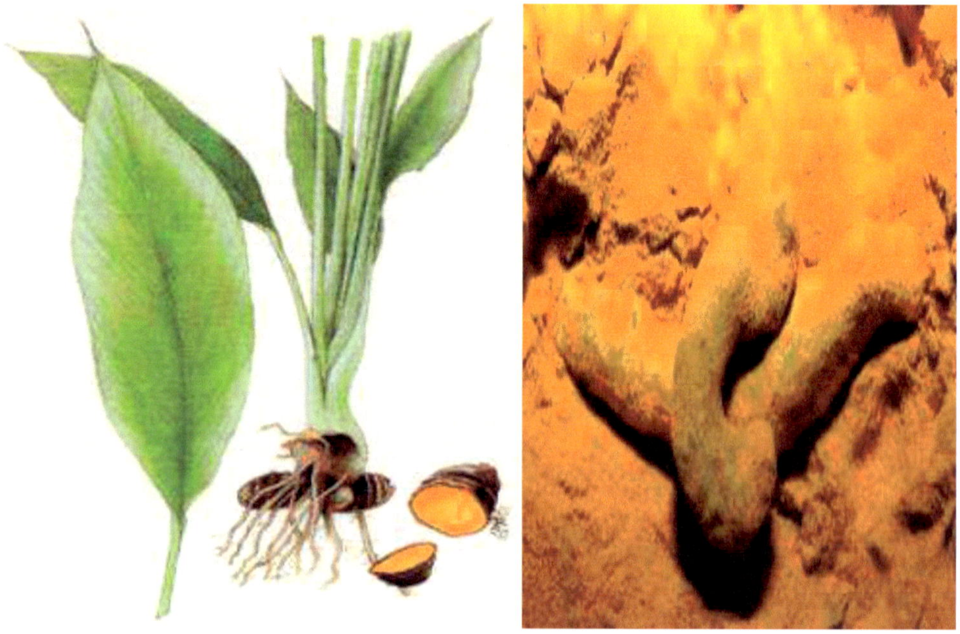

Fig. (9). Turmeric and its plants [69].

Commonly used Traditional immune-boosting recipes

Ayurvedic Herbal preparations like Triphalachurna (Baidyanath), Haritakichurna (Ayurveedya Arkashala) Mahasudarshanchurna (Baidyanath), and Lavanbha-skarchurna (Baidyanath).

The traditional system of medicine like Ayurveda and Siddha system of medicine quoted several traditional immune-boosting recipes like Maha- sudharshnach-oornam, Talisadichoornam, Dhanavantam, Gulika-churnam, and sitophala-dichoornam.

Maha Sudarshan Churna: Maha Sudarshan Churna is a blend of 52 potent Ayurvedic herbs and is employed in Ayurvedic treatments for fever especially of chronic type and associated with diarrhoea, indigestion, cough, cold or allergy. It balances all three doshas (vata, pitta, and kapha), maintains a healthy metabolism, and strengthens the immune system that helps protect the body from allergens and infectious microorganisms. Talisadichoornam: TalisadiChurna is an ayurvedic remedy used to treat coughs and digestive problems such as anorexia and irritable bowel syndrome. It is also useful in the treatment of chronic fever caused by respiratory disorders. The main ingredients of TalisadiChurna are pippali, sonth, black pepper, and talispatra. Within the therapeutic dosage, TalisadiChurna is most likely safe and well-tolerated bymost people. Dhanavantam Gutika-churnam: Dhanwantharam Gutika is an Ayurvedic medicine in the tablet form that is useful in treating digestive disorders such as bloating, flatulence, and gastritis. This Ayurvedic medicine for gastritis is made with traditional ingredients that help ease the discomfort caused by gastric problems and promote optimum digestion. This recipe contains 13 herbs, including cardamom, ginger, terminalia chebula, nutmeg, solanum melongena, swertia chirata, cuminum cyminum, cedrus deodara, eleaocarpus ganitrus, and andrographis paniculata. SitopladiChurna: SitopladiChurna is a unique combination of herbs (Fig. **10**) [71], which acts as a very good antitussive agent and can be used as an expectorant, carminative, and anti-inflammatory digestive agent. It is used in diseases like cough, bronchitis, pneumonia, and tuberculosis. Sitopaladi is an amazing immunomodulator and a super-effective churna that leverages the power of five compounds, such as mishri, vankshalochana (the white part of the bamboo tree), pepper, cardamom, and cinnamon. All these ingredients, taken in the right proportion, are dried and powdered into a churna. Mishri has the potential to balance the Kapha and Vata doshas, and Vankshalochana contains a host of plant compounds that have healing properties. While pepper and cinnamon function as bio-enhancers; cardamom is loaded with antioxidants that prevent free radical damage and possess strong anti-inflammatory properties.

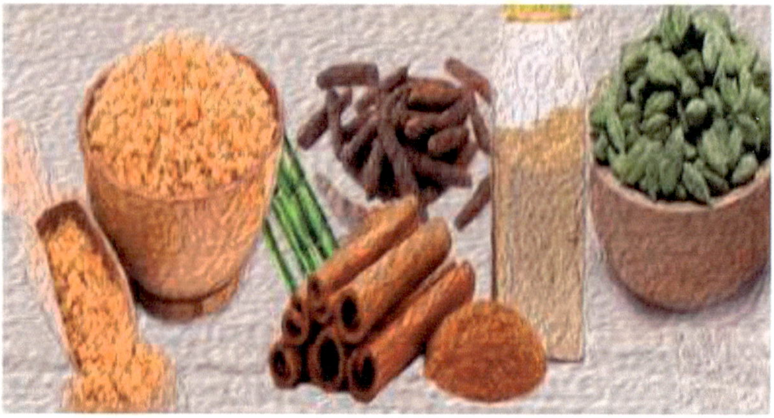

Fig. (10). Traditional preparation of SitopladiChurna [71].

CONCLUSION

The immune system is a complex array of cells and molecules operating in an orchestrated manner in order to protect the host from pathogenic microorganisms and exogenous noxious agents within our environment. However, the destruction of host tissue may occur if the immune response is inadequate due to intrinsic or extrinsic mechanisms in cell function, or if there is a hyper-responsiveness due to dysfunctional regulatory mechanisms. The pathogenesis of disease is clearly of an inflammatory origin and, as such, has a close association with the Immune System. Perfect food is the most important criterion to obtain good health. We have to consume foods which are rich in different compounds responsible for building our immunity. It is very much important to be on a good diet to boost immunity. Several vitamins with trace elements, probiotics, and nutraceuticals are necessary for the proper performance of the immune system. Traditional recipes are rich sources of antioxidants, vitamins, and minerals. A person consuming the required amount of antioxidants, vitamins, and minerals can have the perfect balance of immunity and can fight against diseases.

REFERENCES

[1] Sunil K, Priyanka G, Salini S, Dinesh K. A review on Immunostimulatory Plants. J Chinese Int. Med 2011; 2(9): 117-27.

[2] Available from: https://www.aber.ac.uk/~dcswww/ISYS/immune_system.html

[3] Hunt R. Virology: Microbiology and Immunology Online.

[4] Manjrekar PN, Jolly CI, Narayanan S. Comparative studies of the immunomodulatory activity of *Tinospora cordifolia* and *Tinospora sinensis*. Fitoterapia 2000; 71(3): 254-7. [http://dx.doi.org/10.1016/S0367-326X(99)00167-7] [PMID: 10844163]

[5] Govindan S, Viswanathan S, Vijayasekaran V, Alagappan R. A pilot study on the clinical efficacy of Solanum xanthocarpum and Solanum trilobatum in bronchial asthma. J Ethnopharmacol 1999; 66(2): 205-10.

[http://dx.doi.org/10.1016/S0378-8741(98)00160-3] [PMID: 10433479]

[6] Govindan S, Viswanathan S, Vijayasekaran V, Alagappan R. Further studies on the clinical ef?cacy ofSolanum xanthocarpum andSolanum trilobatum in bronchial asthma. Phytother Res 2004; 18(10): 805-9. [http://dx.doi.org/10.1002/ptr.1555] [PMID: 15551394]

[7] Jain SP, Puri HS. Ethnomedicinal plants of Jaunsar-Bawar hills, Uttar Pradesh, India. J Ethnopharmacol 1984; 12(2): 213-22. [http://dx.doi.org/10.1016/0378-8741(84)90049-7] [PMID: 6521494]

[8] Pandey MM, Rastogi S, Rawat AKS. Indian herbal drug for general healthcare: an overview. Internet Journal of Alternative Medicine 2008; 6(1): 3.

[9] Sachin P, Amit G, Navin S. *Solanum xanthocarpum* (Yellow Berried Night Shade): A review. Pharm Lett 2010; 2(4): 373-83.

[10] Subhose V, Srinivas P, Narayana A. Basic principles of pharmaceutical science in Ayurvĕda. Bull Indian Inst Hist Med Hyderabad 2005; 35(2): 83-92. [PMID: 17333665]

[11] Perumal Samy R, Ignacimuthu S, Sen A. Screening of 34 Indian medicinal plants for antibacterial properties. J Ethnopharmacol 1998; 62(2): 173-81. [http://dx.doi.org/10.1016/S0378-8741(98)00057-9] [PMID: 9741889]

[12] Perumal Samy R, Ignacimuthu S. Antibacterial activity of some folklore medicinal plants used by tribals in Western Ghats of India. J Ethnopharmacol 2000; 69(1): 63-71. [http://dx.doi.org/10.1016/S0378-8741(98)00156-1] [PMID: 10661885]

[13] Kamboj VP. Herbal medicine. Curr Sci 2000; 78(1): 35-9.

[14] Rabe T, van Staden J. Antibacterial activity of South African plants used for medicinal purposes. J Ethnopharmacol 1997; 56(1): 81-7. [http://dx.doi.org/10.1016/S0378-8741(96)01515-2] [PMID: 9147258]

[15] John D. One hundred useful raw drugs of the Kani tribes of Trivandrum forest division, Kerala, India. Int J Crude Drug Res 1984; 22(1): 17-39. [http://dx.doi.org/10.3109/13880208409070646]

[16] Veale DJH, Furman KI, Oliver DW. South African traditional herbal medicines used during pregnancy and childbirth. J Ethnopharmacol 1992; 36(3): 185-91. [http://dx.doi.org/10.1016/0378-8741(92)90043-Q] [PMID: 1434676]

[17] Anesini C, Perez C. Screening of plants used in Argentine folk medicine for antimicrobial activity. J Ethnopharmacol 1993; 39(2): 119-28. [http://dx.doi.org/10.1016/0378-8741(93)90027-3] [PMID: 8412245]

[18] Cox PA.(1990), Ciba Foundation Symposium 154, John Wiley & Sons, Chichester, UK.

[19] Cox PA, Balick MJ. The ethnobotanical approach to drug discovery. Sci Am 1994; 270(6): 82-7. [http://dx.doi.org/10.1038/scientificamerican0694-82] [PMID: 8023119]

[20] Ji BH. Drug resistance in leprosy--a review. Lepr Rev 1985; 56(4): 265-78. [PMID: 3908861]

[21] Manandhar NP. Traditional medicinal plants used by Tribals of Lamjung District, Nepal. Int J Crude Drug Res 1987; 25(4): 236-40. [http://dx.doi.org/10.3109/13880208709055200]

[22] Nair P, Nagar R, Gupta R. Dietary anti-oxidant phenolics and flavonoids in coronary heart disease. Indian Heart J 1996; 48: 545.

[23] Nehir El S, Karakaya S. Radical scavenging and iron-chelating activities of some greens used as traditional dishes in Mediterranean diet. Int J Food Sci Nutr 2004; 55(1): 67-74.

[http://dx.doi.org/10.1080/0963748031000164250 1] [PMID: 14630594]

[24] Tanira MOM, Bashir AK, Dib R, Goodwin CS, Wasfi IA, Banna NR. Antimicrobial and phytochemical screening of medicinal plants of the United Arab Emirates. J Ethnopharmacol 1994; 41(3): 201-5.
[http://dx.doi.org/10.1016/0378-8741(94)90033-7] [PMID: 8176960]

[25] Isbrucker RA, Burdock GA. Risk and safety assessment on the consumption of Licorice root (Glycyrrhiza sp.), its extract and powder as a food ingredient, with emphasis on the pharmacology and toxicology of glycyrrhizin. Regul Toxicol Pharmacol 2006; 46(3): 167-92.
[http://dx.doi.org/10.1016/j.yrtph.2006.06.002] [PMID: 16884839]

[26] Nair S, Nagar R, Gupta R. Dietary anti-oxidant phenolics and flavonoids in coronary heart disease. Indian Heart J 1996; 48: 545.

[27] Balasinor N, Bhan A, Paradkar NS, *et al.* Postnatal development and reproductive performance of F1 progeny exposed in utero to an ayurvedic contraceptive: Pippaliyadi yoga. J Ethnopharmacol 2007; 109(3): 406-11.
[http://dx.doi.org/10.1016/j.jep.2006.08.007] [PMID: 17088035]

[28] Cáceres A, Cabrera O, Morales O, Mollinedo P, Mendia P. Pharmacological properties of Moringa oleifera. 1: Preliminary screening for antimicrobial activity. J Ethnopharmacol 1991; 33(3): 213-6.
[http://dx.doi.org/10.1016/0378-8741(91)90078-R] [PMID: 1921416]

[29] Jain SP, Puri HS. Ethnomedicinal plants of Jaunsar-Bawar hills, Uttar Pradesh, India. J Ethnopharmacol 1984; 12(2): 213-22.
[http://dx.doi.org/10.1016/0378-8741(84)90049-7] [PMID: 6521494]

[30] Dutta R, Khalil R, Green R, Mohapatra SS, Mohapatra S. *Withania Somnifera* (Ashwagandha) and Withaferin A: Potential in Integrative Oncology. Int J Mol Sci 2019; 20(21): 5310.
[http://dx.doi.org/10.3390/ijms20215310] [PMID: 31731424]

[31] Variya BC, Bakrania AK, Patel SS. Emblica officinalis (Amla): A review for its phytochemistry, ethnomedicinal uses and medicinal potentials with respect to molecular mechanisms. Pharmacol Res 2016; 111: 180-200.
[http://dx.doi.org/10.1016/j.phrs.2016.06.013] [PMID: 27320046]

[32] Gupta A, Kumar R, Bhattacharyya P, Bishayee A, Pandey AK. Terminalia bellirica (Gaertn.) roxb. (Bahera) in health and disease: A systematic and comprehensive review. Phytomedicine 2020; 77: 153278.
[http://dx.doi.org/10.1016/j.phymed.2020.153278]

[33] Sharma PC, Yelne MB, Dennis TJ. Database on Medicinal Plants Used in Ayurveda, Central Council for Research in Ayurveda and Siddha Department of ISM & H. New Delhi, India: Ministry of Health and Family Welfare, Government of India 2000; Vol. I: pp. 93-101.

[34] Ghosal S, Chauhan RBPS, Mehta R. Alkaloids of Sida cordifolia. Phytochemistry 1975; 14(3): 830-2.
[http://dx.doi.org/10.1016/0031-9422(75)83057-3]

[35] Zhang M, Chen Y. [Chemical constituents of *Eclipta alba* (L.) Hassk]. Zhongguo Zhongyao Zazhi 1996; 21(8): 480-481, 510.
[PMID: 9642409]

[36] Ahmad F, Khan RA, Rasheed S. Preliminary screening of methanolic extracts of Celastrus paniculatus and Tecomella undulata for analgesic and anti-inflammatory activities. J Ethnopharmacol 1994; 42(3): 193-8.
[http://dx.doi.org/10.1016/0378-8741(94)90085-X] [PMID: 7934089]

[37] Chatterjee A, Dutta CP. Alkaloids of Piper longum Linn. I. Structure and synthesis of piperlongumine and piperlonguminine. Tetrahedron 1967; 23(4): 1769-81.
[http://dx.doi.org/10.1016/S0040-4020(01)82575-8] [PMID: 6047519]

[38] Ghosal S, Singh S, Bhattacharya SK. Alkaloids of Mucuna pruries chemistry and pharmacology.

Planta Med 1971; 19(3): 280-4.
[PMID: 5546268]

[39] Suchita M, Praveen KD. *In vivo* anti inflammatory and anti arthritic activity of ethanolic extract of Asparagus racemosus roots. International Research Journal of Pharmacy 2013; 4(4): 167-72.

[40] Attanayake A, Boralugoda Mudduwa LK, Pathirana C, Wijewardana Jayatilaka KAP. Antioxidant activity of *Gmelina arborea* Roxb. (Verbenaceae) bark extract: *In vivo* and *in vitro* study. Journal of Medical Nutrition and Nutraceuticals 2015; 4(1): 32-8.
[http://dx.doi.org/10.4103/2278-019X.146159]

[41] Sharma U, Bala M, Kumar N, Singh B, Munshi RK, Bhalerao S. Immunomodulatory active compounds from *Tinospora cordifolia.* J Ethnopharmacol 2012; 141(3): 918-26.
[http://dx.doi.org/10.1016/j.jep.2012.03.027] [PMID: 22472109]

[42] Vishnukanta AC. Analgesic and anti-inflammatory activity of hydroalcoholic extract of Plumbago zeylanica leaf extract. Pharmacognosy Magzine 2008; 15: 133-6.

[43] Choudhary GP. Anthelmintic activity of fruits of Embeliaribes Burm. International Journal of Pharmaceutical and Chemical Sciences 2012; 1(4): 1336-7.

[44] Pareek A, Pareek LK. *Commiphora wightii* (Guggal) An Endangered Medicinal Plant of Rajasthan Needs Attention of Biotechnologists for Its Conservation. J. of Pharmaceutical. Biological and Chemical Sciences 2012; 3(1): 83-9.

[45] Shehzad A, Rehman G, Lee YS. Curcumin in inflammatory diseases. Biofactors 2013; 39(1): 69-77.
[http://dx.doi.org/10.1002/biof.1066] [PMID: 23281076]

[46] Suleria HAR, Butt MS, Khalid N, *et al.* Garlic (*Allium sativum*): diet based therapy of 21st century–a review. Asian Pac J Trop Dis 2015; 5(4): 271-8.
[http://dx.doi.org/10.1016/S2222-1808(14)60782-9]

[47] Kannan M, Ranjit A, Narayanan M. Phytochemistry and Ethanopharmacological studies on Rubia cordifolia Linn,(Rubiaceae). Ethanobotanical leaflet 2009; 13: 338-42.

[48] Balasubramani SP, Venkatasubramanian P, Kukkupuni SK, Patwardhan B. Plant-based Rasayana drugs from Ayurveda. Chin J Integr Med 2011; 17(2): 88-94.
[http://dx.doi.org/10.1007/s11655-011-0659-5] [PMID: 21390573]

[49] Upadhya AS, Kambhojkar MS. Studies on Ayurvedic drug Shankhpushpi from Western Maharastra medicobotanical reported aspects. Bullet Med Ethanob Res 1993; 14(1□2): 64-9.

[50] Available from: https://gardenerspath.com/garlic-allium-sativum/

[51] Rana SV, Pal R, Vaiphei K, Sharma SK, Ola RP. Garlic in health and disease. Nutr Res Rev 2011; 24(1): 60-71.
[http://dx.doi.org/10.1017/S0954422410000338] [PMID: 24725925]

[52] Borek C. Garlic reduces dementia and heart-disease risk. J Nutr 2006; 136(3) (Suppl.): 810S-2S.
[http://dx.doi.org/10.1093/jn/136.3.810S] [PMID: 16484570]

[53] Available from: https://www.nexles.com/articles/onion-allium-cepa-treatments-common-dis-ases-pests-vegetable/

[54] Lim T K. Edible Medicinal and Non Medicinal Plants. Switzerland: Springer Nature 2015; Volume 9.

[55] Breu W, Dorsch W. Chemistry, analysis and pharmacology.Economic Medicinal Plant Research. London: Academic Press 1994.

[56] Available from: https://www.123rf.com/photo_89707655_lemon-citrus-limon.html

[57] Klimek-Szczykutowicz M, Szopa A, Ekiert H. *Citrus limon* (Lemon) Phenomenon—A Review of the Chemistry, Pharmacological Properties, Applications in the Modern Pharmaceutical, Food, and Cosmetics Industries, and Biotechnological Studies. Plants 2020; 9(1): 119.
[http://dx.doi.org/10.3390/plants9010119] [PMID: 31963590]

[58] Mustafa N. Citrus essential oils: Current and prospective uses in the food industry. Recent Pat Food Nutr Agric 2015; 7(2): 115-27. [http://dx.doi.org/10.2174/2212798407666150831144239] [PMID: 26321174]

[59] Available from: https://www.flipkart.com/ayansh-plants-ashwagandha-indianginseng/p/itm6d1a6-d9cdf26e

[60] Bhattacharya SK, Bhattacharya A, Sairam K, Ghosal S. Anxiolytic-antidepressant activity of Withania somnifera glycowithanolides: an experimental study. Phytomedicine 2000; 7(6): 463-9. [http://dx.doi.org/10.1016/S0944-7113(00)80030-6] [PMID: 11194174]

[61] Ghosal S, Lal J, Srivastava R, *et al.* Immunomodulatory and CNS effects of sitoindosides IX and X, two new glycowithanolides fromWithania somnifera. Phytother Res 1989; 3(5): 201-6. [http://dx.doi.org/10.1002/ptr.2650030510]

[62] New withanolides from Withania spp. J Nat Prod 1991; 56: 1000-6.

[63] Singh N. *Withaniasomnifera* (Ashwagandha), a rejuvenating herbal drug which enhances survival during stress (an Adaptogen). Pharm Biol 1982; 20(1): 29-35.

[64] Available from: https://nurserylive.com/products/drumsticks-moringa-oleifera-plant

[65] Sharma V, Paliwal R, Sharma S. Phytochemical analysis and evaluation of antioxidant activities of hydro-ethanolic extract of Moringa oleifera Lam. Pods. J Pharm Res 2011; 4(2): 554-7.

[66] Available from: http://bajabeat.com/moringa-tree-of-life/

[67] Gilani AH, Aftab K, Ahmed S. Cholinergic actions of crude saponins from Castanospermum australe. Int J Pharmacol 1994; 32: 209-16.

[68] Available from: https://commons.wikimedia.org/wiki/File:Curcuma_longa_roots.jpg

[69] Cronin JR. Curcumin: Old Spice Is a New Medicine. Biochemistry of Alternative Medicine 2004; 9(1): 34-6.

[70] Available from: https://carebunch.in/product-tag/sitopaladi-churna/

CHAPTER 4

The Indian Cytotoxic Weed Flora and Their Phytochemicals

Prabha Thangavelu[1,*], Jubie Selvaraj[2], Rashmi Saxena Pal[3] and **Vishnu Nayak Badavath[4]**

[1] *Department of Pharmaceutical Chemistry, Nandha College of Pharmacy, Affiliated to The Tamil Nadu Dr. MGR Medical University-Chennai, Erode-638052, Tamil Nadu, India*

[2] *Department of Pharmaceutical Chemistry, JSS College of Pharmacy, Ooty-643001, Tamil Nadu, India*

[3] *Department of Pharmacognosy, School of Pharmacy, Lovely Professional University, Phagwara, Punjab-140118, India*

[4] *Department of Pharmaceutical Chemistry, College of Pharmacy, Chitkara University, Chitkara, Panjab, India*

Abstract: India has rich biodiversity and a large number of medicinal plants that are weeds. Usually, weeds are seen as troublemakers in the yard and interfere with the man's land utilization for a specific purpose. Farmers and field botanists recognized these weeds as medicinal plants such as *Adonis vernalis, Phyllanthus amarus, Eclipta alba, Centella asiatica, etc.* used in folk and indigenous medicines. Most of the plants that are considered weeds have not yet explored phytochemically and pharmacologically. Simultaneously, many of these weeds were reported for their secondary metabolites like alkaloids, glycosides, flavonoids, phenolics, saponins, *etc.* having medicinal values like anticancer, antioxidant, and anti-inflammatory activities. Many therapeutically important weeds are more popular in India, like *Achyranthes bidentata, Artemisia nilagirica, etc.* with preferable medicinal benefits such as a diuretic, anti-malarial, and brain tonic. Weeds are storehouses and chemical libraries with simple to complex bioactive secondary metabolites, which serve as drug leads against several resistance diseases like cancer and tuberculosis. Weed biomolecules like Atropine from *Atropa belladonna*, Berberine from *Berberis vulgaris*, Colchicine from *Colchicum autumnale*, Phenoxodiol from *Glycine max*, Ingenol 3-angelate from *Euphorbia* species, Combretatin from *Combre vulgaris* have been reported. This chapter explains various cytotoxic Indian weed flora, reported phytochemicals, drug leads, ethnomedicinal values, modern pharmacology, mechanism of action and clinical safety and efficacy issues.

[*] **Corresponding author Prabha Thangavelu:** Department of Pharmaceutical Chemistry, Nandha College of Pharmacy, Affiliated to The Tamil Nadu Dr. MGR Medical University-Chennai, Erode-638052, Tamil Nadu, India; E-mail: drtpappa@yahoo.com

Motamarri Venkata Naga Lalitha Chaitanya, Galvina Pereira, & Heyam Saad Ali (Eds.)

Keywords: Anti-cancer, Adonis vernalis, Cancer treatment, Cytotoxicity, Cytotoxic weed, Cancer targets, Centella asiatica, Colchicum autumnale, Combrestatin, Colchicine, Drug, Eclipta alba, Medicinally valued weeds, Phytoconstituents, Phytochemicals, Phyllanthus amarus, Phenoxodiol, Phytochemicals, Secondary metabolites, Weed Flora, Weeds.

INTRODUCTION

On this green planet, there are uncountable plants that are considered wild/weed/unwanted due to a lack of obvious economical value. However, these plants have adapted well to harsh conditions and thrive very well without any special attention. This chapter is focusing on herbaceous weeds which have immense potential in herbal medicine based on traditional knowledge [1]. Around one-quarter of prescription medicines are found to have plant extracts or active ingredients derived from plants. A few essential descriptions of pharmaceutical products extracted from plants are aspirin, atropine, artemisinin, colchicine, digoxin, ephedrine, morphine, physostigmine, pilocarpine, quinine, quinidine, reserpine, taxol, tubocurarine, vincristine, and vinblastine [2]. However, the search for natural promising anticancer lead molecules is in demand as it is possible to investigate the primary view of structure-activity relationships and its potential mechanism of action from these lead molecules [3].

Significance of Weeds

Weeds are the important and unused components of the agricultural ecosystem, *i.e.*, the right plant in the wrong place. However, weeds are beneficial to humans as food, erosion prevention, drugs, aesthetic value, shelter, organic matter supply, and soil mineral nutrients. The utilisation of agricultural weeds is a widespread problem as some of the plants are characterised by high nutritional value and medicinal properties. There is an extensive awareness that weeds are reasonably rich in bioactive molecules, which is therefore very significant for the development of new medicines [4]. Since the weeds are worthless because of a false assumption, most of these weeds really are not phytochemically and biologically examined, but there are many possibilities for researchers to find new leads toward tough diseases such as cancer [5]. India is a major source of medicinally valuable aromatic plants. Among the high biodiversity range of medicinal plants, this book chapter focused on native ethnomedicinal weeds with documented cancer activities [6].

Basic Insight into Cancer

In evaluating the possible toxicity of research material, whether it be plant extracts or bioactive substances that are derived from plants, the cytotoxic activity study is helpful in the early phase. Cytotoxicity assays are a quick way to assess a certain chemical compound's impact on a particular human cell line, help to better assess the antineoplastic characteristics of the plant, and could further help to classify novel anticancer compounds [7]. Despite the illness's high profile, its management has been a major challenge with comparatively poor results.

Surgical extraction and radioactive therapy of the massive cumulative biomass of cancer are currently possible alternatives for cancer treatment, usually accompanied by systemic chemotherapy treatment for prevention. Antimetabolites (*e.g.*, methotrexate), DNA-interactive agents (*e.g.*, cisplatin, doxorubicin), anti-tubulin agents (taxanes), hormones, and molecular targeting agents are the majorly accessible chemotherapy medications.

Traditionally, plants are the principal components of the discovery of natural drug ingredients, and plant-derived products like vinblastine and vincristine, etoposide, paclitaxel, taxol, docetaxel, topotecan, and irinotecan are some of the most effective chemotherapeutics widely accessible for treatment of cancer [8]. Numerous significant chemotherapy substances were previously established from natural origins, including such taxanes, some topoisomerase inhibitors, and Vinca alkaloids [9]. Assessing the anticancer potential of these locally available plants brings us one step closer to discovering an alternative source of chemotherapy against cancer [10]. The chapter highlights current trends involved in the discovery of the cytotoxic potential of weeds containing secondary metabolites (Table **1** and Fig. **1**). This chapter was compiled in order to obtain information precisely about Indian cytotoxic weeds.

Phytochemicals used for cytotoxicity Activity from Weeds

Table 1. The reported cytotoxic weed phytoconstituents

Scientific name of the weed	Major constituents	References
Acalypha Indica linn.	Alkaloids like acalyphine, acalyphamide, amides, quinine, sterols, and cyanogenic glycosides, kaemperol, sitosterol, triacetonamine, auranthiamide and its acetate succinimide, 2-methylanthraquinone, tri-o-methylellagic acid.	[1]
Tridax procumbens linn.	Alkaloids, carotenoids, flavonoids like catechins flavones, fumiric acid, oleanolic acid, saponins, tannins, luteolin, glucoluteolin, and quercetin.	[1]
Leucas aspera **(Willd.)** *linn.*	Alpha-amyrin and alpha-tocopherol, triterpenoids, oleanolic acid, ursolic acid and b-sitosterol, nicotine, sterols, glucoside, diterpenes, phenolic compounds (4-(24-hydroxy-1-oxo-5-n-propyltetracosanyl)-phenol).	[11]
Heliotropium indicum linn.	Heliotrine, lasiocarpine, indicine, 12-acetyl indicine, indicinine, indicine-N-oxide, retronecine, trachelan-thamide, supinidine, and lindelofidine. Echinatine, heleurine, lasiocarpine-N-oxide, supinine, heliotrine, indicine, indicine-N-oxide, and lasiocarpine. Presence of cynoglossine, europine-N-oxide, heleurine-N-Oxide, heliotridine-N-Oxide, heleotrine-N-Oxide, and heliotrine. Other alkaloids such as putrescine, spermidine, homo spermidine, and spermine. Several triterpenes and steroids including b-amyrin, lupeol, chalinasterol, b-sitosterol, stigmasterol and campesterol. Rapanone and hexacosan---ol.	[12]
Cleome rutidosperma linn.	Tannins, lipids, amino acids, flavonoids, cardiac glycosides, alkaloids, steroids, saponins, terpenoids, polyphenols, phlobatannins, pentose, and reducing sugars.	[13]

(Table 1) cont.....

Scientific name of the weed	Major constituents	References
Commelinabenghalensis linn.	n-octacosanol, n-triocotanol, stigmasterol, campesterol, hydrocyanic acid, polyphenols, salicylic acid, p-coumaric acid, 8- hydroxyquinoline, caffeic acid, quinolones, catechol, resorcinol, tannic acid, chlorogenic acid, flavonoids, astringents, saponins, anthocyanin is cyanidin 3, 7, 3- triglucoside. Hydroxycinnamic acids, the flavones C-glycosides, flavonol O-glycosides, and Quercetin.	[1]
Euphorbia hirta linn.	Quercitrin, myricitrin, shikmic acid, tinyatoxin, kaempferol, gallic acid, protocatechuic acid, β-amyrin, and choline.	[1]
Argemone mexicana Linn.	Alkaloids (berberine, protopine, sarguinarine, optisin, and chelerytherin), amino acids, Phenolics and fatty acids (myristic, palmitic, oleic, linoleic acids). N-demethyloxysanguinarine, and pancorine, respectively; three alkaloids of the benzylisoquinoline type, namely, (+)-1,2,3,4-tetrahydro-1-(2-hydroxymethyl-3,4-dimethoxyphenyl-ethyl)-6,7-methylenedioxyisoquinoline, (+)-higenamine, and (+)-reticuline. In addition, N-demethyloxysanguinarine, and (+)-1,2,3,4- tetrahydro-1-(2-hydroxymethyl-3,4-dimethoxy phenyl methyl)-6,--methylenedioxy-isoquinoline.	[14]
Adhatodavasica linn.	Vasicine, Vasicinone, deoxyvasicinone, adhatonine, adhatodine, adhavasinone, peganine, anisotine, vasicinol, lunacrine, and vasicinolone, betaine, steroids, carbohydrates, alkanes, triterpenes, and flavonoids.	[1]
Calotropis procera linn.	Triterpenoids, calotropursenyl acetate, calopfriedelenyl, procerleanol A and B, cardiac glycosides, calotropin, calotoxin, cardenolides, and anthocyanins. Benzoylinesolone and benzoylisolinelone, Calotropin and calotropagenin, Calotropenyl acetate and multiflavenol, and uzarigenin.	[15]
Lantana camara linn.	Alkaloids, essential oils, phenols, flavonoids, iridoid glycosides, phenyl ethanoid, quinine, saponins, steroids, terpens, sesquiterpenoides, and tannins.	[16]
Solanum nigrum linn.	Alkaloids, reducing sugars, gallic acid, flavonoids, phlobatannis, steroids, tannis, catechin, protocatechuic acid, caffeic acid, epicatechin, rutin, and naringenin.	[17]
Parthenium hysterophorus linn.	Parthenin, a sesquiterpenoid flavonoid, terpenoids, alkaloids and cardiac glycosides.	[18]
***Solanum xanthocarpum*Schrad. &Wendl.**	Alkaloids, sterols, saponins, flavonoids, Solasodine glycosides and tomatidenol, glycoalkaloid namely solanacarpine, solanacarpidine, solanine, and solamargine, diosgenin, carpesterol, and coumarins namely scopoletin, esculetin, and esculin. solanacarpine, solanacarpidine, solanine, and solamargine, diosgenin, carpesterol, and coumarins namely scopoletin, esculetin, and esculin.	[19]
***Mikania micrantha* Knuth.**	Terpenoids (sesquiterpene lactones and diterpenes), polyphenols and flavonoids, mikanolide and miscandenin, guaianolide 8-epi-mikanokryptin and the melampolide 11Hβ-11,13-dihydromicrantholide along with known sesquiterpene lactones. Essential oil -sesquiterpene hydrocarbons made of Isoledene, δ-Cadinene, Debromofiliformin, Trans-Caryophyllene, β-Bisabolene, Germacrene-D, and Zingiberene.	[20]
Scoparia Dulcis linn.	Flavonoids and terpenes. Scopadulcic acids A and B, scopadiol, scopadulciol, scopadulin, scoparic acids A□C, and betulinic acid. Scopadulciol, 4-*epi*-scopadulcic acid B, dulcidiol, scopadulcic acid B, hymenoxin, glutinol, eupatilin, and 5-demethylnobiletin. Labdane-derived diterpenes, iso-dulcinol, 4-epi-scopadulcic acid B, dulcidiol, and scopanolal, together with two known diterpenes, dulcinol/scopadulciol and scopadiol.	[21]
Crotalaria retusa linn.	Alkaloids, benzoxazinones, cinnamic acid,, cyanogenic compounds, ethylene, and flavonoids.	
Achyranthes aspera linn.	Saponins, alkaloids (betaine, achyranthine), amino acids, steroids (stigmasterol), triterpenoids (oleanolic acid and its glucoside), phenolic content (indole acetic acid oxidase), and flavonoids. Sterols, alkaloids, saponins, sapogenins, cardiac glycosides, and ecdysterone.	[22]
Launaeaprocumbens Linn.	1-H-pyrazole, β-amyrin, α-amyrin,lupeol, inositol, 1-H-pyrazole, and fructose.	[23]
Ipomoea carnea Jacq.	Glycosides, alkaloids, reducing sugars, flavones, fatty acid, esters, and alcohol, flavonoids and tannins. Hexadecanoic acid, steric acid, 1, 2 diethyl phthalate, n-octadecanol, octacosane, hexatriacontane, tetraacontane, 3-diethylamino-1- propanol.	[24]
Alternanthera sessilis linn.	Flavonols, triterpenoids, steroids, and tannins; β-sitosterol, stigmasterol, campesterol, and lupeol.	[25]
***Alternanthera philoxeroides* (Mart.) Griseb.**	Phaeophytin a, phaeophytin a', oleanolic acid, βsitosterol, 3β-hydroxystigmast-5-en-7-one, α-spinasterol, 24-methylene cycloartanol, cycloeucalenol and phytol. Alternanthin B, and N-trans-feruloyl-3,5-dimethoxytyramine.	[26]
Chromolaena odorata linn.	Monoterpenes, sesquiterpenes hydrocarbons, triterpenes/steroids, alkaloids, and flavonoids like Quercetin, sinensetin, sakuranetin, padmatin, kaempferol, and salvagenin. Sakuranetin, isosakuranetin, kaempferide, betulenol, 2-5-7-3 tetra-o-methyl quercetagetin, tamarixetin, two chalcones and odoratin, essential oils (geyren, bornyl acetate and β-eubeden), saponin triterpenoids, tannins, protocatechuic, p-hydroxybenzoic, p-coumaric, ferulic and vanillic acids) and complex mixtures of lipophilic flavonoid aglycones (flavanones, flavonols, flavones and chalcones, acacetin, dihydrokaempferide, isosakuranetin, and kaempferide.The essential oil -β-caryophyllene, germacrene D, and linalool.	[27]
Cassia tora linn.	Anthraquinone glycosides, naphthopyrone glycosides, phenolic compounds, flavonoids, sennosides, and rubrofusarinetriglucoside.	[28]

(Table 1) cont.....

Scientific name of the weed	Major constituents	References
Ageratum conyzoides linn.	Lycopsamine and echinatine, two isomeric pyrrolizidine alkaloids-friedelin, and the major sterols are sterols---sitosterol. Monoterpenes include sabinene, β-pinene, β-phellandrene, 1,8-cineole and limonene, terpinen-4-ol, α-terpineol, linalool, α-pinene, eugenol, and methyleugenol. Sesquiterpenes hydrocarbons contain β-caryophyllene, caryophyllene epoxide, β-sesquiphellandrene, and δ-cadinene. Chromene, Chromone, Benzofuran, and Coumarin.	[29]
Solanum mauritianum Scop.	Caulophyllumine-A, solasodine, alkaloids, phenolics, flavonoids, and saponins glycoside namely, Tetrahydro---(hydroxymethyl)-6-(octadecahydro-2,7,10a-trimethyl-1propylchrysen-8-yloxy)-2H-Pyran-3,4,5-triol. Saponin glycoside Tetrahydro-2-(hydroxymethyl)-6-(octadecahydro-2,7,10a-trimethyl-1propylchrysen-8-ylox-)-2H-Pyran-3,4,5-triol, Nocturnoside –b, Protodioscine, Paraquisoside –b, Solanine, and Solasodine.	[3]
Cestrum aurantiacum Lindl.	Saponin, phenolic, flavanoid, and alkaloid Steroidal saponins, sterols, catechol tannins, carbohydrates and flavonoids.	[30]
Cytisusscoparius linn.	Quericitin, saponin, Volatile oil, tannin, fat, wax, sugar. Glucoside-Scoparin, alkaloid-Sparteine, Oxysparteine.	[4]
Erigeron karvinkianus DC	Naringenin, 7-Methoxy Hesperetin, Saponins, calenduloside E, and leiocarposide.	[31]
Phytolacca dodecandra L'Her.	Alkaloids, tannins, phenolics, steroids, and triterpenoids, saponins.	[32]
Cnicuswallichi DC	Steroids, triterpenoids, phenolic compounds, flavanoids, tannins, and carbohydrates.	[33]
Achyranthes bidentataBlume	Alkaloids, glycosides, triterpenoids, saponins, flavonoids, and mucilage, phytoecdysteroids, saccharides.	[34]
Artemisia nilagirica linn.	Phenolics, total flavonoids, triterpenoids, tannins, and alkaloids.	[35]
Centella asiatica linn.	Fatty oil consists of glycerides of palmitic, stearic, lignoceric, and oleic acids Glycosides: Asiaticoside A & B, madecassoside & centelloside. Triterpene acids- asiatic, madecassic, terminalic, centic, centellic, centoic acid, betulic, brahmic, and isobrahmic acid. Flanonoids -3-β glucosyl quercetin, 3-β glucosylkaempferol, 7- β-glucosylkaempferol, kaempferol, and quercetin.	[36]
Berberis vulgaris linn.	Berberine, Berlambine, Hydroxycanthine, Isocorydine, (-) Tejedine, Lupeol, Oleanolic acid, Steroids stigmasterol, and Stigmasterol glucoside.	[37]

Glimpses of cytotoxic weed plants in India

Acalypha Indica Linn.

Acalypha Indica linn. belonging to the family Euphorbiaceae, is a weed plant reported for its cytotoxic potency by Amarnath *et al.* [38]. The aqueous ethanol extract of Acalypha indica primed chitosan-casein microparticles in a human prostate cancer cell line (PC3). In the first 24 hours, there were no significant differences between the extract alone and extract loaded chitosan-casein microparticles-treated cells, but after 72 hours, the microparticle demonstrated greater cytotoxicity. The probability percentage of cytotoxic effects was also shown by the LDH test, which revealed concentration-dependent leakage of LDH from free-extract-exposed PC3 cells and extract-loaded chitosan-casein microvesicles. A study by Sudhakar *et al.* [39] emphasised the cytotoxic activity of hexane leaf crude extract (concentrations of 10 g/ml, 25 g/ml, 50 g/ml, and 100 g/ml) of Acalypha indica on MCF-7 cell lines. The maximum inhibitory effect (IC50 value) was found to be 50 g/ml.

Tridax procumbens linn

Tridax procumbens linn. belonging to the family Compositae, is known as Ghamara and is a widespread weed that has been found all through India. The anticancer activity of crude extracts of the leaves of Tridax procumbens, *viz*., methanol, ethanol, and chloroform solvents, was screened for cytotoxicity against two breast cancer cell lines, MCF-7 (benign) and MDA-MB-231 (metastatic) [40]. The chloroform extract was active against MCF-7 and MDA-MB-231 cells at an IC50 value of 136 g/ml and 129 g/ml, respectively, from among the three extracts isolated. Phytochemical analysis revealed the presence of steroids and terpenoids such as 3, 9-Dihydroxy-18 alpha-olean-28-oic acids and 3, 28-Bis (cinnamoyl) betulin.

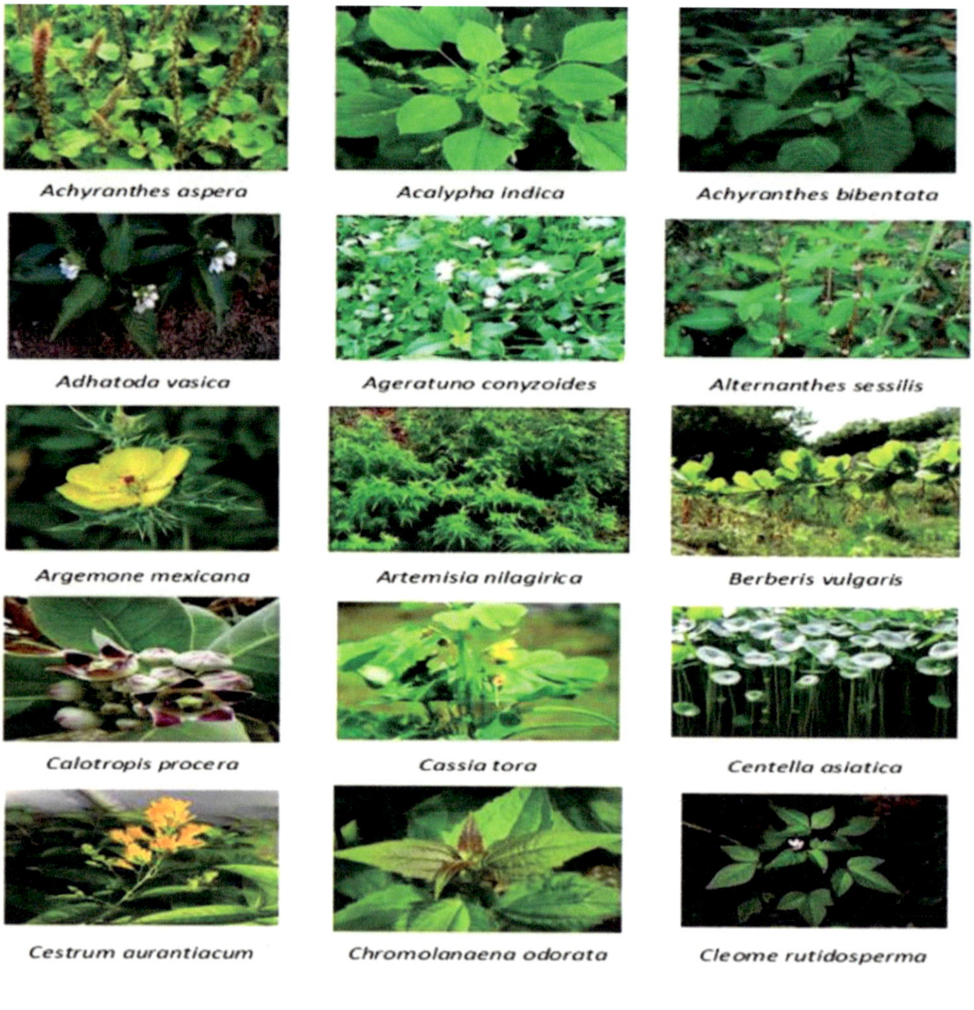

(Fig. 1) contd.....

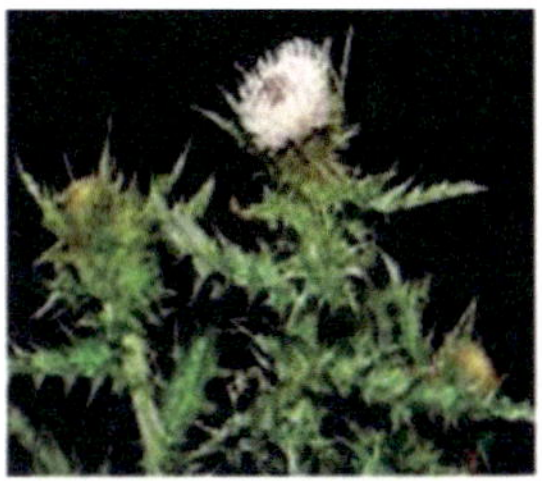

Cnicus wallichi

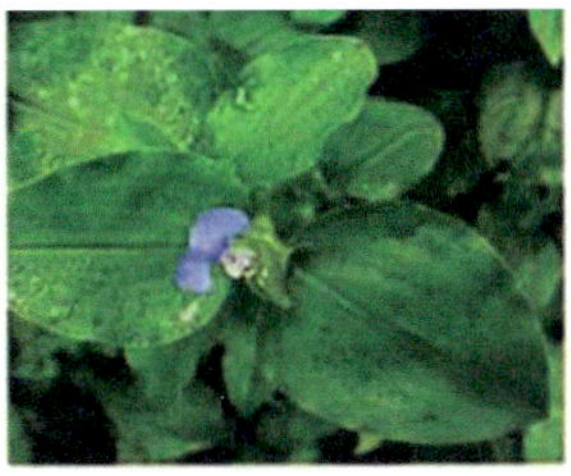

Commelina benghalensis

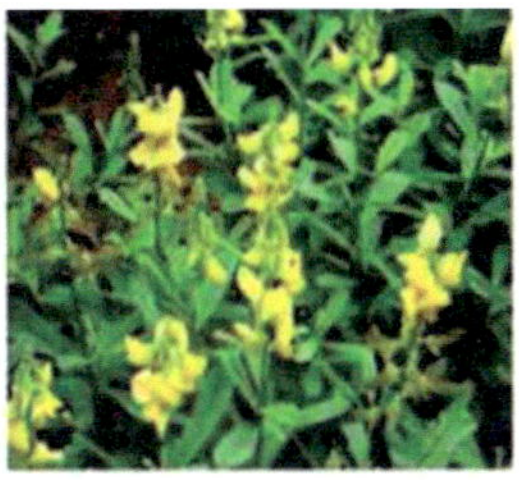

Crotalaria retusa

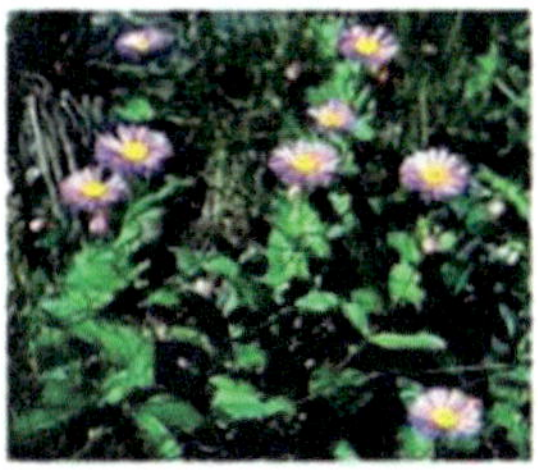

Erigeron karvinkianus

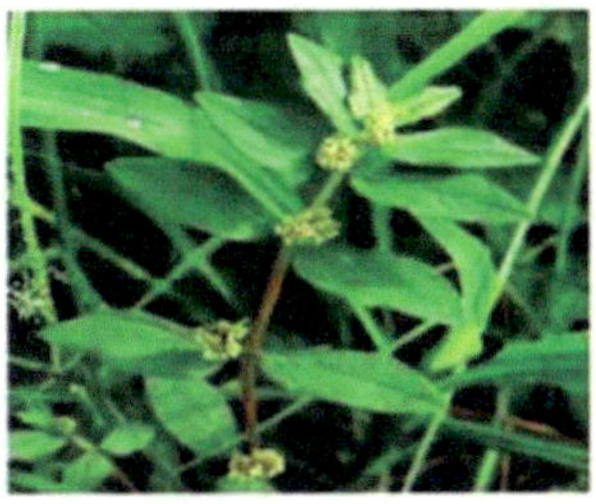

Euphorbia hirta

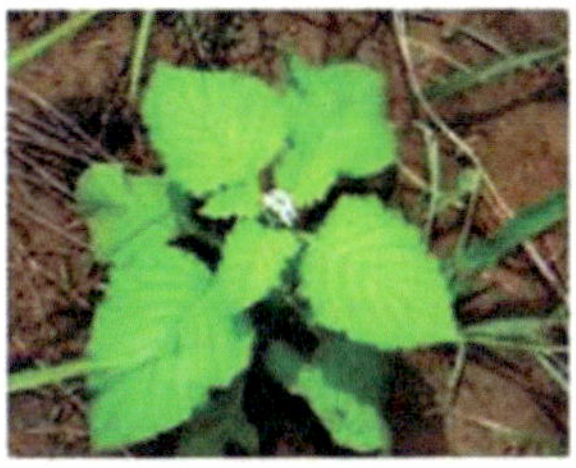

Heliotropium indicum

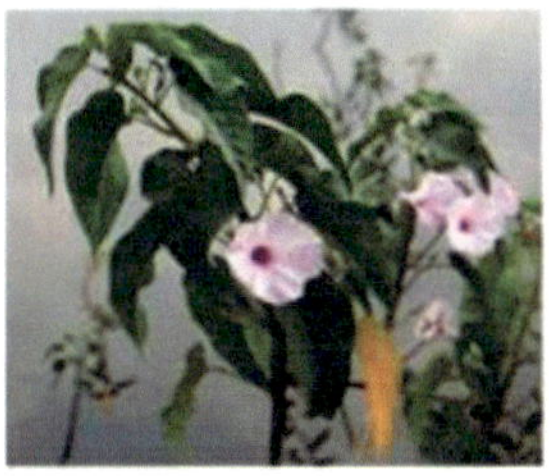

Ipomoae carnae

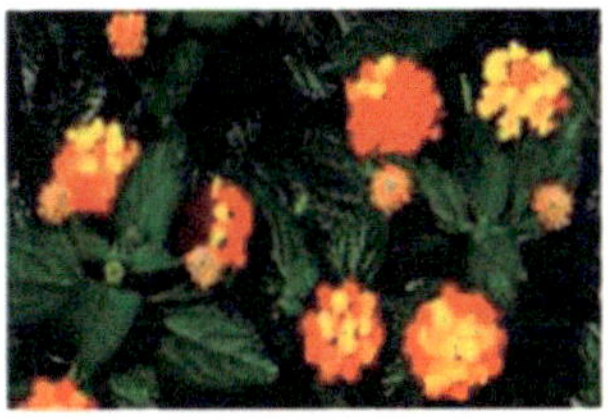

Lantana camara

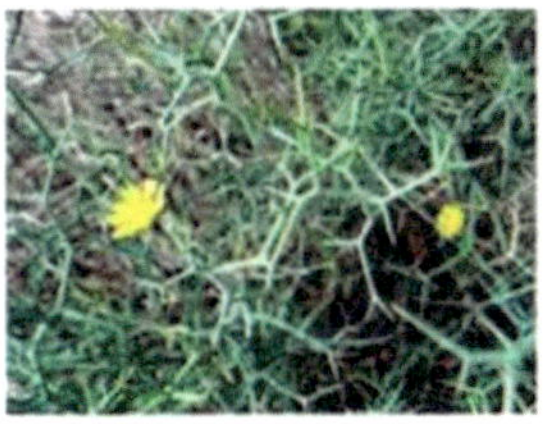

Launaea procumbens

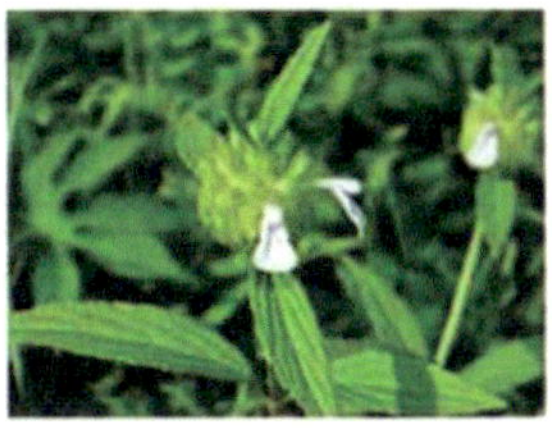

Leucas aspera

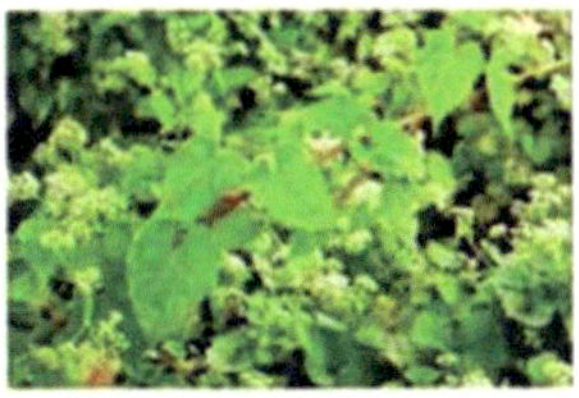

Mikania micrantha

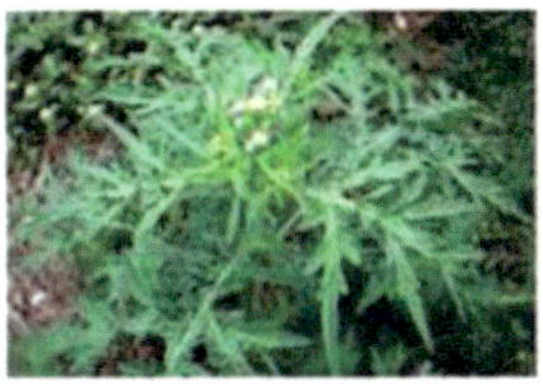

Parthenium hysterophorus

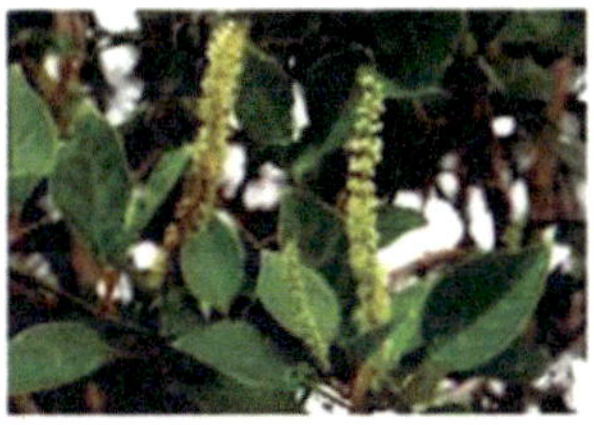

Phytolacca dodecandra

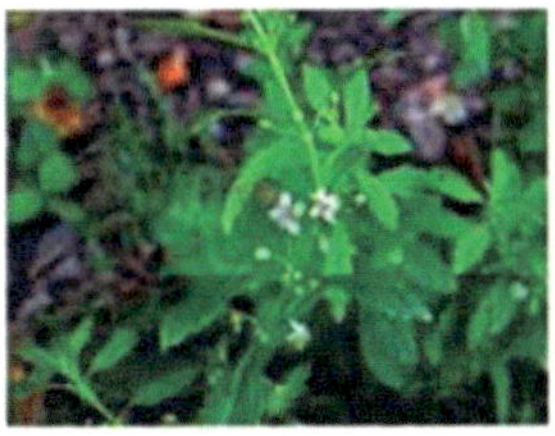

Scaparia dulcis

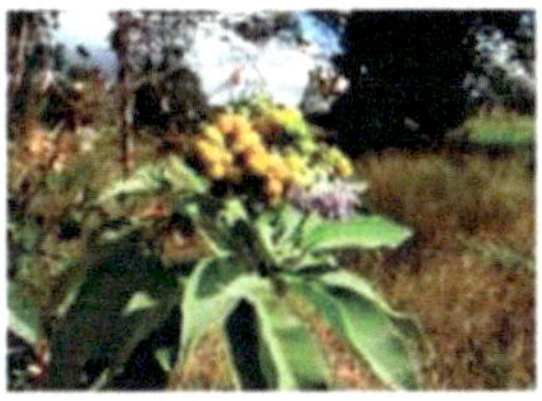

Solanum mauritianum

(Fig. 1) contd.....

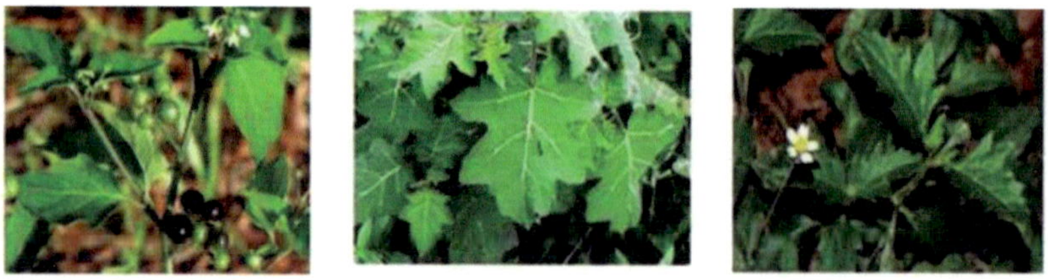

Fig. (1). Cytotoxic weeds profile in India

The author, Vishnu Priya and Srinivasa Rao, 2015 [41] reported the anticancer activity of acetone and ethanol leaf extracts of *T. procumbens* on A549 and Hep G2 human cancerous cell lines showed potent anticancer activity. While the hydroethanolic extract of Tridax procumbens at concentrations of 0–10 g/l was used to assess the cytotoxic effects of HepG2 cells and had no impact on cell survival; however, a small decrease in cell survival was reported at 20 g/l [42]. Lakshmipriya *et al.*, 2019 [43], evolved a bioassay-guided differentiated fraction of the cytotoxic acetone leaf extract upon the growth of MCF-7, Hep G2, and K562 cells, with fraction 15 presenting the maximum antiproliferative effect towards K562 cells, keeping the normal peripheral blood lymphocyte unchanged.

Ikpefan *et al.* [44] investigated the cytotoxicity of Tridoxproumbens methanol extract in Raniceps sranninus tadpoles at concentrations ranging from 10-400 g/ml.The crude methanol extract and the chloroform portion showed maximum cytotoxicity of 63.33 1.33 and 100 percent at 400 g/mL after 24 h, respectively. Moreover, this plant also contains tannins, saponins, flavonoids, cardiac glycosides, and anthraquinone phytoconstituents. The author assessed the cytotoxicity activity on HepG2 and PANC1 cells, which were treated with 20, 50, 100, and 250 g/ml of dimethyl sulfoxide (control), leaf extract, and fractions (n-hexane, dichloromethane, ethyl acetate, aqueous) for 24 and 48 hours. The phytochemical study showed the presence of total flavonoids and phenol. The dichloromethane fraction caused a significant level of cytotoxicity and induction of the activities of ALP, catalase, and caspase 3 as compared to the control and was described as a promising anticancer agent [45]. A lung metastasis essential oil isolated from Tridax procumbens and mediated by B16F-10 melanoma cells in C57BL/6 mice developed 70.2% *in vitro* cytotoxicity for 50 g/ml of cancer cell death at 24 h. Conversely, compared to untreated mice, *in vivo* oil therapy strongly suppressed tumour nodulation by 71.7% [46].

Uzuegbu *et al.*, 2020 [47], reported the cytotoxic activity of the crude alkaloid such as Chloroquine and ethanolic leaf extracts prepared from the selected eight plants *viz. Tridax procumbens*, *Ipomoea purpurea*, *Sida acuta*, *Senna alata*,

Phyllanthus amarus, *Azadirachta indica*, *Nauclea latifolia*, and *Polyalthia longifolia* were tested on L929 animal cell fibroblasts at varying doses (50.00, 25.00 12.50, 6.25, 3.13, and 1.57 μg/ml). The CC_{50} values show that the ethanolic leaf extracts of *T. procumbens* and *S. acuta* demonstrated mild toxicity (CC_{50}=23.99μg/ml for each plant) as compared with the standard (CC_{50}: 30 μg/ml= non-toxic), while others, including the alkaloid extracts, were non-toxic. The leaves, stems, and blossoms of *T. procumbens* were isolated from acetonitrile and a formic acetic acid portion at a 50:1 ratio. The derived SPs were evaluated for their cytotoxic activity response on human breast cancer metastatic cell lines (MDA MB 231). The leaf SPs were studied by Jayanthi *et al.* 2020 [49] who investigated the ethanol extract of Leucas asperaflower against Ehrlich ascetic tumor: an *in vitro* and *in vivo* model of Leucas aspera (Willd.) *linn.* family Lamiaceae.Their *in vitro* cytotoxicity study showed a concentration-dependent increase in the reduced IC_{50} at 4μg/ml of all the evaluated SPs [48].

Leucas aspera (Willd.)linn

Jayanthi *et al.* 2020 [49] investigated the ethanol extract of Leucas asperaflower against Ehrlich ascetic tumor: an *in vitro* and *in vivo* model of Leucas aspera (Willd.) *linn.* family Lamiaceae. Their *in vitro* cytotoxicity study revealed that cytotoxicity increased concentration-dependently up to 200 g/ml, with an IC50 value of 102.14 g/ml. The ethanolic extract of whole Leucas aspera was subjected to a brine shrimp lethality assay. Related to the positive control vincristine sulphate, the LC50 was 0.760.04 g/ml, and the extract showed that the LC50 value was statistically relevant (P 0.01) as 181.682.15 g/ml [50].

In order to evaluate a substance's capacity to eliminate cancer cells, the bioassay for brine shrimp lethality provides an impressive means of testing and evaluating the biological properties. In another study by Sayed *et al.*, 2014 [51], the dichloromethane fraction displayed the greatest cytotoxic effect towards A. salina (LC50 = 268 ppm), accompanied by methanol extract (LC50 = 327 ppm), while being less cytotoxic than gallic acid (LC50 = 4.12 ppm), a positive control. Related toxicities were seen in the hexane and ethyl acetate fractions (LC50 = 364 and 388 ppm, respectively). The researchers then looked into the cytotoxicity of alpha-amyrin and alpha-tocopherol and discovered that alpha-tocopherol (LC50 = 195 ppm) was more toxic than alpha-amyrin (LC50 = 241 ppm), both of which were extracted from the dichloromethane fraction.

Cleome rutidosperma linn

Cleome rutidosperma linn. belongs to the family *Cleomeceae*. Prabha *et al.*, 2017 [52], prepared hexane, ethyl acetate, and methanol extracts from the leaf of *C.*

rutidosperma and confirmed the presence of phytoconstituents such as flavonoids, tannins, saponins, alkaloids, steroids, proteins and polyphenols in these extracts. *In vitro* cytotoxicity by MTT assay of methanol extract exhibited significant anticancer activities.

Commelina benghalensis linn

Commelina benghalensis linn. belongs to the family *Commelinaceae*, generally referred to as Bengal dayflower, utilized for the prevention of headache, fever, leprosy, constipation, jaundice, and snakebite. The essential antioxidant, anticancer, and antitumor activities were documented for this weed [53]. In 2018, research by Birendra *et al.* [54], stated that at doses of 200 mg/kg and 400 mg/kg, the anticancer activity study substantially decreased the total cell count and tumor volume relative to the control group of EAC. Percentage TCI, the percentage inhibition of tumor volume was observed to be 79.92% and 78.81%, respectively for 200 mg/kg, and was 89.51% and 94.77%, respectively, for 400 mg/kg.

The anticancer activity of methanol, ethanol, chloroform, and hexane extracts of *Commelinabenghalensis* on MDA-MB-231cell lines was evaluated based on IC_{50} values, the highest anticancer effect was observed in MDA-MB-231 cells by chloroform extract that showed IC_{50} of 134 µg/ml at 24 h treatment and 79 µg/ml at 48 h treatment. In contrast, hexane extract presented a weaker inhibitory effect for cell mortality as compared to other tested extracts of *C. benghalensis* with an IC_{50} of 219 µg/ml at 24 h and 185 µg/ml at 48 h treatment of cancer cells. Whereas, ethanol and methanol extracts showed considerable inhibitory action in breast cancer cells. Moreover, chloroform extract showed significant activity in the inhibition of Hep-2 cell proliferation with an IC_{50} of 111 µg/ml. In other words, benzene extract was more active on DU-145 cell inhibition with an IC_{50} of 173 µg/mL at 24 h [55].

Kgomotso *et al.* (2014) [56] carried out the effect of sub-fractions of acetone extracts of the stem against growth-related molecular pathways of the Jurkat-T (JT) cell division process and cell apoptosis. Concentration- and time-dependent multiplication and survival of JT cells were inhibited by the F1 and F2 fractions, with IC50 values of 32.5 g/ml and 56 g/ml, respectively. In 2015, Chowdhury *et al.* [57] stated that the methanol crude extract of C. benghalensis had a significant cytotoxic impact on the brine shrimp survivability bioassay (LC50 = 278.69 g/ml) relative to normal vincristine sulphate (LC50 = 0.512 g/ml).

The authors, Vusi *et al.* (2008) [58], evaluated the growth inhibitory and apoptosis-inducing effects of a crude methanolic stem extract of C. benghalensis (0-600 g/ml) on Jurkat T cells. The extract resulted in a dose-dependent and time-dependent cell proliferation reduction accompanied by a consequent reduction in cell survival. Proma Roy *et al.* (2018) [59] showed that at a concentration of 278.68 g/ml after 24 h, the methanolic extract exhibited considerable cytotoxic effects against the brine shrimp lethality assay. The authors also performed research in which hydroethanolic leaf extracts were used. However, despite the large dose of 2000 mg/kg, no toxic reactions or deaths were observed, and therefore the LD50 of hydroethanolic extracts of Commelina benghalensis should be more than 2000 mg/kg.

Euphorbia hirta linn

Euphorbia hirta linn. family *Euphorbiaceae*, a pantropical weed, often seen invading waste disposal spaces and farmlands, public roads, and sidewalks. The tannins, sterols, alkaloids, glycosides, triterpenoids, flavonoids, and polyphenols are found in *E. hirta* leaves. It's being used in the conventional medical system to treat a range of diseases like asthma, coughs, warts, diarrhea, and dysentery [1]. A variety of cytotoxicity studies were reported by many scientists on this weed. Anitha *et al.* 2014 [60], reported the ethanol leaf extract of *Euphorbia hirta* on Carcinoma cell lines (DLA and EAC), and its cytotoxic IC_{50} value was found to be 560.83 µg/ml and 384.7 µg/ml, respectively.

In addition, a dose-dependent decrease in multiplication and apoptosis induction was noticed. Hydromethanol extracts of leaf of *Euphorbia hirta* were shown to have antiproliferative activity against prostate cancer LNCaP cell lines with 251.15 ± 6.5 µg/ml. This effect may be explained by the occurrence of phenolic compounds in *Euphorbia hirta*. Moreover, anticancer activities have been documented for terpene, polyphenols, and sterols [61].

Yuet Ping *et al.* 2016 [62], studied a cytotoxicity effect on MCF-7 breast cancer cells showed substantial suppression of MCF-7 cell survival and IC_{50} values of 25.26 mg/ml at 24 h. The microscopy and flow cytometry tests, furthermore, displayed significant morphological features characteristics of cell death. Of all the fractions measured with an IC_{50} value of 10.01mg/ml at 24 h, the hexane fraction (HF sub4 fraction) exhibited the greatest activity.

The cytotoxic activity of the methanol extract of leaves on Hep-2 cells from human epithelium of the larynx was investigated and showed a dose-dependent anti-proliferative activity, IC_{50} at 625µg/ml of crude extract [63]. Brindha *et al.*, 2010 [64], by using a human liver-derived HepG2 cell line assessed the level of cytotoxic effects of this weed extract by measuring the viability of cells (MTT assay). A dose-dependent improvement in percentage survival was reported when HepG2 cells subjected to anti-tubercular drugs were treated to various plant extract concentrations (125, 250, 500, and 1000 μg/ml). At 1000 μg/ml concentration, the maximum percentage viability of HepG2 was reported. The findings indicate that *E. hirta* defends against *in vitro* cytotoxicity induced by anti-tubercular drugs.

A report by Pranabesh *et al.*, 2020 [65], revealed a greater proportion of polyphenols, flavonoids, and tannins isolated from the water extract of five weeds namely *Heliotropium indicum*, *Tridax procumbens*, *Cleome rutidosperma*, *Commelinabenghalensis*, and *Euphorbia hirta*, from West Bengal, India. While 70% ethanol extract shows excellent alkaloid and cardiac glycoside content. The study of HPLC-DAD relates to 10 prominent phenolic constituents. *Euphorbia hirta* extract exhibited minimal cytotoxic effects (apoptosis ~2.5% and 4% in water and 70% ethanol extract, respectively), while ethanol extracts of *Cleome rutidosperma* and *Tridax procumbens* exhibited significant apoptosis related to the control (cell apoptosis ~10-12%) (~13% and 28%, respectively).

Argemone Mexicana linn

Argemone Mexicana *linn.* a member of the Papaveraceae family, is known as prickly poppies in English and grows as a roadside weed in almost every part of India.The two aliphatic substances extracted from the leaves, namely, mexicanol and mexican acid, have a promising pharmacological profile [1].

The ethyl acetate flower portion of A. mexicana has been evaluated for its cytotoxicity on HepG2 cell lines (liver cancer) at different concentrations. The IC50 value was reported as 72 1.7 g/ml on the HepG2 cell line [66]. Yuh-Chwen *et al.*, 2003 [67], demonstrated that the sub-fraction of the chloroform extract from the aerial portion of Argemone mexicana succeeded in the isolation of benzophenanthridine-type alkaloids. In order to emphasise their greater efficacy on human nasopharyngeal carcinoma (HONE-1) and human gastric cancer (NUGC) cell lines, a cytotoxicity test was carried out on these isolated alkaloids. The HeLa and MCF-7 cells were exposed to a methanolic extract of the leaves of Argemone Mexicana; a phytochemical study revealed the flavonoids contents, with IC50 values ranging from 1.35 g/l to 1.2 g/l. The nature of cytotoxic activity is found to be apoptotic rather than necrotic by the Hoechst test [68]. Further research performed by Nilesh *et al.* in 2016 [69] on both cold aqueous and methanolic stem and leaf extracts had quite a cytotoxic effect on immortalised cell lines A549, SiHa, and KB, which was close to berberine.

Adhatoda vasica linn

Adhatoda vasica linn. a weed in the *Acanthaceae* family, is traditionally used to treat asthma, cough, bleeding piles, and to turn sputum into liquid. The bitter principle, namely vasicine, and other phytoconstituents include betaine, steroids, carbohydrates, alkanes, triterpenes, and flavonoids [1]. The anticancer-cytotoxic effect of Adhatodavasica ethanol extract was examined in various cancer cell lines, such as MCF-7, MDA-MB-231, Hela, and HepG2, through an *in vitro* study by Nirmala *et al.*, in 2019 [70]. The active constituents such as carbohydrates, steroids, alkaloids, tannins, flavonoids, saponins, gums, and mucilage were found in this weed plant. Their outcome demonstrated strong cytotoxicity in Hela, HepG2, MCF-7, and MDA-MB-231 cells at 24 h, which were found to be 60%, 60%, 85%, and 65%, respectively. Significant cytotoxic effects towards seven distinct forms of leukaemia cells, including CEM, NB-4, MOLM-14, Jurkat, IM-9, K562, and HL-60, were also evaluated for an isolated alkaloid, 2-acety--benzylamine, from Adhatodavasica, reported by Balachandran *et al.*, 2017 [71]. Relative to other tested cells, 2-acetyl-benzylamine displayed remarkable cytotoxic activity on MOLM-14 and NB-4 cells, with IC50 values of 0.40 and 0.39 mM at 24 h, respectively.

Calotropis procera linn.

Milkweed, *Calotropis procera linn.* (*Asclepiadaceae*), is primarily found in India. Hassan *et al.*, 2017 [72], showed the cytotoxicity of a methanol extract of C. procera towards the MCF7 breast cancer cell line at concentrations of 5, 10, and 25 l. The MTT assay revealed that the total extract significantly reduced cell viability (p 0.05) by more than 70% after 48 hours.In addition, further work was done by the authors to assess the cytotoxic effects of C. proceramethanolic extract on T47D breast cancer cell lines at 5, 10, and 25 g concentrations. As the concentration of C. procera improved, the number of viable cells was observed to be reduced. The total extract of C. procera was able to significantly reduce cell viability by more than (p 0.05) for T47D.

The *C. procera* root extract was shown to have major cytotoxicity on COLO 320 tumor cells [73]. In the human xenograft models of nude mice, the hemi synthetic cardenolide derivative collected from the root bark displayed elevated cytotoxic effects on several human cancer lines, strong *in vivo* tumor growth susceptibility, and prolonged survival period [74]. Suraj *et al.*, 2015 [75], isolated a fraction from chloroform extract which showed positive results in the brine shrimp experiment and shows a LC50 of 5 mg/ml benzene extract while the petroleum ether extract revealed LC50 at 20 mg/ml. Cell culture experiments by Choedon *et al.*, 2006 [76] showed that in both Huh-7 and COS-1 cells the methanol extract of dried latex of *Calotropis procera* and its portion 8 triggered substantial cell death whereas, AML12 cells were preserved. This was accompanied by considerable fragmentation of DNA in Huh-7 and COS-1 cells. Fortunately, the rates of canonical cell death markers, including Bcl2 and caspase 3, have not been altered.

Five of those extracts, namely, hexane, dichloromethane, ethyl acetate, acetone, and methanolic extracts of Calotropis procera, demonstrated higher IC50 cytotoxic cancer cell effects ranging from 0.8 to 4.4 g/ml, while the methanolic extract was clumsily cytotoxic. Cytotoxic extracts have frequently been shown to inhibit cell division, implying IC50 values less than 5 g/mL. In the *in vivo* anti-tumor experiments, ethyl acetate and acetone-treated animals showed tumour growth inhibition levels of 64.3 and 53.1%, respectively. Application of various root extracts (viz., methanolic (CM), hexane (CH), aqueous (CW), and ethyl acetate (CE)) of Calotropis procera weed at concentrations of 1, 5, 10, and 25 g/ml revealed that CM, CH, and CE were cytotoxic, whereas CW wasn't really cytotoxic. At 48 h after treatment, CE (10 g/ml) exhibited the greatest cytotoxicity (96.3%) against Hep2, while CM and CH exhibited 72.7 and 60.5% cytotoxicity, respectively. Standard morphological alterations of cell death were displayed by extract-treated cells. Findings from Mathur *et al.* 2009 [77] indicate that the development of Hep2 cells *via* apoptosis and cell cycle degradation-focused mechanisms is inhibited by root extracts of C. procera.

An ethanolic extract of the stem and leaves was tested *in vitro* against the HCT-15 (colon) cancer cell line at concentrations of 10, 30, and 100 g/ml, and it was discovered that the 100 g/ml concentration inhibited HCT-15 growth by 50% [78]. A cardiac glycoside extract derived from the latex of *C. procera* was tested for its anticancer activity against breast cancer cells, MCF-7. The extract strongly suppressed MCF-7 cell proliferation (P 0.05) and enhanced this activity with increased concentration. There have also been structural morphological variations in treated cells when compared to normal cells [79].

Lantana camara linn

Lantana camara linn. (*Verbenaceae*), called as Wild sage and Spanish flag. The isolated Oleanonic acid from *L. camara* produced the anti-cancer on the murine tumor (Ehrlich ascites carcinoma) and three human cancer cell lines, including A375 (malignant skin melanoma), Hep2 (epidermoid laryngeal carcinoma) and U9375 (lymphoma). Moreover, the isolated oleanonic acid has shown good cytotoxic effects on cells of A375 [80]. L. camara leaf methanol extract showed an antiproliferative effect on HEp-2 (laryngeal cancer) and NCI-H292 (lung cancer) cell lines. The number of living cells was noted to be 25.8 0.19, as reported by Sanjeeb *et al.*, 2012 [81]. Research by Raghu *et al.*, in 2004 [82], found comparatively greater cytotoxic effects in five methanol extracts obtained from various parts of Lantana camara: leaf, root, stem, fruit, and flowers. The lung carcinoma cell line, A-549, was observed to be more vulnerable with a CTC50 level of 48.1–58.5 mg/ml extract. The other four extracts exhibited lesser activity, as indicated by the comparatively higher CTC50 values. Methanol root extracts at 191.5 5.1 g/ml and leaves at 219.5 8.4 g/ml have displayed mild activity against DLA cells after 3 h of exposure in short-term toxicity studies. Extracts of Lantana camara stem, fruit, and flowers reported reduced activity with CTC50 values of 268.7 10.2, 492.7 14.4, and > 1000 g/ml, respectively. Patil *et al.* [83] synthesised silver nanoparticles in 2017, which were tested for dose-dependent cytotoxic effects on A. nauplii salina. The LC50 value was calculated to be 514.50 g/ml for AgNPs.

Solanum nigrum linn

Solanum nigrum linn. (*Solanaceae*), a weed, called makoi or black nightshade. The author Lai *et al.*, 2016 [84] shared cytotoxic findings indicating that the aqueous extracts of *Solanum nigrum* significantly suppressed the cell viability of MCF-7 *via* initiation of apoptosis and cell cycle arrest induced by caspase-3 activation and development of reactive oxygen species.

Research on the impact of *Solanum nigrum* extract on methylation status of the genes VIM and CXCR4 in breast cancer cell lines was carried out by Atefeh *et al.* in 2020 [85]. Their findings indicated that the management of MCF-7 with an extract of 0.1 mg/ml hypermethylated the genes VIM and CXCR4, and reduced considerably their mRNA expression levels ($P<0.05$). In addition, the aqueous extract of *S. nigrum* was analyzed by Binbing *et al.*, 2019 [86] at a concentration of 10 g/l, which demonstrated a 43% cytotoxic effect towards the cell line MCF-7, prevented proliferation, and reduced the functions of hexokinase and pyruvate kinase towards the MCF7 cells by around 30% and 40%, respectively.

The cytotoxic activity of varying proportions of hydro-alcoholic extracts of Cucurbita pepo and *S. nigrum* was tested against standard cell lines (Chinese hamster ovarian cells and rat fibroblast) and on cancer lines (HepG2 and CT26). The findings suggested that IC_{50} of *S. nigram* extract was noticeably smaller than *C. pepo* extract on all four cell lines, ($P< 0.05$) [87]. The 80% methanol and chloroform extracts of the leaves and stems of *Solanum nigrum* were evaluated for *in vitro* cytotoxic effects by Ehssan *et al.*, in 2014 [88] towards PC-3, Hela, 3T3, and CC-1 cancer cell lines. Both 100 µg/ml extracts had anticancer effects on PC-3 and Hela, and the highest rate of growth inhibition from stem methanol extracts on Hela was 91.11%, followed by leaf and stem methanol extracts on PC-3 (74.28% and 80.49%, respectively). The results generated for cytotoxic effects suggested that both extracts had a non-toxic action on CC-1 and 3T3 cell lines with IC50 values > 100 g/ml, other than that the leaf methanol extract displayed the greatest percent inhibitory activity on 3T3, 85.63% with an IC50 of 17.37 g/ml. The effect of the compound solanine on the anti-tumor effect was measured in 2007 by Ji YB *et al.* [89]. Their findings reported that the IC50 was 14.47, >50, and >50 g/ml for HepG-2, SGC-7901, and LS-174, respectively. It was observed that the proportion of cell death in solanine-induced HepG-2 cells was 6.0, 14.4, 17.3, 18.9, and 32.2%, respectively. The author concluded that the effect was due to the target of solanine in the inhibition of Bcl-2 protein expression. Research was performed by Lee *et al.* in 2004 [90] to explore the cytotoxic activity of HCT-116 cells with a 150-kDa glycoprotein obtained from Solanum nigrum. At small doses, the glycoprotein had extraordinary, dose-dependent cytotoxic and apoptosis-inducing results. Son YO *et al.*, 2003 [91], studied an ethanol extract from fruited Solanum nigrum for growth-inhibitory activity towards MCF-7. The results showed that the proliferative potential of MCF-7 cells was strongly inhibited in the presence of ethanol extract. The effect of the aqueous extract of Solanum nigrum (SNL-AE) on tumour growth was examined, and the findings showed that SNL-AE affected the formation of cervical carcinoma (U14) and expanded the number of subsets of CD4+ T lymphocytes as well as the CD4+/CD8+ T lymphocyte ratio and lowered the number of subsets of CD8+ T lymphocytes in tumor-bearing mice [92]. The apoptosis effects of glycoproteins (carbohydrate 69.74% and protein -30.26%) extracted from Solanum nigrum in human cervical cancer cells revealed that SNL glycoprotein at 50 g/ml has a stimulating effect on cytochrome c escape into the cytosol, caspase-8, -3 activation, and PARP cleavage in HeLa cells [93]. Various organic solvents and aqueous extracts collected from Solanum nigrum berries for leukemic cell line antiproliferative activity, namely Jurkat and HL-60 cell lines, were assessed by Gabrani *et al.* in 2012 [94] and showed increased cytotoxicity with increased concentration of the extract. On both cell lines, comparative analysis revealed that the LC50 value of the methanol extract was the lowest. A strong cytotoxic effect towards MCF-7 and HepG-2 cancer cell lines with IC50 values of 12.7 and 16.6 g/ml, respectively, was reported by the ethanol extract of green fruits, as stated by El-hawary *et al.*, 2015 [95]. The higher concentration of steroidal glycoalkaloids in unripe green fruits of S. nigrum is related to this activity. Another study by Patel *et al.*, 2009 [96], found that the methanolic extract had a significant cytotoxicity effect and inhibitory action against the HeLa cancer cell line at 10–0.0196 mg/ml. The IC50 values of HeLa cells and Vero cells were 847.8 and 9088, respectively, by SRB assay. The MTT assay reported an IC50 value of 265.0 for HeLa cells and 6.862 for Vero cells.Their study revealed that the methanol extract of these drugs induced a higher effect on HeLa cell lines and a lower effect on Vero cell lines. Solanum nigrum extract showed the strongest cytotoxic activity against U266 cells.were reported by Wang *et al.* 2005 [97]. The IC_{50} was found to be 117 mg/l after treatment of drug on the U266 cells for 48 h. The percentage of apoptosis improved with risinf in the dosage of the drug treatment. In addition, its cell death triggering activity could be identified by the antineoplastic effects of drugs. In the brine shrimp lethality test, the ethanol extract of the ripened fruit of *Solanum nigrum* exhibited substantial cytotoxic effects with LC50 at 63.10 µg/ml and LC_{90}= 160 µg/ml [98].

Parthenium hysterophorus Linn

Parthenium hysterophorus linn. (*Asteraceae*), known as carrot grass, bitter weed, *etc.* is an aggressive ubiquitous annual noxious weed, spotted on roadsides, parks, and mostly in fields with crops [18]. Shashank Kumar *et al.*, in 2013 [99], confirmed the cytotoxic effect of *P. hysterophorus* leaf extracts towards cancer cell lines, including DU-145, MCF-7, and THP-1 at a concentration of 100 µg/ml employing SRB assays. The ethanol fraction displayed significant cytotoxicity (81-85%), whereas the DU-145 cell line exhibited lower activity. In the MTT assay, the same extract showed growth inhibition of 17-98% on HL-60 cancer cell lines, indicating dose-dependent performance. Ethanol extract induced a 12% decrease in mitochondrial function and a 10% increase in the sub G1 group of HL-60 cell lines. The research demonstrates that *Parthenium hysterophorus* leaves have profound cytotoxicity. Results from Sharma *et al.*, 2015 [100], exhibited substantial cytotoxic activity of methanol leaf extracts with significant suppression (80-90%) of HeLa cell lines. The CC_{50} on the HeLa cell line was identified and revealed that the percentage of growth inhibition value gradually increased as the extract concentration increased to 30, 55, 78, 82% for concentrations of 125, 250, 500, 1000 µg/ml, respectively.

A comprehensive research on the cytotoxic effect of the leaf, herb, and root extracts were examined towards various cell lines of cancer at a dose level of 100 µg/ml by Shashank Kumar *et al.*, 2014 [101]. The leaf extract was examined on HOP-62 and IGR-OV1 cell lines, while cytotoxicity of flower and root fractions on cancer cell lines A-549 and HCT-116 were investigated. The ethanol portion of the leaf extracts showed substantially cytotoxic effects towards the test cell lines. Ethanol extract has exhibited 95 and 55% growth inhibition against IGR-OV-1 and HOP-62 cell lines, respectively. 2-50% cytotoxicity on test cell lines was shown in the majority of the leaf fractions. There was significant inhibitory ability noted for most of the flower extracts. Benzene, chloroform, ethanol, and acetone flower extracts displayed 84-90% cytotoxicity on the cell lines of A549 and HCT-116. The aqueous fraction demonstrated 100% cytotoxic effects against the cell line of HCT-116. In addition to this, the hexane and ethanol root extracts of *P.*

hysterophorus demonstrated significant action (99% and 93%) towards HCT-116 cells. Hexane, Benzene, and chloroform portions displayed toxicity on A549 cell lines of 76%, 74%, and 65%, respectively. The remaining fractions were responsible for reduced activity.

Parthenin the compound was tested for cytotoxicity activity using MBMD231, breast cancer cell line showed very low cytotoxicity [18]. A phytochemical and cytotoxic analysis by Durga *et al.*, 2013 [102] showed a significant cytotoxic concentration (CC_{50}) of 230± 0.00 and 183.00± 5.8 on the CHOK-1 and A-549 cell lines, respectively. As the concentration of the extract was raised by 62.5, 125, 250, 500, 1000 μg/ml, however, there was also a rise in the result on growth inhibition as 25.19, 27.30, 55.55, 77.34, and 80.26%, respectively for CHOK 1 cell line, and by 12.49, 33.24, 75.68, 78.95, and 81.95%, respectively for A-549 cell line.

The cytotoxic activity of methanolic extract increased with an increase in the concentration 36, 70, and 82% for MCF-7 and 80% for HeLa cell lines at concentrations of 5, 10, and 15 M respectively. IC_{50} values for MCF-7 and HeLa cell lines were 30.81±0.09 and 5.35±0.03ng/mL respectively [103]. The descriptive study was performed by Raies *et al.* 2011 [104], on various methanol, ethanol, chloroform, and water extracts for cytotoxicity on human cancer cell lines, such as IGROV-I, A-549, PC-3, MCF-7, and SF-295 with the exception of HOP-62. The methanol extract was demonstrated to display the maximum cytotoxic effects towards PC-3 with an IC_{50} of 0.11μM. While three other extracts exhibited substantial cytotoxic effects, however, a normal pattern was not followed.

A study by Ali Ahsan *et al.*, 2020 [105] on the viability of NIH3T3 fibroblasts was adversely and progressively affected by raising the leaf extract concentrations. Shoot and root extracts, however, had no major activity on cell viability, despite root extracts supporting cell viability (14%) at the lowest dose (0.0625 mg/ml) related to the untreated control. The maximum decrease in cell viability was triggered by leaf extracts (90%), accompanied by root extracts (22%) and shoot extracts (11%).

*Solanum xanthocarpum*Schrad. &Wendl.

Solanum xanthocarpumSchrad. & Wendl., (Solanaceae), yellow-berried nightshade, is a nontoxic weed on roadsides and wastelands. The capacity of different compounds from S. xanthocarpum to induce apoptosis in the human colon carcinoma cell line HCT116 was reviewed and reported on by Bhutani *et al.*, 2010 [106]. Two of the compounds, solamargine and solasonine, were strongly cytotoxic. Moreover, no induction of ccCK18 was observed at cytotoxic doses of 4–10 mM. Therefore, cell death at elevated doses was not due to apoptosis induction but also to necrosis. Diosgenin and solasodine compounds were weakly cytotoxic (70-80% cell viability at 50 mM), and these compounds triggered 2-fold background levels of ccCK18 [106]. The acetone leaf extract treated wells showed 625 g/ml as the effective drug concentration and were nontoxic to Vero cells; however, they caused more than 50% cytotoxicity to HEp-2 cells [107].

Solanum xanthocarpum (Sx) leaf extract was used to synthesize gold nanoparticles (AuNPs) by Pengfei *et al.*, 2018 [108], which mediated C666-1 cell line apoptosis. Upon treatment with Sx-AuNPs, there was a decrease in both cell viability and colony formation of C666-1 cells. Significant anticancer ability was shown by the non-polar extracts including hexane, benzene, chloroform, and ethyl acetate, showing 85-91% reduction in the growth of the THP-1 cell line, whereas benzene and chloroform fractions controlled for about 70% cytotoxic activity on the HOP-62 cancer cell line [1]. leaf extract was used to synthesise gold nanoparticles (AuNPs) by Pengfei *et al.* (2018) [108], which mediated C666-1 cell line apoptosis. Upon treatment with Sx-AuNPs, there was a decrease in both cell viability and colony formation in C666-1 cells. Significant anticancer ability was shown by the non-polar extracts, including hexane, benzene, chloroform, and ethyl acetate, showing an 85–91% reduction in the growth of the THP-1 cell line, whereas the benzene and chloroform fractions controlled for about 70% cytotoxic activity on the HOP-62 cancer cell line. Mikania micranthaKnuth. Mikania micrantha Knuth: belonging to the family *Asteraceae*, identified as "mile---minute weed," the decoction of the leaves has been used for the treatment of tumours [109]. Isolated compounds from the aerial parts of Mikania micrantha and Mikania cordifolia were guaianolide, 8-epi-mikanokryptin, and melampolide, 11H-11,13-dihydromicrantholide, along with established sesquiterpene lactones. In human cancer cell lines, the investigator screened for antiproliferative activity, and they reported modest activity [110]. The n-butanolic extracts of leaves of M. micrantha were used at doses of 250, 500, and 1000 mg/kg/day p.o. to significantly decrease the tumour volume (3.23 0.20 ml and 4.02 0.36 ml), increase the life span (58.81% and 54.37%), and significantly decrease the tumour mass (1.92 0.067 g) as compared with control [109]. Matawali *et al.*, 2016 [111], studied the four extracts from M. micrantha, *viz.*, methanol, ethanol, ethanolic fraction 1, and ethanolic fraction 2, against HL-60 cells. The cell's viability was vigorously reduced even at a lower concentration of 20 g/ml of extracts (*i.e.*, fractions 1 and 2). Different types of human cancer cell lines, K562 and Hela, were used in *in vitro* experiments to evaluate the anti-tumor effect of aqueous extracts. The study found that when administered with an aqueous extract at 20 mg/ml after 48 h, the growth of K562 and Hela was improved. However, the other concentrations, such as 50, 100, 200, and 400 mg/mL, prevented all forms of cells from proliferating. The IC50 values for K562 and Hela were found to be 167.16 and 196.27 mg/ml at 48 h and 98.07 and 131.56 mg/ml at 72 h, respectively [112]. The LC50 values were revealed at 7.51 l/ml in an experiment by Sabreena *et al.*, 2019 [113] on the cytotoxic activity assay of the plant extract, while the positive control revealed 124.13 l/ml. Human cervical cancer (Hela) cells were treated with methanol extracts of Mikania micrantha, Allium hookeri, Eryngium foetidium, and Alpinia galangal, which showed increased cytotoxic effects with higher concentrations. Their IC50 values were, respectively, 49.02, 138.5, 199.7, and 209.4 g/ml. The leaves' anticancer activity was linked to their flavonoid material [114]. Essential oil is mainly obtained from the M. micrantha flower as sesquiterpene hydrocarbons made of isolédene, -cadinene, debromofiliformin, trans-caryophyllene, -bisabolene, germacrene-D, and zingiberene. Saikia *et al.*, 2020 [115], measured the cytotoxic effect of essential oil in cervical, ovarian, and pancreatic cell lines. The researcher noted that oil has excellent cytotoxic effects on the cell lines HeLa with an IC50 of 5.44 1.33 g/ml and PA1 with an IC50 of 10.57 1.44 g/ml.

Scoparia Dulcis linn

Scoparia dulcis linn.Plantaginaceae family, a sweet broom weed. A cytotoxic study by Abu Hasanat *et al.*, 2011 [116], of ethanolic extracts on brine shrimp lethality bioassay, showed the LC_{50} value at 40.39 µg/ml. Sung Le *et al.*, 2019 [117], reported the *in vitro* antioxidant, HepG2 and A549 growth inhibitory effect of the ethanol extracts. The rutin and rosmarinic acid were newly identified from the *Scoparia Dulcis*. The extract could induce HepG2, and A549 growth inhibition with IC_{50} at 553.32 ± 14.46 µg/ml and 446.35± 0.9 µg/ml at 48 h, respectively. The cytotoxic activity of the glutinol obtained from the fraction of petroleum ether and crude extracts of *Scoparia dulcis* was carried out by Monira *et al.* 2014 [118]. The isolated compounds glutinol had to possess the cytotoxic ED50 values of ranged from 140.91 to 215.44 µM whereas, the crude extracts showed 17.13 to 92.03% cell mortality at 500 µg/ml on the tested cell lines.

Scopadulciol, a scopadulan variety diterpenoid, was isolated and the cytotoxic activity effect on human AGS gastric adenocarcinoma cells showed that compound-treated AGS cells exhibited reduced β-catenin levels, impaired their nuclear localization and also suppressed TOP activity in AGS cells and decreased cyclin D1 and c-Myc protein levels [119]. The identified active constituents examined for cytotoxicity towards four cancers and two kidney cell lines were established by Nur-e-Alam *et al.*, in 2020 [120]. Scopadulciol, 4-epi-scopadulcic acid B, and dulcidiol were shown to have major cytotoxicity on cancer cell lines with IC_{50} values of 3.8 to 42.3 μM accompanied by 5-demethylnobiletin with values of IC_{50}: 30.9 to >64.4 μM). The effects of tumor promoter 12--tetradecanoylphorbol-13-acetate (TPA) were blocked by scopadulcic acid B, a tetracyclic diterpenoid, in both *in vitro* and *in vivo* trials. The intensity was showed to be greater than that of other natural antitumor-promoting terpenoids, such as glycyrrhetinic acid [121].

Achyranthes aspera linn

A roadside weed is *Achyranthes aspera linn.* (*Amaranthaceae*).Significant inhibitory effects of the methanol extract and its alkaloid, non-alkaloid, and saponin fractions were seen at a dose level of 100 g on the early activation of the Epstein-Barr virus antigen caused by the carcinogen 12-Otetradecanoylphorbo--13-acetate in Raji cells. The non-alkaloid fraction, consisting of predominantly non-polar compounds, displayed the most important inhibitory behaviour in the *in vitro* analysis. The methanol extract had a high cytotoxic effect in the *in vivo* mouse skin carcinogenesis test [122]. The anticancer efficiency of an ether extract of A. aspera was evaluated in Swiss albino mice treated with mineral oil to induce cancer. After 15 days of treatment (3 mg/ml), it was found that none of the mice had the symptoms of cancer [123].

The research aimed to thoroughly understand the anti-proliferative effects of methanol-extracted Achyranthes aspera leaves (LE) against human cancer cells. Pancreatic cancer cells were slightly more susceptible to LE relative to colon, breast, lung, and prostate cancer cells. Preliminary experiments showed that the transcription of metalloproteases (MMP inhibitors) and angiogenic factors were selectively inhibited by LE [124]. A cytotoxicity test of a leaf methanolic extract of A. aspera on brine shrimp lethality bioassay showed the highest percentage of mortality (90%) at 1250 g/ml and a LC50 value of 50.12 g/ml. This effect can be attributed to due to the presence of primary phytoconstituents like alkaloids, glycosides, cardiac glycosides, flavonoids, tannins, terpenoids, *etc* [125]. Ethyl acetate, acetone, ethanol, and methanol fractions were individually extracted from the powdered leaf, stem, and root biomass. For cytotoxic effects, each extract was evaluated on the HeLa cell line, but the root-acetone extract was found to be more cytotoxic. This extract revealed 11 bands, besides the fact that more than 90% suppression of HeLa cells was shown by the solution obtained from the ninth band (Rf = 0.870.06) [126]. The numerous extracts from wheatgrass, Achyranthes aspera roots, various forms of mushrooms, and a homoeopathic drug, Ruta graveolens (Ruta), were used as CAM treatments by the Arora *et al.*, 2014 [127] for studying their therapeutic potential. The criteria selected for this analysis focused on the antiproliferative and cytotoxic effects of normal and epithelial kidney cells (NRK-52E). The findings showed that, compared to 5-FU, treatment of normal cells with CAM therapies resulted in decreased cell damage. The pharmacological research study by Rishikesh *et al.*, 2013 [128], comprises thrombolytic and cytotoxic activity of Achyranthes aspera methanol extract that revealed considerable cytotoxic impact in the bioassay of brine shrimp lethality and demonstrated LC50 = 3.80 g/ml and LC90 = 7.04 g/ml (after 18 h); LC50 = 3.31 g/ml and LC90 = 6.36 g/ml (after 21 h); LC50 = 2.18 g/ml and LC90 = 6.

Launaeaprocumbens Linn

Launaea procumbens linn. belongs to the family *Asteraceae*, commonly known as jangalibooti, and is found as a weed in India. Rawat *et al.* in 2016 [23] reported phytochemical analysis and cytotoxicity of methanolic extracts of Launaea procumbens towards K562, HeLa, MIA-Pa-Ca-2, and MCF-2 cancer cell lines by SRB assay. Ethyl acetate extract exhibits significant cytotoxic effects towards cell lines of human leukaemia (K562), cervix (HeLa), and breast (MCF-7), and the IC50 values were found to be 25.300.50, 19.800.10, and 36.904.90 g/ml, respectively.

In comparison, for hexane extract, a lower cytotoxic activity of 418 and 48.200.50 g/ml was found for leukaemia (K562) and breast (MCF-7) cancer cell lines, respectively. The findings of the MTT assay revealed that the plant's methanolic extract and methanol and petroleum ether fractions demonstrated additional safety at concentrations of 500 g/ml that have already been proven to be bactericidal [129]. Khan *et al.*, 2016 [130], analysed the antitumor activity of six different Launaea procumbens extracts at different concentrations (10, 100, and 1000 ppm). Amongst them, the methanolic fraction showed maximum suppression of tumours of the crown gall induced by *Agrobacterium tumefaciens*, followed by the butanol fraction. Their findings revealed the presence of bioactive components, which are important for tumour suppression, in the methanolic and butanol fractions. The number of tumours were counted, and their IC50 order was calculated as follows: methanol (13 0.2) > butanol (55 2.3) > water (58 1.6) > chloroform (65 1.9) > hexane (325 5.7) > ethyl acetate (495 6.2), respectively.

Heliotropium indicum linn

Heliotropium indicum linn. (Boraginaceae), known as “Indian heliotrope,” is found as a weed in wasteland. The analysis of methanol extracts of Heliotropium indicum (*Boraginaceae*) on the human cancer cell line (HeLa) showed that the stem and leaf of Heliotropium indicum had a reasonable amount of antitumor efficacy for both extracts; IC50 was obtained as 200 g/ml. While stem extracts demonstrated outstanding behaviour at 200 g/ml up to 64.5%, they were accompanied by leaf extract at 200 g/ml up to 49.67% [131]. In 2016, Chunthorngorn *et al.* [132] studied the cytotoxic effects of Heliotropium indicum extracts on two types of lung cancer cell lines (A549 and NCI-H226). Ethanol extracts showed cytotoxicity primarily against NCI-H226 (IC50 = 51.90 2.35 g/ml), whereas water extracts showed no cytotoxicity against either A549 or NCI-H226 (IC50 > 100 g/ml).

The methanol extracts of the leaf and stem of H. indicum showed considerable activity against the tumour cell lines (HeLa) at concentrations of 200–1000 g/ml. The relative death percentages of leaf extracts were 49.67% and 14.82% at 200 and 400 g/ml, respectively. whereas stem extracts ranged from 64.52% to 16.11% in an inversely dose-dependent manner at 200-1000 g/ml.The IC50 value of leaf and stem extracts was shown to be 200 g/mL [131]. Jitpisute *et al.* (2016) [133] investigated the effects of ethanol extracts on cytotoxic effects on two types of lung cancer cell lines (A549 and NCI-H226), finding that cytotoxicity was mostly against NCI-H226 (IC50 = 51.90 + 2.35 g/ml), while aqueous extracts had no cytotoxic activity on A549 or NCI-H226 (IC50 > 100 g/ml).

Aqueous extract of leaves showed cytotoxicity on MCF-7 cell lines, with 1000 g/ml extract showing the highest inhibition of 84.75% and the lowest percentage of 44.83 at 62.5 g/ml.The inhibition action may be due to the presence of phytochemicals such as alkaloids, flavonoids, and terpenoids. The inhibitory concentration (CTC50) for 50% of cells was determined to be 97.54 g/mL [134]. For cytotoxic testing of dichloromethane extract, the brine shrimp lethality bioassay was employed, and the study found that the number of dead shrimps was just one at concentrations of 10 g/ml and 100 g/ml. Nevertheless, the number of dead shrimps was 23 when the concentration of the measured sample rose to 1000 g/ml, yet only 7 shrimps lived. Therefore, an LD50 of 462 g/ml relative to the reference agent (etoposide) was determined from the data reported above, resulting in an LD50 of 7.46 g/ml [135]. The methanol extract of the dried roots showed lethality against the brine shrimp nauplii. It showed LC50 and LC90 were deduced to be 47.86 g/ml and 75.85 g/ml, respectively. The most prominent cytotoxicity in Artemia salina brine shrimp was developed by the crude extract (LC50 = 47.86 g/ml and LC90 = 75.85 g/ml) [136]. The extract fractions (aqueous, chloroform, and hexane) of Solanum nigrum, Phyllanthus amarus, and Heliotropium indicum have been tested against three cervical cancer cell lines: HeLa (HPV-18 positive), SiHa (HPV-16 positive), and C33A (HPV negative). The determined IC50 doses were discovered to be non-toxic to the normal mouse embryonic cell line NIH3T3.However, the fractions that showed anti-proliferative activity at low dose level were considered effective. Among the medicinal plant The chloroform fractions of Solanum nigrum, Phyllanthus amarus, and both the chloroform and hexane fractions of Heliotropium indicum were found to be most efficient in inhibiting cell growth and inducing apoptosis [137]. An extract of ethanol from the whole plant of H. indicum exhibited notable anti-proliferative activity on the cell line of SK-BR-3, a human breast adenocarcinoma. In comparison with the standard drug used, the IC50 value of the extract was found to be 34 9.09 g/ml, while paclitaxel had an IC50 value of 22.20 2.30 g/ml [138].

Ipomoea carnea Jacq

Ipomoea carnea Jacq.(*Convulvulaceae*), common weeds in India have been identified and confirmed as a poisonous plant [139]. Sivajothi *et al.*, 2015 [24] conducted the anticancer activity of Monochoria Vaginalis, Ipomea Carnia, and NardostachysJatamansi against HeLa cells. At varying concentrations of 200-1000 µg/ml, the cytotoxicity demonstrated acceptable activity at 200 µg/ml. For the four plants chosen, namely, *Dovyaliscaffra*, *Gingko biloba*, *Ipomoea carnea*, and *Lonchocarpus*, the methanol extracts had remarkable cytotoxicity (about 75%) on MCF-7, HCT-116, HepG2, and A-549 cell lines, respectively. The LC_{50} ranged in breast, colon, liver, and lung, respectively, from 11 to 37.3, 9.7 to 25.7, 12.6 to 43.3, and 15.5 to 31.9. To measure their SI values, these four plant extracts were additionally exposed to the human standard cell line (BJ-1). In contrast to the existing cell lines, the extracts of Ginkgo biloba leaves, *Ipomoea carnea* leaves, and Lonchocarpusspeciosus bark displayed comparatively high cytotoxic specificity (SI= 3.9, 3, and 3.9, respectively) on colon cancer cells [140].

The cytotoxicity activity of methanolic leaf extracts showed an IC50 value of 1 mg/ml. The cytotoxic activity was higher for Ipomoea extracts as compared to Alternanthera extracts [141]. Considerable toxicity was found in the different leaf fractions of Ipomoea carnea, *viz.*, hexane (LC50: 141.4 g/ml), chloroform (LC50: 211.28 g/ml), and ethyl acetate (LC50: 307.28 g/ml), and the positive control demonstrated the LC50 value was less than 100 g/ml on the bioassay of brine shrimp lethality [100]. Ethanol extract of Ipomoea carnea leaves was tested for *in vivo* anticancer activity on mice with Ehrlich ascites carcinoma (EAC), and the results revealed an increased life span, decreased viable cell counts, and increased ascites fluid volume.The extract therapy also reduced the content of nucleic acid and the level of glycoprotein in the tumor-bearing animals [142].

In-vitro anticancer activity of the hydroalcoholic extract exhibited significant cytotoxicity against EAC cell lines at different concentrations of 250 and 500 mg/kg. The criteria analysed were the percentage of cell viability and cytotoxicity, which were compared with untreated cells. Dose-dependent reduction in viability and a rise in cytotoxic effects of hydroalcoholic extract leaves were found in EAC cell lines; however, a substantial reduction in cell viability (p 0.001) was detected for hydroalcoholic extracts at 1000, 500, 250, and 100 g/ml doses [143]. Sharma *et al.*, 2013 [100] proposed that hexane fractions have cytotoxic activity., chloroform, and ethyl acetate of I. carnea with 141.4 g/ml, 211.28 g/ml, and 307.28 g/ml LC50 values, respectively. Swainsonine, an isolated natural alkaloid from I. carnea, was documented in many mouse models of cancer and human carcinomas to exhibit anti-cancer activity. This compound prevents the development of cells by causing apoptosis in the A549 line of human lung cancer cells [144].

Crude water leaf extracts had maximum cytotoxicity against the HepG2 cell line and exhibited a maximum inhibitory effect on the A549 cell line. I. cairica was the largest growth inhibitor (GI50 at 30.6 g/mL) for the HepG2 cell line. Considering the A549 cell line, at 80 g/ml, the extracts exhibited GI50 suppression [145]. The greatest free radical scavenging effect (IC50 of 61.22 g/ml) was expressed by the ethanol-chloroform root extract, whereas 94.64% of the extracts demonstrated cytotoxic effects on the brine shrimp lethality assay. In 2019, Waqaret al [146]. published a study on ethanolic leaf extract, and the results demonstrated remarkable behaviour on the THP-1 cell line with an IC50 of 8 0.05 g/ml and a protein kinase line (31 mm phenotype bald zone).

Alternanthera sessilis Linn

Alternanthera sessilis linn. is an *Amaranthaceae* weed.It is popularly known as water amaranth. The cytotoxicity of A. sessilis plant parts on HT-29 and 3T3 cell lines was investigated at concentrations of 25–500 g/ml for 24, 48, and 72 h. The cytotoxicity of aerial and leaf extracts of A. sessilis (IC50 200 g/mL) was better than stem extract (IC50 > 500 g/mL) on the HT-29 cell line. When tested against normal fibroblast cell 3T3, the extracts exhibited selective cytotoxicity, indicating that all extracts of A. sessilis plant parts were nontoxic to 3T3 with IC50 > 500 g/mL.HT-29 cells responded to the cytotoxic effects in a dose- and time-dependent fashion [147]. Various concentrations of Alternanthera sessilis and Alternanthera philoxeroides crude ethanolic leaf extracts were investigated for their anticancer effect on the human osteosarcoma cell line, MG63. The extract of Alternanthera philoxeroides demonstrated substantial antiproliferative activity relative to Alternanthera sessilis. Maximum inhibition of 67.37% was recorded for Alternanthera philoxeroides and 47.7% for Alternanthera sessilis at 300 g/ml [25].

The use of a water extract of Alternanthera sessilis (1-15 mg/ml) for 24 h incubation significantly reduced cell viability in HeLa cells with increased AuNP concentrations [148].The synthesised nanosilver using Alternanthera sessilis was analysed at various concentrations (1.56, 3.12, 6.25, 12.5, and 25 l/ml) for its cytotoxicity on prostate cancer cells (PC3). At the maximum concentrations (12.5 and 25 l/ml) of AgNPs compared to placebo, a decrease in the number of PC3 cancer cells was observed. Compared to silver ions (14.62 g/ml), the IC50 value of AgNPs was identified at 6.85 g/ml. The findings indicated that the nanosilver-assisted Alternanthera sessilis could exert its cytotoxicity against prostate cancer cells through an apoptosis-dependent mechanism [149].

In a research work conducted by Sherine *et al.*, 2010 [150], 44 specific extracts of medicinal plants were tested for cytotoxic effects on the PANC-1, a pancreatic adenocarcinoma cell line. A further two pancreatic carcinoma cell lines, including Mia Paca-2 and Capan-1, and a fibroblast cell line, Hs68, were tested for the top known cytotoxic extracts. The results indicated that three cancer cell lines with IC50 values ranging from 20.3 to 31.4 g/ml, 13.08 to 34.9 g/ml, and 42.8 to 49.8 g/ml had cytotoxic effects in crude extracts of Petunia punctata, Alternanthera sessilis, and Amoorachittagonga, respectively. Besides, it was found that the treatment of PANC-1 cells with Petunia punctata increased the activity of caspase-3, suggesting that the reported cytotoxic effect was regulated by apoptosis. Compared to that of normal cisplatin, the cytotoxic action of biosynthesized silver nanoparticles on the MCF-7 cell line demonstrated significant cytotoxicity with an IC50 value of 3.04 g/ml. However, complete cell depletion (99%) of MCF7 was reported at a maximum level of 25 g/mL [151].

Alternanthera philoxeroides (Mart.) Griseb.

Alternanthera philoxeroides Mart. & Griseb. (*Amaranthaceae*) is an aquatic plant known as alligator weed. The ethanolic leaf extract of A. philoxeroides showed percentage inhibition concentrations of 37.5 g, 75 g, 150 g, and 300 g on the MG-63 cell line. The inhibition concentrations of A. sessilis at 37.5 g, 75 g, 150 g, and 300 g were found to be an extent of 0.58, 0.36, 5.81, 15.2, and 47.71, respectively, on the MG-63 cell line. The IC50 values for A. philoxeroides and A. sessilis were found to be 249.2 and 314, respectively. The antitumor metabolites alternanthin B and N-transferuloyl-3, 5-dimethoxytyramine were extracted from the aerial portions of the plant A. philoxeroides. Cytotoxic activities towards SK-N-SH and HL60 cell lines were demonstrated by pentacyclic triterpene saponins (philoxeroides A–D) extracted from the plant. The 3-O--D-glucuronopyranoside oleanolic acid derived from the plant's n-butyl extract inhibited the Hela and L929 cell lines strongly. From the result of Sunmathi and Sivakumar's 2016 study [25], it was reported that both plant extracts displayed mild cytotoxicity on the MG-63 cell line. Jiang *et al.*, in 2005 [152], examined the cytotoxic effects of Alternanthera philoxeroides on C6/36 cell lines and its impact on the dengue virus. The author's findings revealed that none of the extracts showed apparent cytotoxic effects at diverse concentrations in the cells, except for the overdose at 320 g/mL. Philoxeroides A, B, C, and D, the four new pentacyclic triterpene saponins, were extracted from the aerial sections of Alternanthera philoxeroides and displayed cytotoxic activity towards SK-N-SH and HL60 cell lines [153].

Chromolaena odorata linn

Chromolaena odorata *linn*. (*Asteraceae*), Siam weed (prolific weed).The varieties of flavanone components were isolated from flowers by Suksamrarn et al. 2004 [154]. Among those flavanones, compound 7 (acacetin) demonstrated mild cytotoxic effects with a MIC value of 24.6 M towards human small cell lung cancer (NCI-H187) cells, while compound 8 (luteolin) showed reasonable toxicity on NCI-H187 cells and weekly toxicity on human breast cancer cells with a MIC value of 19.2 and 38.4 M, respectively. From the dichloromethane extract of C. odorata, four active principle components were obtained through bioactive guided fractionation: acacetin, isosakuranetin, kaempferide, and dihydrokaempferide. The preliminary cytotoxic evaluation on the HeLa cell line was the most sensitive to kaempferide (IC50: 16 M), followed by acacetin (174 M), dihydrokaempferide (> 200 M), and isosakuranetin (> 200 M) [155].

The essential oil of triterpene derivatives isolated from the fresh leaves resulted in a significant cytotoxic effect on the HepG2 cancer cell line in a dose-dependent manner, and the IC50 value was determined as 206.7 g/ml. However, the previous study by the researcher on cytotoxic effect revealed a reasonable effect against HeLa, NIH 3T3, and Hep-2 cell lines, and its IC50 values were 60.3, 67.5, and 72.0 g/ml, respectively [156]. The ethanol extract was evaluated on MCF-7, HeLa, and HCT116 tumour cells by Jaganathan *et al.* 2020 [157], which showed maximum growth inhibition at 8, 16, 24, 30, 70, and 100 g/ml concentrations. However, the cytotoxic effect has been observed at a lower concentration of 1.5 g/mL. The EC50 value for cell mortality in the MCF-7 cell line after exposure for 24 h was found to be 91.51 0.43 g/mL. The antiproliferative effect on the lung cancer cell line HeLa showed moderate activity. The EC 50 value for cell mortality in A549 cell lines after exposure to ethanol extract for 24 h was found to be 89.13 0.43 g/ml. Koba *et al.* (2011) [158] performed the cytotoxicity bioassays against the human HaCaT cell line, and the results revealed that there was no toxicity exhibited up to 3000 l/ml of essential oil, which is separated from the weed.

However, the pure commercial -caryophyllene and germacrene D standards appeared to be almost non-toxic (IC50 > 3000 l/ml), demonstrating that the major phytoconstituents played a significant role in total cell viability [158].The findings of the brine shrimp lethality assay revealed that the average LD50 was 2154 and >5000 mg/kg for aqueous and ethanol extracts, respectively, while the LC50 levels were 324 and 392 ppm for aqueous and ethanol extracts, respectively [159]. Acacetin from Chromolaena odorata exhibited mild cytotoxicity for human small cell lung cancer (NCI-H187) cells with a MIC of 24.6 M, whereas luteolin exhibited moderate toxicity for NCI-H187 cells and weekly toxicity for human breast cancer cells with MICs of 19.2 and 38.4 M, respectively [160].

The findings of Adeolu *et al.*, 2016 [161], showed that the concentrations of methanolic leaf extract (100–700 g/ml) alone induced pronounced inhibition against HT29 cell lines after 72 h. However, the effect on the cell line was that of proliferation in the presence of mitogens (VEGF and ET-1), suggesting that mitogens interacted with the effectiveness of the plant extract to induce cell line inhibition.

Cassia tora Linn

Cassia tora linn. (Caesalpinaceae), a weed found during the rainy season. The effect of cytotoxicity on brine shrimp was also observed with the LD50 value less than 100 g/mL, which can be beneficial in the treatment of various cancers and tumours [28]. The hexane extract of leaves and stems was examined for cytotoxic effect on six human cancer cell lines, including breast cancer cells such as BT-549, MDA-MB-468, and MCF-7, and colon cancer cells such as SW48, LoVo, and HT-29. The study results revealed that Cassia tora is a potential source of palmitic acid and exhibits significant cytotoxic activity [162]. Col320 cell line therapy with ANPs covered with *C. tora* leaf extract, when compared to the untreated cells, inhibited the cell viability of cancer cells up to 71.2% at 75 g levels [163]. Methanol, ethyl acetate, and petroleum ether extracts of leaves were tested for antiproliferative activity on HCT15 and HepG2 cell lines. At a concentration of 100 g/ml, all the samples produced a cytotoxic effect, as evidenced by the increased number of dead cells. Extract cytotoxicity was reduced by reducing extract concentrations to 50, 25, and 10 g/ml [164].

The antitumor effect in mice fed low levels (50 mg/kg) of C. tora was associated with high tumour weight and increased concentrations (100 and 200 mg/kg), which were correlated with tumours of lower weight. This proliferation rate was higher than the rates obtained with C. tora therapy at 100 and 50 mg/kg.A high concentration of C. tora [200 mg/kg] raised the levels of tumour necrosis factor-alpha and interleukin-1 beta cytokines substantially (P 0.05) relative to the mice treated with 100 and 50 mg/kg C. tora [165].

Ageratum conyzoides Linn

Ageratum conyzoides linn. (*Asteraceae*) is a weed that has become invasive. The cytotoxicity of the hydroalcoholic extract of Ageratum conyzoides and their pyrrolizidine alkaloids was very close at 500 and 1000 mg/kg, and they could induce toxicity effects after the 90-day treatment [166]. An *in vitro* study by Adebayo *et al.* (2010) [167] on ethanol, petroleum ether, ethyl acetate, butanol, and water extract of A. conyzoids on the cytotoxic activity against A-549, HT-29, SGC-7901, U-251, MDA-MB-231, DU-145, BEL-7402, and P-388 cancer cell lines was studied. The report showed that the ethyl acetate extract demonstrated the highest cytotoxic activity on A-549 and P-388 cancer cells, with IC(50) values of 0.68 and 0.0003 g/ml, respectively. Furthermore, kaempferol was isolated from the ethyl acetate extract. The ethanolic extracts could induce cell death in HeLa cells, as reported by Rahmawati *et al.* 2012 [168]. The smallest concentration, 0.016 mg/ml, showed the lowest death cell percentage, *i.e.*, 23.93%, and the increased concentration of 2 mg/ml increased the death cell percentage to 57.06%. The LC50 value of 855 g/mL obtained was the sample concentration that could kill 50% of HeLa cell lines.

The crude methanolic stems extract on a cytotoxic study by brine shrimp lethality bioassay exhibited promising LC 50 value 1.32μg/ml, comparing with the LC 50 (0.689μg/ml) values of vincristine sulphate [169]. The cytotoxicity of crude extracts and fractions of A. conyzoides hydroethanolic leaf extracts was tested on all four cell lines: leukemic (Jurkat), prostate cancer (LNCap), breast cancer (MCF-7) and normal human prostate (PNT2).The leaf, flower, and whole plant extracts were slightly cytotoxic (p 0.0001) at the concentration range of 0-1000 g/ml compared to curcumin, 0-100 g/ml [170].

***Solanum mauritianum*Scop.**

Bugweed is *Solanum mauritianum* Scop. (Solanaceae).A research study carried out by Jayakumar and Murugan in 2017 [171] revealed that the solasodine isolated from this weed was treated on MCF-7 cells, and the results showed varying degrees of cellular damage. Besides, solasodine-treated MCF-7 cells showed a significant decline in the expression of Bcl-2 and Bcl-xL (anti-apoptotic proteins) after 48 h, with an increase in Bax and Bak (pro-apoptotic proteins) expression. The isolated alkaloids caulophyllumine-A and solasodine from S. mauritianum were evaluated for their antiproliferative potential against MCF-7 cells. The development of MCF-7 cell lines was interrupted by both alkaloids, but the most active of them was solasodine, with impressive IC50 values. A study by Chaitanya *et al.* (2016) [3] identified the secondary metabolites from this plant, like alkaloids, phenolics, flavonoids, and saponins. The isolated compound named

CH1 also showed good CTC50 values on A-549 (53.71.7), MCF-7 (64.61.2), and HCT-116 (72.80.6) when compared to standard quercetin.

Cestrum aurantiacum Lindl

Cestrum aurantiacum Lindl., (*Solanaceae*), commonly known as Orange Cestrum, found as an invasive weed. The authors investigated the cytotoxic activity of 70% hydro alcohol, water, ethyl acetate, chloroform, petroleum ether, and saponin rich portions isolated from the aerial parts of *Cestrum aurantiacum* and *Solanum mauritianum*. The cytotoxic effect of saponin portion on MCF-7 and HCT-116 cell lines showed significant action at 212±0.23 µg/ml and 67±1.32 µg/ml on MCF-7 cell lines, and with HCT-116 cell lines showed action at 208±0.34 µg/ml and 308±0.47 µg/ml [30].

Cytisus scoparius Linn

Cytisusscoparius linn. (*Fabaceae*), commonly known as Scotch broom, a non-regulated Class B noxious weed. *In vitro* cytotoxic studies on Vero, A-549, MCF-7, and HCT-116 cell lines were carried out which was compared with reference quercetin. The saponin-rich portions named CH-2 was showed potent anti-cancer action [4].

Erigeron karvinkianus DC

Erigeron karvinkianus DC., (*Asteraceae*), a prominent weed commonly identified as Mexican fleabane. The saponin portion isolated was subjected to *in vitro* cytotoxic screening showed excellent results in *in vitro* antioxidant and cytotoxic effect [31].

Phytolacca dodecandraL'Her

*Phytolacca dodecandra*L'Her., family *Phytolaccaceae*, and *in vitro* cytotoxic experiments were conducted using the Brine shrimp lethality study in favor of *Gymnemasylverstre*, *Phytolacca dodecandra*, *Cynoglossum geometrium*, *Leonotisnepetifolia*, and *Ocimumfilamentosum* plant extracts. The cytotoxic effect of all plant extracts on brine shrimp was higher than that of the normal potassium permanganate. With an LC_{50} of 4.57 µg/ml, *P. dodecandra* leaf extract exhibited the highest cytotoxic effects. *O. filamentosum*, *P. dodecandra*, and *C. geometrium* with LC_{50} values of 28.08, 34.74, and 71.09 µg/ml, respectively, were active on brine shrimps. The existence of alkaloids, terpenes, tannins, phenols, flavonoids, saponins, and glycosides was shown by a phytochemical screening of the plant species [172].

Cytotoxic action of identified mother tincture of homeopathic medicinal products and their ultramolecular dilution (*i.e.* 30C, 200C, 1M, and 10M) towards tumor-derived cell lines of various organs, such as *Sarsaparilla* against ACHN cells, *Ruta graveolens* against COLO-205 and *Phytolacca decandra* against MCF-7 reported by Arora *et al.*, 2013 [173] was, however, evaluated against the normal monkey's kidney (MDCK) cells of Madin-Darby (a non-malignant cell line). In the corresponding cancer cell lines, the mother tincture and ultra-diluted formulations of the three homeopathic drugs had relatively significant effects, causing cytotoxic effects and a reduction in cell proliferation.

An ethanolic extract of Phytolacca decandra was tested for its possible anticancer potential. The cytotoxicity of the drug was tested on both normal and A375 cells. Results revealed that Phytolacca decandra administration, without exhibiting many cytotoxic effects on peripheral mononuclear blood cells, induced a surprising decrease in A375 cell proliferation. In Phytolacca decandra-treated cells, the generation of ROS and DNA damage that rendered the cancer cells vulnerable to apoptosis was found to be increased [174].

Cnicuswallichi DC

Cnicus wallichi DC. (*Asteraceae*) is commonly found as a weed, and an ethyl acetate extract of this weed demonstrated antitumor activity at 175 mg/ml [33].

Achyranthes bidentataBlume

Achyranthes bidentataBlume (*Amaranthaceae*), an ethanolic extract of the leaves, was used to investigate the *in vitro* anticancer activity of various concentrations (10 g/ml to 200 g/ml) against DAL and EAC cell lines. The report on the experiment reveals significant anticancer activity at 200 g/ml for the ethanolic extract. But the alcoholic extract showed a remarkable increase in the percentage of DAL (95.5%) and EAC (96%) cancer dead cells compared to the ethyl acetate extract [175]. The compound ginsenoside Ro specifically inhibited the metastatic dissemination capability of colon cancer cells HT29, including their migration and invasion abilities and their adhesion to human endothelium *via* inhibiting integrin v6, MMP-2, MMP-9, and ERK phosphorylation. Pretreatment of nude mice with oral ginsenoside Ro followed by HT29 intravenous inoculation significantly prevented lung metastasis with downregulation of integrin v6 and no toxicity [176]. Achyranthes bidentata polysaccharides (ABPS) and their anti-tumor effect on LTEP-a-2 cells were investigated by Yang *et al.*, 2018 [177]. LTEP-a-2 cells were treated with various concentrations of ABPS (0, 0.2, 0.4, 0.6, 0.8, and 1 mg/mL) for 48 h. Furthermore, ABPS significantly inhibited the proliferation and induced the apoptosis of LTEP-a-2 cells.

Artemisia nilagiricalinn

Artemisia nilagirica linn. (*Asteraceae*) is locally known as "Indian wormwood." The Artemisia nilagirica and Murrayakoenigii extracts were extracted from ethanol, petroleum ether, and water and evaluated on mouse macrophage RAW 264.7 cells for their cytotoxic activities. By contaminating RAW 264.7 cells with M. smegmatis, an intracellular viability assay was conducted prior to and after the treatment of extracts. Ethanol extracts of M. koenigii leaf extract induced more cytotoxicity (IC50, 20 g/ml), genotoxicity, and apoptosis in the mouse macrophage RAW 264.7 cell line than Artemisia nilagirica [178]. The ethanolic extract was further fractionated into butanol (AR-02), ethyl acetate (AR-03), hexane (AR-04), and water (AR-05) to test their anticancer activity. The cytotoxicity was evaluated against three different human cancer cell lines, including DLD-1, A-549, and MCF-7. The results showed that the cytotoxic effects of AR-03 and AR-04 fractions on tested cells were significant, particularly in colon cancer cell lines (DLD-1).Moreover, the sub-fractions were further studied against the same cell lines along with one more colon cancer cell line, HT-29. The ethyl acetate (AR-03) and hexane (AR-04) fractions were found to be the most potently cytotoxic on all cell lines tested.At 100 g/ml concentrations, more specific cytotoxicity on DLD-1 cancer cell lines was also observed in their sub-fractions [179].

The treatment of methanolic extract has decreased the tumor volume, packed cell volume and viable tumor cell count in a dose-dependent manner while compared to EAC control mice. The median life period in EAC control mice was 22±0.25 days, while the median survival time was marginally increased (24±0.33, 29±0.49, and 31±0.55) with various concentrations of 150 mg/kg, 250 mg/kg, and the reference drug vincristine at 30 mg/kg, respectively [180].

Centella asiatica linn

Centella asiatica *linn.* (Apiaceae) is a weed in rice paddies. The cytotoxic activities of an aqueous extract of leaves were investigated against B16F1, MDA-MB-231, and C6 cell lines, with IC50 values of 698.0, 648.0, and 1000.0 g/ml, respectively [181]. The aqueous leaf extract of Andrographis paniculata and the methanolic leaf extract of Centella asiatica were evaluated against the Hela, MCF-7, DLA, and EAC cancer cell lines and showed significant activity against the tested cancer cell lines [182].

Berberis vulgaris linn

Berberis vulgaris linn. (Berberidaceae), a common barberry, is found as an environmental weed. The research was conducted to examine the cytotoxic effect of ethanol and ethyl acetate extracts of Moroccan Berberis vulgaris and its principal component, berberine, in association with S-nitroso-N-acetyl-penicillamine (SNAP), a donor of nitric oxide (NO), on the MCF-7 cell line. The investigator recorded that ethanol extract has marginal cytotoxicity greater than ethyl acetate, with IC50 = 3.54 μg/ml and 596.71 μg/ml, respectively. However, against normal cells, no cytotoxic activity was found. Furthermore, various concentrations of berberine, when mixed with the NO donor, produced complementary cytotoxicity (IC30) at concentrations varying from 8.40 M to 33.60 M, as confirmed by the resulting combination index values.

The cytotoxic effects of *B. vulgaris* were compared to those of berberine on promastigotes of Leishmania major and Leishmania tropica, and it was discovered that berberine had the highest cytotoxic effect, with CC50 values ranging from 27.3 to 362.6 g/ml, indicating increasing cytotoxicity on murine macrophages [183].The antioxidant activity and cytotoxic effect of Berberis vulgaris fruit extract on the human liver cancer cell line (HepG2) displayed an IC50 of 106.0 10.1 g/ml at a concentration of 5–140 g/ml. The crude extract was able to increase the intracellular protein content in the cell cancer line by one-fourth, in addition to reducing cell proliferation [184].

CONCLUSION

This chapter has importance regarding the medicinal value of the weeds. In the quest and emergence of new pharmacological standards, medicinal plants remain a key source. One of the key assets of the discovery of medicinal plant-based drugs is the presence of ethnopharmacological knowledge that offers perfect opportunities to restrict the enormous range of potential findings to much more interesting candidates. Based on the survey, India has a rich source of weed flora, hence the current chapter provides a platform to expose the phytochemical and biological documentation of these weed flora as an important bio-prospecting tool for drug discovery of novel anticancer leads.

Some plants considered as weeds are not phytochemically and pharmacologically explored in India, yet these weed plants also produce essential secondary metabolites such as alkaloids, glycosides, flavanoids, phenolics, and saponins. The literature report collected from elsewhere showed that the biological screening of the isolated secondary metabolites proved that they are good cytotoxic molecules and found to act through a possible apoptotic mechanism.

In recent years, the anticancer and chemopreventive properties of phytochemicals are attracting interest from oncology researchers due to their low intrinsic toxicity in normal cells but prominent effects in cancerous cells. In this chapter, an attempt has been made to provide a database of weed phytochemicals that are used as cytotoxic substances. This information will be extremely useful to identify a series of additional weed-derived drugs to treat cancer. The report presents the results observed from various research works submitted worldwide with exciting information along with phytoconstituents obtained from these weed flora. However, further research is needed on these weed derived metabolites and the whole weeds in order to make the clinical significance through structural modification, possible mechanisms, *etc.*

Declarations

ABBREVIATIONS USED IN THIS CHAPTER

Table 2. Abbreviation of diverse cancer cell lines used particularly in this chapter

Abbreviation	Full-form	Abbreviation	Full-form
3T3	Mouse fibroblast	IGROV-1	Human ovarian cancer
A375	Human skin malignant melanoma	IM-9	Human B lymphoblast peripheral blood multiple myeloma
A549	Human epithelial lung carcinoma	Jurkat-T	Human T lymphocytes
ACHN	Human kidney renal cell adenocarcinoma	K-562	Human bone marrow chronic myelogenous leukemia
AGS	Human stomach gastric adenocarcinoma	KB	Human HeLa contaminant carcinoma
AML12	Mouse normal liver hepatocyte	L929	Normal fibroblast cell
B16-F1/B16-F10	Mouse skin melanoma	LNCaP	Human prostate carcinoma
Bcl2	Human T lymphocyte peripheral blood acute T cell leukemia	LTEP-A2	Human lung adenocarcinoma
BEL-7402	Human papillomavirus-related endocervical adenocarcinoma	MDCK	Normal dog kidney
BT-549	Human epithelial breast ductal carcinoma	MG-63	Human bone osteosarcoma
MDA-MB-468/ MCF7/MDA MB-231/ SK-BR-3	Human breast metastatic adenocarcinoma	MIA-Paca2/Capan-1	Human epithelial cell pancreatic carcinoma
C-33 A	Human epithelial cervix carcinoma	MOLM-14	Human acute myeloid leukemia

(Table 2) cont.....

Abbreviation	Full-form	Abbreviation	Full-form
C57BL/6	Mouse embryonic stem cell embryo	NB4	Human acute promyelocytic leukemia
C6	Rat glial cell brain glioma	NCI-H187	Human retinoblastoma lung carcinoma
C6/36	Aedes albopictus larva clone	NCI-H226	Human lung squamous cell carcinoma
C666-1	Nasopharyngeal carcinoma	NRK-52E	Rat epithelial kidney cells
CC-1	Normal liver cells of a male Wistar rat	NUGC	Human gastric cancer
ccCK18	caspase cleaved Cytokeratin 18	P388D1	Mouse macrophage lymphoma
CD4+ T/ CD8+ T	Lymphocytes	PA-1	Human ovary teratocarcinoma
CEM/C1	Human T lymphoblast peripheral blood acute lymphoblastic leukemia	PANC-1	Human pancreas epithelioid carcinoma
CHO-K1	Chinese hamster ovary	PC-3	Human prostate adenocarcinoma
COLO 320/ COLO 205/ LS 174T/ SW48/LoVo	Human colorectal adenocarcinoma	PNT2	Human normal prostate epithelial cell
COS-1	Fibroblast-like cell lines derived from monkey kidney tissue	RAW 264.7	Mouse murine macrophage
CT26	Mouse fibroblast colon carcinoma	SF295	Human glioblastoma
CXCR4	C-X-C chemokine receptor type 4	SGC-7901	Human gastric carcenoma
DLA	Dalton's Lymphoma Ascites	SiHa	Human cervix squamous cell carcinoma
DLD-1/ HT-29	Human epithelial colorectal adenocarcinoma	SK-N-SH	Human brain neuroblastoma
DU 145	Human brain carcinoma	T-47D	Human mammary gland ductal carcinoma
EAC	Ehrlich ascites carcinoma	THP-1	Human acute monocytic leukemia
HCT 116/HCT-15	Human colorectal carcinoma	U14	Human cervix carcinoma
HeLa	Human epitheial cervix adenocarcinoma	U-251	Human glioblastoma astrocytoma
Hep G2	Human liver hepatocellular carcinoma	U266B1	Human B lymphocyte peripheral blood myeloma
Hep-2	Human HeLa contaminant carcinoma	U-937	Human myeloid histiocytic lymphoma

(Table 2) cont.....

Abbreviation	Full-form	Abbreviation	Full-form
HL-60	Human peripheral blood acute promyelocytic leukemia	WRL 68	Human HeLa contaminant normal
HONE-1	Human nasopharyngeal carcinoma	PCNA	Proliferating cell nuclear antigen
HOP-62	Human lung carcinoma	PARP	Poly ADP ribose polymerase
Hs68	Human skin fibroblast	MMP	Matrix metaloproteas
Huh-7	Hepatocyte derived cellular carcinoma	LDH	Lactate dehydrogenase

REFERENCES

[1] Shashank K, Abhayp K. Pharmacological Activities Of Some Common Indian Weeds: A Review. Mintage Journal Of Pharmaceutical & Medical Sciences 2014; 3(1): 12-7.

[2] Sekar T, Ayyanar M, Gopalakrishnan M. Medicinal Plants And Herbal Drugs. Curr Sci 2010; 98: 1558-9.

[3] Chaitanya MVNL, Dhanabals P, Duraiswamy B, Dhamodaran P, Sameer V. Isolation Of Weed Dual Topopoisons (I& Ii) From Solanum Mauritianumscop. Indoamerican Journal Pharmaceutical Science 2016; 3(8)

[4] Anushi J, Soumenr AJ, Nitesh J. Evaluation Of In-Vitro Cytotoxic And Antioxidant Activity Of Methanolic Extracts Of *Ipomoea Carnea*and *Alternanthera Sessilis.* Int J Bioassays 2016; 4763-6.

[5] Chaitanya MVNL, Dhanabals P, Jubie S, Pavithra M. Phytochemical, Cytotoxic Investigation And Molecular Docking Studies Of Cytisusscoparius Link For Its Dual Human Topo Poisoning (I& Ii) Activity. Journal Of Harmonized Research In Pharmacy 2016; 5(1): 16-35.

[6] Ghosh P, Das C, Biswas S, *et al.* Phytochemical composition analysis and evaluation of in vitro medicinal properties and cytotoxicity of five wild weeds: A comparative study. F1000 Res 2020; 9: 493. [Version 1; Peer Review: 1 Approved, 2 Approved With Reservations]. [http://dx.doi.org/10.12688/f1000research.22966.1]

[7] Lyndy J. 8 - Cytotoxicity Of African Medicinal Plants Against Normal Animal And Human Cells. Toxicological Survey Of African Medicinal Plants. Elsevier 2014; pp. 181-233.

[8] Choudhari AS, Mandave PC, Deshpande M, Ranjekar P, Prakash O. Phytochemicals in Cancer Treatment: From Preclinical Studies to Clinical Practice. Front Pharmacol 2020; 10: 1614. [http://dx.doi.org/10.3389/fphar.2019.01614] [PMID: 32116665]

[9] Célia C, Thomas E, Isabel PM, Patricia S, Marcol FL. Natural Products As A Source For New Leads In Cancer Research And Treatment. Evidence-Based Complementary And Alternative Medicine. Article Id 2018; 8243680: 2.

[10] Mathiast A, Cristopher L, Reginaa O, Isaac T, Kofib AO, Abigail A. Phytochemical, Antioxidant And Cytotoxicity Of Hydroethanolic Extracts Of *Crotalaria Retusa* L. World J Pharm Res 2016; 5(2): 162-79.

[11] Shah MB, Prajapati MS, Patel JB, Modi K. Leucas aspera: A review. Pharmacogn Rev 2010; 4(7): 85-7. [http://dx.doi.org/10.4103/0973-7847.65330] [PMID: 22228946]

[12] Dash GK. And Abdullah M. S. A Review On *Heliotropium Indicum* L. (Boraginaceae). International Journal Of Pharmaceutical Sciences And Research. 2013; 4(4), 1253-1258. Pranabesh G, Swagata B, Alolika D, Maitrayeeb D, Chandrima D, Chandreyi G, Sirshendu C. Evaluation Of Phytochemical

Constituents And Antioxidant Property Of Leaf Acetone Extracts Of Five Herbaceous Medicinal Weeds. Pharm Sci & Res 2019; 11(8): 2806-13.

[13] Ghosh P, Chatterjee S, Das P, Karmakar S, Mahapatra S. Natural Habitat, Phytochemistry And Pharmacological Properties Of A Medicinal Weed-Cleome Rutidosperma DC.(Cleomaceae): A Comprehensive Review. Int J Pharm Sci Res 2019; 10(4): 1605-12.

[14] Chang YC, Chang FR, Khalil AT, Hsieh PW, Wu YC. Cytotoxic benzophenanthridine and benzylisoquinoline alkaloids from Argemone mexicana. Z Naturforsch C J Biosci 2003; 58(7-8): 521-6.
[http://dx.doi.org/10.1515/znc-2003-7-813] [PMID: 12939038]

[15] Hassan SA, Safara A, Mohamedr R. Study Of The Cytotoxic Effect Of *Calotropisprocera*on Breast Cancer Cell Line T47d *In vitro*: A Traditional Remedy. International Journal Of Scientific Innovations 2019; 7(01): 107-12.

[16] Sanjeeb K, Gaurav K, Loganathan K, Kokativ BR. A review on medicinal properties of lantana camara Linn. Research J Pharm And Tech 2012; 5(6)

[17] Lai YJ, Tai CJ, Wang CW. Anti-Cancer Activity Of Solanum Nigrum (Aesn) Through Suppression Of Mitochondrial Function And Epithelial-Mesenchymal Transition (Emt).Breast Cancer Cells Molecules 2016; 21(5): 553.

[18] Pande Roshani A, Gole Akshata R, Sankpal Rohan V, Jadhav Pallavi B. Waghmode Meghmala S1 And Patil Neha N. Bioactive Potential Of Parthenium Hysterophorus And Cytotoxicity Assay Of Parthenin. International Journal Of Pharmacy And Biological Sciences-IJPBSTM 2019; 9(3): 296-313.

[19] Verma SP, Tripathi VC, Das P. Asparagus racemosus leaf extract inhibits growth of UOK 146 renal cell carcinoma cell line: simultaneous oncogenic PRCCTFE3 fusion transcript inhibition and apoptosis independent cell death. Asian Pac J Cancer Prev 2014; 15(5): 1937-41.
[http://dx.doi.org/10.7314/APJCP.2014.15.5.1937] [PMID: 24716915]

[20] Sheam M, Haque Z, Nain Z. Towards the antimicrobial, therapeutic and invasive properties of Mikania micrantha Knuth: a brief overview. Journal of Advanced Biotechnology and Experimental Therapeutics 2020; 3(2): 92-101.
[http://dx.doi.org/10.5455/jabet.2020.d112]

[21] Nur-e-Alam M, Ahmed S, Yousaf M, Khan SI, Mothana RA, Al-Rehaily AJ. Isolation and characterization of cytotoxic and anti-inflammatory constituents from *Scoparia dulcis* L. J Chem Res 2020; 44(7-8): 381-7.
[http://dx.doi.org/10.1177/1747519819901100]

[22] Gulab CM, Sharmal N, Rajendra PP, Nagendra S. Anti–cancer activity of common herbs in ayurvedic perspective. International Ayurvedic Medical Journal 2017; 5(5)

[23] Rawat P, Saroj LM, Kumar A, Singh TD, Tewari SK, Pal M. Phytochemicals and Cytotoxicity of *Launaea procumbens* on Human Cancer Cell Lines. Pharmacogn Mag 2016; 12(4) (Suppl. 4): S431-5. [PMID: 27761070]

[24] Sivajothi V, Shruthis D, Bhargavic H, Muthukumar A. Evaluation Of In-Vitro Cytotoxicity Of Monochoria Vaginalis, Ipomoea Carnea, Nardostachysjatamansi Extracts On Hela Cells. Res J Pharm Biol Chem Sci 2015; 6: 698-703.

[25] Sunmathi D, Sivakumar R. *In vitro* Cytotoxicity Of Ethanolic Leaf Extract Of *Alternanthera Sessilis*(L.) R.Br. Ex Dc And *Alternanthera Philoxeroides*(Mart.) Griseb Against Human Osteosarcoma Cell Line Mg-63. European Journal Of Biomedical And Pharmaceutical Sciences 2016; 3(3): 416-20.

[26] Pulipati S, Babu S, Devi PBS, Devi GR, Bhanuja M. Pharmacognostic Studies Of Alternanthera Philoxeroides (Mart.) Griseb. J Pharmacogn Phytochem 2015; 4(2): 202-4.

[27] Kavitha V, Johanna R, Syedn BB, Badra S, Mohammeda S. A Neglected Weed With A Wide Spectrum Of Pharmacological Activities Review. Mol Med Rep 2017; 15: 1007-16.

[http://dx.doi.org/10.3892/mmr.2017.6133] [PMID: 28112383]

[28] Ansari A, Bhot M. Evaluation Of Phytochemicals Of *Cassia Tora*linn And Its Cytotoxicity Assay Using Brine Shrimp. International Journal Of Pharmacognosy And Phytochemical Research 2017; 9(4): 587-95.

[29] Kamboj A, Saluja AK. Ageratum conyzoides L.: A review on its phytochemical and pharmacological profile. International Journal of Green Pharmacy 2008; 2(2): 59-68 [http://dx.doi.org/10.4103/0973-8258.41171]

[30] Chaitanyam VNL, Dhanabals P, Pavithra N, Ramasatyanarayanaraju K, Jubie S. Phytochemical Analysis And In-Vitro Antioxidant And Cytotoxic Activity Of Aerial Parts Of *Cestrum Aurantiacum*and *Solanum Mauritianum*(Solanaceae Weeds Of Niligiris). Helix 2015; (3): 683-7.

[31] Chaitanya MVNL. Dhanabal, Jawahars P, Jubie, Prakash J, Unni R. International Journal Of Green And Herbal Chemistry Section B: Herbal Chemistry Molecular Docking Studies, Phytochemical And Cytotoxic Investigation On *Erigeron Karvinkianus*dc As A Dual Topoi& Ii Poisons. International Journal Of Green And Herbal Chemistry 2015; 444: 359-78.

[32] Desta KT, Abd El-Aty AM. Triterpenoid and Saponin Rich *Phytolacca dodecandra* L'Herit (Endod): A Review on Its Phytochemistry and Pharmacological Properties. Mini Rev Med Chem 2021; 21(1): 23-34.
[http://dx.doi.org/10.2174/1389557520666200617110241] [PMID: 32552643]

[33] Vijaylakshmi S, Nanjan MJ, Suresh B. In vitro anti-tumour studies on *Cnicus wallichi* DC. Anc Sci Life 2009; 29(1): 17-9.
[PMID: 22557338]

[34] Zhang M, Zhou ZY, Wang J, *et al.* Phytoecdysteroids from the roots of *Achyranthes bidentata* Blume. Molecules 2012; 17(3): 3324-32.
[http://dx.doi.org/10.3390/molecules17033324] [PMID: 22418932]

[35] Mohanty B, Puri S, Kesavan V. A Review on Therapeutic Potential of Artemisia nilagirica. J Plant Biochem Physiol 2018; 6(1): 205-10.
[http://dx.doi.org/10.4172/2329-9029.1000205]

[36] Rashmi SP, Yogendra P. Pharmacognostic Review And Phytochemical Screening Of *Centella Asiatica* Linn. Journal Of Medicinal Plants Studies 2016; 4(4): 132-5.

[37] Furrianca M, Marysol Alvear Z, Tomás B, Leticia F, Victor S. Luis. Medicinal Value Of The Berberis Genus As Hypoglycemic Agent. Bol Latinoam Caribe Plantas Med Aromat 2015; 14: 423-41.

[38] Amarnath K, Dhanabal J. Agarwali, Seshadry S. Cytotoxicity Induction By Ethanolic Extract Of Acalypha Indica Loaded Casein-Chitosan Microparticles.Human Prostate Cancer Cell Line In vitro. Biomedicine & Preventive Nutrition 2014; pp. 445-50.

[39] Chekuri S, Panjala S, Anupalli RR. Cytotoxic activity of Acalypha indica L. hexane extract on breast cancer cell lines (MCF-7). Journal of Phytopharmacology 2017; 6(5): 264-8.
[http://dx.doi.org/10.31254/phyto.2017.6502]

[40] Rai V, Pai VR, Duwal SR. Triterpenoids with Cytotoxic Potential from the Leaves of Tridax procumbens L. Int J Phytomed 2017; 9(4): 597-604.
[http://dx.doi.org/10.5138/09750185.2109]

[41] Vishnu PP, Srinivasar A. Evaluation Of Anticancer Activity Of *Tridax Procumbens* Leaf Extracts On A549 And Hep G2 Cell Lines. Asian J Pharm Clin Res 2015; 8(3): 129-32.

[42] Omedine K, Cokoua PD, Esperance M, *et al.* Chemical Profile, Cytotoxicity Anti-Radical And Hypolipidemic Activities Of *Tridax Procumbens* Of Benin. Res J Pharm Biol Chem Sci 2015; 6(4): 1441-9.

[43] Lakshmipriya T, Soumya T, Jayasreep R, Kumarp RM. Cytotoxic And Apoptogenic Effects Of A Bioactive Fraction Isolated From The Leaves Of A Traditional Medicinal Plant Tridax Procumbens.

Int J Pharm Sci Res 2019; 10(11): 5075-86.

[44] Ikpefane O, Fajana A, Olowojobaj I. Cytotoxic And Growth Inhibitory Effects Of The Methanol Extract Of *Tridax Procumbens* Linn (Asteraceae). J Pharmacogn Phytochem 2013; 1(2): 26-32.

[45] Samuel ES, Akinolat J, Tosh D, Odunolao A. The Antioxidant And Cytotoxic Properties Of Tridax Procumbens Leaf Extract On Liver And Pancreatic Cancer Cell Lines. The Faseb Journal 2019; 33

[46] Manjamalai A, Kumar MJM, Grace VMB. Essential oil of *Tridax procumbens* L induces apoptosis and suppresses angiogenesis and lung metastasis of the B16F-10 cell line in C57BL/6 mice. Asian Pac J Cancer Prev 2012; 13(11): 5887-95. [http://dx.doi.org/10.7314/APJCP.2012.13.11.5887] [PMID: 23317275]

[47] Uzuegbuu E, Opajobio E, Utalorj E, Elu CO. Onyesomi. Cytotoxicity And Antiplasmodial Activity Of Alkaloid Extracts Prepared From Eight African Medicinal Plants Used In Nigeria. Thaiphesatchasan 2020; 44(4): 237-44.

[48] Choppavarapu H, Kasturi K. *In vitro* Anticancer Activity Of Small Peptides From Tridax Procumbens. Int J Biosci 2018; 3(13): 180-4.

[49] Jayanthi MK, Shabeenab N, Ramith R. Evaluation Of Anticancer Activity Of Ethanol Extract Of *Leucas Aspera* Flower. International Journal Of Green Pharmacy 2020; 14(3): 126.

[50] Rahman MA, Islam MS. Antioxidant, antibacterial and cytotoxic effects of the phytochemicals of whole *Leucas aspera* extract. Asian Pac J Trop Biomed 2013; 3(4): 273-9. [http://dx.doi.org/10.1016/S2221-1691(13)60062-3] [PMID: 23620850]

[51] Alam MS, Saha S, Lee DU. Antibacterial and *In vivo* cytotoxic activities of the leaves of Leucas aspera. J Korean Soc Appl Biol Chem 2014; 57(5): 551-4. [http://dx.doi.org/10.1007/s13765-014-4202-1]

[52] Prabha SB, Rao M, Kumar MRR. Evaluation of *in vitro* Antioxidant, Antibacterial and Anticancer activities of leaf extracts of *Cleome rutidosperma*. Research Journal of Pharmacy and Technology 2017; 10(8): 2492-6. [http://dx.doi.org/10.5958/0974-360X.2017.00440.1]

[53] Pranabesh G, Swagata B, Alolika D, *et al.* Evaluation Of Phytochemical Constituents And Antioxidant Property Of Leaf Acetone Extracts Of Five Herbaceous Medicinal Weeds. Pharm Sci & Res 2019; 11(8): 2806-13.

[54] Birendran K, Tanushree S, Tapank M, *et al.* Evaluation Of Anticancer Activity Of Methanol Extract Of *Commelinabenghalensis*linn, Against Ehrlich Ascites Carcinoma In Albino Mice. International Journal Of Green Pharmacy 2018; 12(1): S160.

[55] Riffat B, Ejaz A. Javedi, Hina S, Benny K.H.T, Saira T, Tariq M. *In vitro* Antioxidant And Anti-Cancer Activities And Phytochemical Analysis Of *Commelinabenghalensis*l. Root Extracts. Asian Pac J Trop Biomed 2020; 10(9): 417-25. [http://dx.doi.org/10.4103/2221-1691.290133]

[56] Kgomotso WL, Matlou PM, Victor PB, *et al.* Leseilane M. Semi-Purified Extracts Of Commelinabenghalensis(Commelinaceae) Induce Apoptosis And Cell Cycle Arrest In Jurkat-T Cells. Bmc Complementary And Alternative Medicine 14-65.

[57] Chowdhury TA, Hasanat A, Jakaria M, *et al.* Thrombolytic and cytotoxic activity of methanolic extract of *Commelina benghalensis* (Family: Commelinaceae) Leaves. Journal of Scientific and Innovative Research 2015; 4(2): 100-4. [http://dx.doi.org/10.31254/jsir.2015.4210]

[58] Vusi G. Mbazima, Matlou P, Mokgotho, Faghri F, Jasper R.G, Leseilane J, Mampuru. Alteration Of Bax-To-Bcl-2 Ratio Modulates The Anticancer Activity Of Methanolic Extract Of *Commelinabenghalensis*(Commelinaceae) In Jurkat T Cells. Afr J Biotechnol 2008; 7(20): 3569-76.

[59] Proma RO, Hosnej S, Tanzim K, Sadmans BRPD. A Comprehensive Review On *Commelina benghalensis*l (Commelinaceae). International Journal Of Pharmacognosy 2018; 5(10): 637-45.

[60] Anitha P, Geegi PG, Yogeswari J, Anthonis A. *In vitro* Anticancer Activity Of Ethanolic Extract Of Euphorbia Hirta(L). Science, Technology And Arts Research Journal 2014; 3(1): 01.

[61] Bayala B, Zohoncon TM, Djigma FW, *et al.* Antioxidant and antiproliferative activities on prostate and cervical cultured cancer cells of five medicinal plant extracts from Burkina Faso. Int J Biol Chem Sci 2020; 14(3): 652-63.
[http://dx.doi.org/10.4314/ijbcs.v14i3.1]

[62] Yuet PK, Tamio S. Darahi, Faisalm SAL, Cherne O, Yeng C, Subramanion L, Jothy, Jagat R, Kanwar, Sreenivasan S. Evaluation Of The Cytotoxicity Cell-Cycle Arrest And Apoptotic Induction By Euphorbia Hirtain Mcf-7 Breast Cancer Cells. Pharm Boil 2016; 54(7): 1223-36.

[63] Raja SR, Dineshm G, Jayalakshmi ET. An *In vitro* Study Of Cytotoxic Activity Of *Euphorbia Hirta*on Hep2 Cells Of Human Epithelioma Of Larynx. Int J Pharm Pharm Sci 2011; 3(3): 101103.

[64] Brindha D, Saroja S, Jeyanthi GP. Protective Potencial of Euphorbia hirta Against Cytotoxicity-Induced in Hepatocytes and a Hepg2 Cell Line. J Basic Clin Physiol Pharmacol 2010; 21(4): 401-13.
[http://dx.doi.org/10.1515/JBCPP.2010.21.4.401] [PMID: 21305854]

[65] Ghosh P, Das C, Biswas S, *et al.* Phytochemical composition analysis and evaluation of in vitro medicinal properties and cytotoxicity of five wild weeds: A comparative study. F1000 Res 2020; 9: 493. [Version 1; Peer Review: 1 Approved, 2 Approved With Reservations].
[http://dx.doi.org/10.12688/f1000research.22966.1]

[66] D P, Mm S, A R. Anticancer Activity Of *Argemone Mexicana*l (Flowers) Against Human Liver Cancer (Hepg2) Cell Line. Asian J Pharm Clin Res 2017; 10(10): 351-3.
[http://dx.doi.org/10.22159/ajpcr.2017.v10i10.20744]

[67] Chang YC, Chang FR, Khalil AT, Hsieh PW, Wu YC. Cytotoxic benzophenanthridine and benzylisoquinoline alkaloids from Argemone mexicana. Z Naturforsch C J Biosci 2003; 58(7-8): 521-6.
[http://dx.doi.org/10.1515/znc-2003-7-813] [PMID: 12939038]

[68] Kiranmayi G, Ramakrishnani G, Kothai R, Jaykar B. *In vitro* Anti-Cancer Of Methanolic Extract Of Leaves Of *Argemone Mexicana*linn. Int J Pharm Tech Res 2011; 13(3): 1329-33.

[69] More N, Kharat A. Antifungal and Anticancer Potential of *Argemone mexicana* L. Medicines (Basel) 2016; 3(4): 28.
[http://dx.doi.org/10.3390/medicines3040028] [PMID: 28930138]

[70] Nirmala S, Nadana Sabapathi P, Sudhakar M. Naveen Bathula, Sravanthi Y. Investigation Of *In vitro* Anti-Cancer Property Of Adhatoda Vasica In Hela, Hepg2, MCF-7, MDAMB-231 Cell Lines. Res J Pharmacognosy And Phytochem 2019; 11(4): 212-6.

[71] Balachandran C, Arun Y. Sangeetha, Duraipandiyan V, Awale S, Emi N, Ignacimuthu S, Perumal P.T. In-Vitro And In-Vivo Anticancer Activity Of 2-Acetyl-Benzylamine Isolated From *Adhatodavasica*l. Leaves. Biomed Pharmacother 2017; 93: 796-806.
[http://dx.doi.org/10.1016/j.biopha.2017.06.096] [PMID: 28715864]

[72] Hassans A, Mohamed M, Jamal S, Kulvinders S, Walieda M, Mohamed R. Rizgallah. Anticancer And Antibacterial Activity Of *Calotropisprocera*leaf Extract. J Basic Appl Sci Res 2017; 7(12): 18-25.

[73] Smit HF, Woerdenbag HJ, Singh RH, Meulenbeld GJ, Labadie RP, Zwaving JH. Āyurvedic herbal drugs with possible cytostatic activity. J Ethnopharmacol 1995; 47(2): 75-84.
[http://dx.doi.org/10.1016/0378-8741(95)01255-C] [PMID: 7500639]

[74] Van Quaquebeke E, Simon G, André A, *et al.* Identification of a novel cardenolide (2''-oxovoruscharin) from *Calotropis procera* and the hemisynthesis of novel derivatives displaying potent *in vitro* antitumor activities and high *in vivo* tolerance: structure-activity relationship analyses. J Med

Chem 2005; 48(3): 849-56.
[http://dx.doi.org/10.1021/jm049405a] [PMID: 15689169]

[75] Surajs K, Padma C. Brine Shrimp Cytotoxic Activity Of 50% Aqueous Ethanolic Leaf Extract Of *Calotropisprocera*r. *Br.* Asian J Pharm Clin Res 2015; 8(8): 215-7.

[76] Choedon T, Mathan G, Arya S, Kumar VL, Kumar V. Anticancer and cytotoxic properties of the latex of *Calotropis procera* in a transgenic mouse model of hepatocellular carcinoma. World J Gastroenterol 2006; 12(16): 2517-22.
[http://dx.doi.org/10.3748/wjg.v12.i16.2517] [PMID: 16688796]

[77] Mathur R, Gupta SK, Mathur SR, Velpandian T. Anti-tumor studies with extracts of Calotropis procera (Ait.) R.Br. root employing Hep2 cells and their possible mechanism of action. Indian J Exp Biol 2009; 47(5): 343-8.
[PMID: 19579799]

[78] Madhulika B. Anticancer Activity Of Arka (Calotropis Procera) On HCT-15 Cancer Cell Line. International Journal Of Medical Sciences 2010; 2(2): 152-4.

[79] Al-Qahtani M, Farahm A, Abou-Tarbousf M, Al-Anazik M, Al-Harbin O, Alim A. Q. Hailanw A. Anticancer Effects Of *Calotropisprocera*latex Extract In Mcf-7 Breast Cancer Cells. Pharmacogn Mag 2020; 16: 550-6.
[http://dx.doi.org/10.4103/pm.pm_156_20]

[80] Ghosh S, Das Sarma M, Patra A, Hazra B. Anti-inflammatory and anticancer compounds isolated from *Ventilago madraspatana* Gaertn., *Rubia cordifolia* Linn. and *Lantana camara* Linn. J Pharm Pharmacol 2010; 62(9): 1158-66.
[http://dx.doi.org/10.1111/j.2042-7158.2010.01151.x] [PMID: 20796195]

[81] Sanjeeb K, Gaurav K, Loganathan K, Kokativ BR. A review on medicinal properties of lantana camara linn. Research J Pharm And Tech 2012; 5(6)

[82] Raghuc Ashok G. *In vitro* Cytotoxic Activity Of *Lantana Camara* Linn. Indian J Pharmacol 2004; 36(2): 93-5.

[83] P PS, T KS. Antioxidant, antibacterial and cytotoxic potential of silver nanoparticles synthesized using terpenes rich extract of *Lantana camara* L. leaves. Biochem Biophys Rep 2017; 10: 76-81.
[http://dx.doi.org/10.1016/j.bbrep.2017.03.002] [PMID: 29114571]

[84] Lai YJ, Tai CJ, Wang CW. Anti-Cancer Activity Of Solanum Nigrum (Aesn) Through Suppression Of Mitochondrial Function And Epithelial-Mesenchymal Transition (Emt). Breast Cancer Cells Molecules 2016; 21(5): 553.

[85] Shirkavand A, Boroujeni ZN, Aleyasin SA. *Solanum nigrum* Anticancer Effect Through Epigenetic Modulations in Breast Cancer Cell Lines. Curr Cancer Ther Rev 2020; 16(2): 121-6.
[http://dx.doi.org/10.2174/1573394715666190101114541]

[86] Ling B, Xiao S, Yang J, Wei Y, Sakharkar MK, Yang J. Probing the Antitumor Mechanism of *Solanum nigrum* L. Aqueous Extract against Human Breast Cancer MCF7 Cells. Bioengineering (Basel) 2019; 6(4): 112.
[http://dx.doi.org/10.3390/bioengineering6040112] [PMID: 31835887]

[87] Shokrzadeh M, Azadbakht M, Ahangar N, Hashemi A, Saravi SSS. Cytotoxicity of hydro-alcoholic extracts of Cucurbita pepo and *Solanum nigrum* on HepG2 and CT26 cancer cell lines. Pharmacogn Mag 2010; 6(23): 176-9.
[http://dx.doi.org/10.4103/0973-1296.66931] [PMID: 20931075]

[88] Ehssanh O. Moglad, Omer A.M, Kokow S, Saadabia M. *In vitro* Anticancer Activity And Cytotoxicity Of *Solanum Nigrum* On Cancers And Normal Cell Lines. International Journal Of Cancer Research 2014; 10(2): 74-80.
[http://dx.doi.org/10.3923/ijcr.2014.74.80]

[89] Ji YB, Gao SY, Ji CF, Zou X. Induction of apoptosis in HepG2 cells by solanine and Bcl-2 protein. J Ethnopharmacol 2008; 115(2): 194-202. [http://dx.doi.org/10.1016/j.jep.2007.09.023] [PMID: 18022776]

[90] Lee SJ, Oh PS, Ko JH, Lim K, Lim KT. A 150-kDa glycoprotein isolated from *Solanum nigrum* L. has cytotoxic and apoptotic effects by inhibiting the effects of protein kinase C alpha, nuclear factor-kappa B and inducible nitric oxide in HCT-116 cells. Cancer Chemother Pharmacol 2004; 54(6): 562-72. [http://dx.doi.org/10.1007/s00280-004-0850-x] [PMID: 15349752]

[91] Son YO, Kim J, Lim JC, Chung Y, Chung GH, Lee JC. Ripe fruits of Solanum nigrum L. inhibits cell growth and induces apoptosis in MCF-7 cells. Food Chem Toxicol 2003; 41(10): 1421-8. [http://dx.doi.org/10.1016/S0278-6915(03)00161-3] [PMID: 12909277]

[92] Li J, Li Q, Feng T, Li K. Aqueous extract of *Solanum nigrum* inhibit growth of cervical carcinoma (U14) *via* modulating immune response of tumor bearing mice and inducing apoptosis of tumor cells. Fitoterapia 2008; 79(7-8): 548-56. [http://dx.doi.org/10.1016/j.fitote.2008.06.010] [PMID: 18687388]

[93] Oh PS, Lim KT. HeLa cells treated with phytoglycoprotein (150 kDa) were killed by activation of caspase 3 via inhibitory activities of NF-κB and AP-1. J Biomed Sci 2007; 14(2): 223-32. [http://dx.doi.org/10.1007/s11373-006-9140-4] [PMID: 17192825]

[94] Gabrani R, Jain R, Sharma A, Sarethy I, Dang S, Gupta S. Antiproliferative effect of *Solanum nigrum* on human leukemic cell lines. Indian J Pharm Sci 2012; 74(5): 451-3. [http://dx.doi.org/10.4103/0250-474X.108421] [PMID: 23716874]

[95] El Hawary SM, Rabab Z. Samehr, Mostafa S, Ahmed. Cytotoxicity Of *Solanum Nigrum* L Green Fruits On Breast (Mcf-7) And Liver (Hepg-2) Cancer Cell Lines. Pharma Innovation Journal 2015; 87: 87-9.

[96] Patels S, Gheewala N, Suthar A, Shah A. In-Vitro Cytotoxicity Activity Of *Solanum Nigrum* Extracts Againsthela Cell Lines And Vero Cell Lines. Int J Pharm Pharm Sci 2009; 1(1): 38-46.

[97] Wang W, Lu DP. [An *in vitro* study of cytotoxic and antineoplastic effect of *Solanum nigrum* L extract on U266]. Beijing Da Xue Xue Bao 2005; 37(3): 240-4. [PMID: 15968310]

[98] Bhatia N, Maiti PP, Kumar A, Tuli A, Ara T, Khan MU. Evaluation Of Cardio Protective Activity Of Methanolic Extract Of Solanum Nigrum L. In Rats. International Journal Of Drug Development & Research 2011; 3(3): 139147.

[99] Shashank K, Gousia C, Ajits K, Abhayp K. Article Id 2013; 810734: 11.

[100] Sharma N, Gupta PC, Singh A, Raoc V. Brine Shrimp Bioassay Of Pentapetesphoenicealinn. And *Ipomoea Carnea*jacq. Leaves. Pharm Lett 2013; 5: 162-7.

[101] Shashank K, Sanjay P, Abhayp K. Article Id 2014; 495154: 10.

[102] Sesha Sai Durga M, Satyavathi K, Bhojaraju P, *et al.* Venkatesh Prasad D And Lakshmi Kanta Kanthal. Cytotoxic And Anthelmintic Activities Of Methanolic Extract Of *Parthenium Hysterophorus* L. Pharmacophore 2013; 4(6): 275-9.

[103] Anup R, Sainathr T, Padma S, Sukumaranm K. *In vitro* Cytotoxic Activity Of Methanolic Extract Of *Parthenium Hysterophorus*flowers On Mcf-7 And Hela Cell Lines. Int J Curr Microbiol Appl Sci 2015; 4(8): 710-5.

[104] Raiesh M, Syma A, Malik CP, Ajazg A, Umesh S. *In vitro* Cytotoxicity Of *Parthenium Hysterophorus*extracts Against Human Cancerous Cell Lines. J Chem Pharm Res 2011; 3(6): 601-8.

[105] Ali AB, Paul A. Weston, Saliya G, Sajid L, Steve W, Adkinsl A. Weston Toxic Potential And Metabolic Profiling Of Two Australian Biotype; Ls Of The Invasive Plant Parthenium Weed (*Parthenium Hysterophorus*l). Toxins (Basel) 2020; 12: 447. [http://dx.doi.org/10.3390/toxins12070447] [PMID: 32664345]

[106] Bhutani KK, Paul AT, Fayad W, Linder S. Apoptosis inducing activity of steroidal constituents from *Solanum xanthocarpum* and Asparagus racemosus. Phytomedicine 2010; 17(10): 789-93. [http://dx.doi.org/10.1016/j.phymed.2010.01.017] [PMID: 20176464]

[107] Raja SR, Dneshm G, Jayalakshmig T, Shafeer S, Kansrajh C. Antibacterial, Antifungal And Cytotoxic Studies On Leaf And Seed Extracts Of *Solanum Xanthocarpum*shrad And Wendl. International Journal Of Phytopharmacology 2011; 2(2): 61-5.

[108] Zhang P, Wang P, Yan L, Liu L. Synthesis of gold nanoparticles with *Solanum xanthocarpum* extract and their in vitro anticancer potential on nasopharyngeal carcinoma cells. Int J Nanomedicine 2018; 13: 7047-59. [http://dx.doi.org/10.2147/IJN.S180138] [PMID: 30464458]

[109] Dasgupta D, Dash S, Chakraborty J. Evaluation Of Anticancer Activity Of *Mikania Micrantha* Kunth (Asteraceae) Against Ehrlich Ascites Carcinoma In Swiss Albino Mice. International Journal Of Pharmaceutical Research And Allied Sciences 2014; 2(3): 9-18.

[110] Ríos V E, León A, Chávez MI, *et al.* Sesquiterpene lactones from *Mikania micrantha* and Mikania cordifolia and their cytotoxic and anti-inflammatory evaluation. Fitoterapia 2014; 94: 155-63. [http://dx.doi.org/10.1016/j.fitote.2014.02.006] [PMID: 24565963]

[111] Matawali A, Chin LP, Engh S, Boon LH, Gansauj A. In-Vitro Evaluation Of Anti-Kinase, Anti-Phosphatase And Cytotoxic Activities Of *Mikania Micrantha* H.B.K. (Asteraceae) From Malaysia. J Chem Pharm Sci 2016; 9(2): 696-701.

[112] Dou X, Zhang Y, Sun N, Wu Y, Li L. The anti-tumor activity of *Mikania micrantha* aqueous extract *in vitro* and *in vivo.* Cytotechnology 2014; 66(1): 107-17. [http://dx.doi.org/10.1007/s10616-013-9543-9] [PMID: 23397444]

[113] Sabreenac R, Sadia AM, Mominurr MR, Arifur R. Assessment Of Phytochemical, Cytotoxic, Anthelmintic And Thrombolytic Activity Of *Mikania Micrantha* Leaves: A New Addition In Phytomedicine. Pharmacologyonline 2009; 1: 246-55.

[114] Barbhuiyas MAA, Devis HV. In-Vitro Comparative Anticancer Activity Study Of Methanolic Extract Of Traditionally Used Medicinal Plant Of Mizoram. Int J Pharm Sci Res 2019; 10(7): 3295-9.

[115] Saikia S, Tamuli KJ, Narzary B, Banik D, Bordoloi M. Chemical characterization, antimicrobial activity, and cytotoxic activity of *Mikania micrantha* Kunth flower essential oil from North East India. Chem Pap 2020; 74(8): 2515-28. [http://dx.doi.org/10.1007/s11696-020-01077-6]

[116] Abu HMD. Zulfiker, Masuma S, Laizumann MD, Razibul H, Nizam U, Nahidh MD, Sohel R. Invitro Antibacterial, Antifungal Cytotoxic Activity Of *Scoparia Dulcis* L. Int J Pharm Pharm Sci 2011; 3(2): 198-203.

[117] Sung LE, Horng L, Lay WU, Ming C. Phenolic Composition, In vitro Antioxidant And Anticancer Activities Of Hypericum Japonicum Thunb And Scoparia Dulcis L. Herbal Medicines Journal 2019; 4.

[118] Monira A, Fatemat Z, Sheikh NI. Cytotoxicity Of *Scoparia Dulcis* On Human Cancer Cell Lines. Indian Journal Of Pharmaceutical Science & Research 2014; 4(1): 9-11.

[119] Fuentes RG, Toume K, Arai MA, Sadhu SK, Ahmed F, Ishibashi M. Scopadulciol, Isolated from *Scoparia dulcis*, Induces β-Catenin Degradation and Overcomes Tumor Necrosis Factor-Related Apoptosis Ligand Resistance in AGS Human Gastric Adenocarcinoma Cells. J Nat Prod 2015; 78(4): 864-72. [http://dx.doi.org/10.1021/np500933v] [PMID: 25793965]

[120] Nur-e-Alam M, Ahmed S, Yousaf M, Khan SI, Mothana RA, Al-Rehaily AJ. Isolation and characterization of cytotoxic and anti-inflammatory constituents from *Scoparia dulcis* L. J Chem Res 2020; 44(7-8): 381-7. [http://dx.doi.org/10.1177/1747519819901100]

[121] Nishino H, Hayashi T, Arisawa M, Satomi Y, Iwashima A. Antitumor-promoting activity of scopadulcic acid B, isolated from the medicinal plant Scoparia dulcis L. Oncology 1993; 50(2): 100-3. [http://dx.doi.org/10.1159/000227156] [PMID: 8451033]

[122] Chakraborty A, Brantner A, Mukainaka T, *et al.* Cancer chemopreventive activity of *Achyranthes aspera* leaves on Epstein–Barr virus activation and two-stage mouse skin carcinogenesis. Cancer Lett 2002; 177(1): 1-5.
[http://dx.doi.org/10.1016/S0304-3835(01)00766-2] [PMID: 11809524]

[123] Geetha P, Narayanank R, Murugesana G. Screening The Anti-Cancerous Efficacy Of *Achyranthes Aspera* Linn Using Animal Model Swiss Albino Mice. J Biomed Sci And Res 2010; 2(4): 231-5.

[124] Subbarayan PR, Sarkar M, Impellizzeri S, *et al.* Anti-proliferative and anti-cancer properties of Achyranthes aspera: Specific inhibitory activity against pancreatic cancer cells. J Ethnopharmacol 2010; 131(1): 78-82.
[http://dx.doi.org/10.1016/j.jep.2010.06.002] [PMID: 20541002]

[125] Hossain MJ, Khaleda L, Chowdhury AMMA, Arifuzzaman M, Al-Forkan M. Phytochemical Screening And Evaluation Of Cytotoxicity And Thrombolytic Properties Of Achyranthes Aspera Leaf Extract. J Phar Biol Sci 2013; 6: 30-8.

[126] Omidiani N, Datkhile KD, Barmukh RB. Anticancer potentials of leaf, stem, and root extracts of *Achyranthes aspera* L. Not Sci Biol 2020; 12(3): 546-55.
[http://dx.doi.org/10.15835/nsb12310764]

[127] Arora S, Tandon C, Tandon S. Evaluation of the cytotoxic effects of CAM therapies: an *in vitro* study in normal kidney cell lines. ScientificWorldJournal 2014; 2014: 1-11.
[http://dx.doi.org/10.1155/2014/452892] [PMID: 24672319]

[128] Rishikesh MD, Moshfiqur R, Rashefulg MD, Muhammadr MA, Parbotir D, Abdullaha MMD. Phytochemical And Pharmacological Investigation Of *Achyranthes Aspera* Linn. Sch Acad J Pharm 2013; 2(2): 74-80.

[129] Khomayezian M, Rahimifard N, Mojab F, Bagheri F, Pakzad S. Cytotoxicity Evaluation Of Launaea Procumbens On Two Cell Lines. Research Journal Of Pharmacognosy. 2017; pp. 6-6.

[130] Khan RA, Khan MR, Shah NA, Sahreen S, Elahi SN. Antitumor characterization of various fractions of *Launaea procumbens*. Toxicol Ind Health 2016; 32(1): 188-91.
[http://dx.doi.org/10.1177/0748233713500823] [PMID: 24097358]

[131] Sivajothi V, Shruthis D, Jasmins R. Cytotoxic Effect Of *Heliotropium Indicum* Extracts On Hela Cell Line. Int J Pharma Sci 2015; 7(6): 412-4.

[132] Chunthorng-Orn J, Dechayont B, Phuaklee P, Prajuabjinda O, Juckmeta T, Itharat A. Cytotoxic, Anti-inflammatory and Antioxidant Activities of *Heliotropium indicum* Extracts. J Med Assoc Thai 2016; 99 (Suppl. 4): S102-9.
[PMID: 29919994]

[133] Chunthorng-Orn J, Dechayont B, Phuaklee P, Prajuabjinda O, Juckmeta T, Itharat A. Cytotoxic, Anti-inflammatory and Antioxidant Activities of Heliotropium indicum Extracts. J Med Assoc Thai 2016; 99(4) (Suppl. 4): S102-9.
[PMID: 29919994]

[134] Aswini R, Murugesan S, Murugesh S. Preliminary Phytochemical, Antibacterial And *In vitro* Anticancer Activity Of Methanolic Extracts Of (Leaf And Stem) *Heliotropium Indicum* Linn. World J Pharm Res 2016; 6(1): 524-35.

[135] Khurm M, Chaudhry B, Uzair M, Janbaz K. Antimicrobial, Cytotoxic, Phytotoxic and Antioxidant Potential of Heliotropium strigosum Willd. Medicines (Basel) 2016; 3(3): 20.
[http://dx.doi.org/10.3390/medicines3030020] [PMID: 28930129]

[136] Rahman MA, Miam A. Shahidl I.Z. Pharmacological And Phytochemical Screen Activities Of Roots Of *Heliotropium Indicum* Linn. Pharmacologyonline 2011; 1: 185-92.

[137] Paul S, Chakraborty S, Mukherjee A, Kundu R. Evaluation Of Cytotoxicity And Dna Damaging Activity Of Three Plant Extracts On Cervical Cancer Cell Lines. Int J Pharm Sci Rev Res 2015; 31(1): 183-9.

[138] Moongkarndi P, Kosem N, Luanratana O, Jongsomboonkusol S, Pongpan N. Antiproliferative activity of Thai medicinal plant extracts on human breast adenocarcinoma cell line. Fitoterapia 2004; 75(3-4): 375-7.
[http://dx.doi.org/10.1016/j.fitote.2004.01.010] [PMID: 15158999]

[139] Nguldes L, Tijjanim B, Giwai MN. Sokoto J Vet Sci 2016; 14(1): 1-9.
[http://dx.doi.org/10.4314/sokjvs.v14i1.1]

[140] Sehamm MA, Bassemm M, Gamilaw M, Khaled M, Marwa MM. Screening Of Some Plants In Egypt For Their Cytotoxicity Against Four Human Cancer Cell Lines. Int J Pharm Tech Res 2014; 6(3): 1074-84.

[141] Anushi J, Soumenr AJ, Nitesh J. Evaluation Of In-Vitro Cytotoxic And Antioxidant Activity Of Methanolic Extracts Of *Ipomoea Carnea*and *Alternanthera Sessilis*. Int J Bioassays 2016; 4763-6.

[142] Ramalingam S, Adithiya R A, Joseph A, Saravanan R. Anticancer activity of *Ipomoea carnea* on Ehrlich Ascites Carcinoma bearing mice. Indian Journal of Pharmaceutical Education and Research 2019; 53(4): 703-9.
[http://dx.doi.org/10.5530/ijper.53.4.134]

[143] Anand G, Sumithira G, Chinnar R, Muthukumar A, Vidhya G. *In vitro* And *In vivo* Anticancer Activity Of Hydroalcoholic Extract Of *Ipomoea Carnea*leaf Against Ehrlich Ascites Carcinoma Cell Lines. International Journal Of Advanced Pharmaceutical Genuine Research 2013; 1(1): 39-54.

[144] Li Z, Xu X, Huang Y, *et al.* Swainsonine activates mitochondria-mediated apoptotic pathway in human lung cancer A549 cells and retards the growth of lung cancer xenografts. Int J Biol Sci 2012; 8(3): 394-405.
[http://dx.doi.org/10.7150/ijbs.3882] [PMID: 22393311]

[145] Rane VA, Patelb B. In-Vitro Cytotoxic Activity Of Leaf Extracts Of Ipomoea Jacq. Species Against A 549 And Hep-G2 Cell Lines. Int J Pharm Sci Res 2015; 6(1): 294-9.

[146] Ahmad W, Zahir A, Nadeem M, Zia M, Hano C, Abbasi BH. Thidiazuron-induced efficient biosynthesis of phenolic compounds in callus culture of Ipomoea turbinata Lagasca and Segura. In Vitro Cell Dev Biol Plant 2019; 55(6): 710-9.
[http://dx.doi.org/10.1007/s11627-019-10027-1]

[147] Arulselvan P, Gothai S, Muniandy K, Mohd Esa N, Subbiah SK. Anticancer potential of *Alternanthera sessilis* extract on HT-29 human colon cancer cells. Asian Pac J Trop Biomed 2018; 8(8): 394-402.
[http://dx.doi.org/10.4103/2221-1691.239427]

[148] Qian L, Su W, Wang Y, Dang M, Zhang W, Wang C. Synthesis and characterization of gold nanoparticles from aqueous leaf extract of *Alternanthera sessilis* and its anticancer activity on cervical cancer cells (HeLa). Artif Cells Nanomed Biotechnol 2019; 47(1): 1173-80.
[http://dx.doi.org/10.1080/21691401.2018.1549064] [PMID: 30942109]

[149] Firdhouse MJ, Lalitha P. Biosynthesis of silver nanoparticles using the extract of *Alternanthera sessilis*—antiproliferative effect against prostate cancer cells. Cancer Nanotechnol 2013; 4(6): 137-43.
[http://dx.doi.org/10.1007/s12645-013-0045-4] [PMID: 26069509]

[150] George S, Bhalerao SV, Lidstone EA, *et al.* Cytotoxicity screening of Bangladeshi medicinal plant extracts on pancreatic cancer cells. BMC Complement Altern Med 2010; 10(1): 52.
[http://dx.doi.org/10.1186/1472-6882-10-52] [PMID: 20849608]

[151] M JF, P L. Apoptotic efficacy of biogenic silver nanoparticles on human breast cancer MCF-7 cell lines. Prog Biomater 2015; 4(2-4): 113-21.
[http://dx.doi.org/10.1007/s40204-015-0042-2] [PMID: 26566469]

[152] Jiang WLL, Luo XL, Kuang SJ. [Effects of Alternanthera philoxeroides Griseb against dengue virus in vitro]. J First Mil Med Univ 2005; 25(4): 454-6.
[PMID: 15837655]

[153] Fang JB, Yao Z, Chen JC, Liu YW, Takaishi Y, Duan HQ. Cytotoxic triterpene saponins from *Alternanthera philoxeroides*. J Asian Nat Prod Res 2009; 11(3): 261-6.
[http://dx.doi.org/10.1080/10286020802684656] [PMID: 19408151]

[154] Suksamrarn A, Chotipong A, Suavansri T, *et al.* Antimycobacterial activity and cytotoxicity of flavonoids from the flowers ofChromolaena odorata. Arch Pharm Res 2004; 27(5): 507-11.
[http://dx.doi.org/10.1007/BF02980123] [PMID: 15202555]

[155] Nath LR, Gorantla JN, Joseph SM, *et al.* Kaempferide, the most active among the four flavonoids isolated and characterized from Chromolaena odorata, induces apoptosis in cervical cancer cells while being pharmacologically safe. RSC Advances 2015; 5(122): 100912-22.
[http://dx.doi.org/10.1039/C5RA19199H]

[156] Prabhu V, Ravi S. Isolation of a novel triterpene from the Essential oil of fresh leaves of Chromolaena odorata and its in-vitro cytotoxic activity against HepG2 cancer cell line. J Appl Pharm Sci 2012; 2(9): 132.
[http://dx.doi.org/10.7324/JAPS.2012.2926]

[157] Jaganathan SS. Cytotoxicity Effects On Negative Breast And Colon Cancer Cell Lines Of Chromolaena Odorata. J Adv Compos 2020; 1(13): 223-43.

[158] Koba K, Nénonéné AY, Catherine G, *et al.* Chemical Composition and Cytotoxic Activity of Essential Oil of *Chromolaena odorata* L. Growing in Togo. J Essent Oil-Bear Plants 2011; 14(4): 423-9.
[http://dx.doi.org/10.1080/0972060X.2011.10643597]

[159] Asomugha RN, Ezejiofor AN, Okafor PN, Ijeh II. Acute and Cytotoxicity Studies of Aqueous and Ethanolic Leaf Extracts of *Chromolaena odorata.* Pak J Biol Sci 2014; 18(1): 46-9.
[http://dx.doi.org/10.3923/pjbs.2015.46.49] [PMID: 26353417]

[160] Anupc K, Sujit R, Umeshk P. *Chromolaena Odorata,* An Overview. J Pharm Res 2011; 4(3): 573-6.

[161] Adeolua A, Ademolao A, Olusegunf A, Temidayoo A, Momohy A. Evaluation Of The Anticancer Properties Of The Methanol Leaf Extract Of *Chromolaena Odorata* On Ht-29 Cell Line. J Pharmacogn Phytochem 2016; 5(2): 52-7.

[162] Shipra S. Cytotoxic Activity Of *Cassia Tora*grown In Different Geographical Area. International Conference On Pharmaceutical Chemistry.

[163] Abel EE, John Poonga PR, Panicker SG. Characterization and *in vitro* studies on anticancer, antioxidant activity against colon cancer cell line of gold nanoparticles capped with *Cassia tora* SM leaf extract. Appl Nanosci 2016; 6(1): 121-9.
[http://dx.doi.org/10.1007/s13204-015-0422-x]

[164] Rao S, Suresh C. *In vitro* and *In vivo* Effects of the Leaf Extracts of *Cassia tora* and Cassia sophera in Reducing the Cytotoxicity and Angiogenesis. Br Biotechnol J 2013; 3(3): 377-89.
[http://dx.doi.org/10.9734/BBJ/2013/4244]

[165] Chen S, Li G, Zhu K, Sun P, Wang R, Zhao X. Antitumor activities of Juemingzi (*Cassia tora* L.) on Balb/c sarcoma 180-injected mice. Oncol Lett 2014; 7(1): 250-4.
[http://dx.doi.org/10.3892/ol.2013.1647] [PMID: 24348858]

[166] Diallo A, Eklug K, Amegbor K, *et al. In vivo* And *In vitro* Toxicological Evaluation Of The Hydroalcoholic Leaf Extracts Of Ageratum Conyzoidesl. (Asteraceae). J Ethnopharmacol 2014; 155(2): 1214-8.

[167] Tan NH, Akindahunsi AA, Zeng GZ, Zhang YM, Adebayo AH. Anticancer and antiradical scavenging activity of *Ageratum conyzoides* L. (Asteraceae). Pharmacogn Mag 2010; 6(21): 62-6. [http://dx.doi.org/10.4103/0973-1296.59968] [PMID: 20548938]

[168] Rahmawati N, Kuswandi M. Cytotoxic Effect Of Etanolic Extract Of Ageratum Conyzoides, L Against Hela Cell Line International Conference: Research And Application On Traditional Complementary And Alternative Medicine In Health Care (TCAM). Surakarta Indonesia. 2012; pp. 48-50.

[169] Nasrin F. Antioxidant and cytotoxic activities of *Ageratum conyzoides* stems. Int Curr Pharm J 2013; 2(2): 33-7.
[http://dx.doi.org/10.3329/icpj.v2i2.13195]

[170] Acheampong F, Larbie C, Appiah-Opong R, Arthur F, Tuffour I. In vitro Antioxidant and Anticancer Properties of Hydroethanolic Extracts and Fractions of Ageratum conyzoides. European J Med Plants 2015; 7(4): 205-14.
[http://dx.doi.org/10.9734/EJMP/2015/17088]

[171] Jayakumar K, Murugan K. Purified solasodine from *Solanum mauritianum* Scop. and its molecular mechanism of antimetastatic potential. Journal of Phytopharmacology 2017; 6(4): 251-9. [http://dx.doi.org/10.31254/phyto.2017.6409]

[172] Qwarse M, Sempombe J, Mihalem J, Henry L, Mugoyela V, Sunghwa F. Ctotoxicity, Antibacterial And Antifungal Activities Of Five Plant Species Used By Agro-Pastoral Communities In Mbulu District, Tanzania. Int J Res Pharm Chem 2017; 7(1): 1-14.

[173] Arora S, Aggarwal A, Singla P, Jyoti S, Tandon S. Anti-proliferative effects of homeopathic medicines on human kidney, colon and breast cancer cells. Homeopathy 2013; 102(4): 274-82. [http://dx.doi.org/10.1016/j.homp.2013.06.001] [PMID: 24050774]

[174] Ghosh S, Bishayee K, Paul A, *et al.* Homeopathic mother tincture of Phytolacca decandra induces apoptosis in skin melanoma cells by activating caspase–mediated signaling *via* reactive oxygen species elevation. J Integr Med 2013; 11(2): 116-24.
[http://dx.doi.org/10.3736/jintegrmed2013014] [PMID: 23506692]

[175] Kotas B, Sivakumar P, Karthiyayini T, Rajkumar M, Kumark L. *In-Vitro* Anti Cancer Activity Of Ethanolic Extract Of The Leaves Of Achyranthes Bidentata (Blume) 2012; pp. 519-23.

[176] Jiang Z, Qian J, Dong H, *et al.* The traditional Chinese medicine *Achyranthes bidentata* and our de novo conception of its metastatic chemoprevention: from phytochemistry to pharmacology. Sci Rep 2017; 7(1): 3888.
[http://dx.doi.org/10.1038/s41598-017-02054-y] [PMID: 28634392]

[177] Yang L, Shen Y, Wang F. Study on the Extraction and Antitumor Activity of Achyranthes Bidentata Polysaccharide. Int J Biol 2018; 10(2): 23.
[http://dx.doi.org/10.5539/ijb.v10n2p23]

[178] Naik SK, Mohanty S, Padhi A, Pati R, Sonawane A. Evaluation of antibacterial and cytotoxic activity of Artemisia nilagirica and Murraya koenigii leaf extracts against mycobacteria and macrophages. BMC Complement Altern Med 2014; 14(1): 87.
[http://dx.doi.org/10.1186/1472-6882-14-87] [PMID: 24597853]

[179] Sahu N, Meena S, Shukla V, *et al.* Extraction, fractionation and re-fractionation of Artemisia nilagirica for anticancer activity and HPLC-ESI-QTOF-MS/MS determination. J Ethnopharmacol 2018; 213: 72-80.
[http://dx.doi.org/10.1016/j.jep.2017.10.029] [PMID: 29109061]

[180] Devmurariv P, Jivanin P. Anticancer Evaluation Of Artemisia Nilagirica. Int J Pharm Tech Res 2010; 2(2): 1603-8.

[181] Pittella F, Dutra R, Junior D, Lopes MT, Barbosa N. Antioxidant and cytotoxic activities of Centella asiatica (L) Urb. Int J Mol Sci 2009; 10(9): 3713-21.

[http://dx.doi.org/10.3390/ijms10093713] [PMID: 19865514]

[182] Nivedheedha M, Sivasubramaniyan C. Cytotoxicity studies on various extracts of andrographispaniculata and centella asiatica against human cancer cell lines. Indoamerican Journal Of Pharmaceutical Research 2017; 7(4)

[183] Mahmoudvand H, Ayatollahi Mousavi SA, Sepahvand A, *et al.* Antifungal, Antileishmanial, and Cytotoxicity Activities of Various Extracts of *Berberis vulgaris* (Berberidaceae) and Its Active Principle Berberine. ISRN Pharmacol 2014; 2014: 1-6. [http://dx.doi.org/10.1155/2014/602436] [PMID: 24977052]

[184] Hanachi P, Golkho S. Assessment of Soy Phytoestrogens and Exercise on Lipid Profiles and Menopause Symptoms in Menopausal Women. J Biol Sci (Faisalabad, Pak) 2008; 8(4): 789-93. [http://dx.doi.org/10.3923/jbs.2008.789.793]

CHAPTER 5

High Throughput Screening Techniques in Anticancer Drug Discovery and Development from Botanicals

Madhavi Patel[1,*] and **Vishal Patel**[2]

[1] *Parul Institute of Pharmacy, Parul University, Limda, Vadodara, Gujarat, India*

[2] *Vasu Research Centre, A Div. of Vasu Healthcare Pvt. Ltd., Vadodara, Gujarat, India*

Abstract: Botanicals obtained from nature are the major source of therapeutic medicines for humans. Utilization of botanicals for a variety of diseases is not mysterious, and a rapid increase in such therapeutic substances is observed due to their efficacy and long-term safety. Cancer, as a leading cause of disease worldwide, piques the interest of researchers seeking novel anticancer agents. Till date, the major share of cancer medicines is occupied by natural products, and the drug discovery process is rapidly going on. However, traditional anticancer drug discovery is time-consuming and herculean. High-throughput screening (HTS) is a tool to make natural product library screening easy and fast. The advancement of extraction, isolation, and structure characterization of Phyto actives obtained from botanicals, provides a large number of compounds for testing *via* HTS. High-density well plates, a liquid handling platform, automation, and robotics allow the screening of 100,000 compounds per day. Anticancer screening of botanicals by HTS can be performed on various cancer cell lines along with molecular targets, enzyme or protein interaction assays, or the capacity of the extract to induce apoptosis. After the replication of identified extracts, further assays are performed for more precise results. HTS screening and computational methods provide speed and a high degree of sensitivity for anticancer agents and compress the time required for drug discovery. Advances in HTS technology, such as ultra-HTS and the use of 3-D cultures, will speed up the process of discovering anticancer drugs from botanicals. Advanced detection techniques for HTS assays, as well as instrumental techniques for identified lead compound separation, help to ensure that the results are neat.

Keywords: Assay, Anticancer, Automization, Apoptosis, Botanicals, Cell proliferation, Dereplication, Drug Discovery, Extracts, High Throughput Screening (HTS), Hit, Lead, Liquid handling platform, Molecular assay, Miniaturization, Natural products, Phytoconstituents, Target identification.

* **Corresponding author Madhavi Patel:** Parul Institute of Pharmacy, Parul University, Limda, Waghodia, Vadodara, Gujarat, India; E-mail: madhavii10@yahoo.co.in

Motamarri Venkata Naga Lalitha Chaitanya, Galvina Pereira, & Heyam Saad Ali (Eds.)

PREAMBLE

Nature is a mine of medicinal substances obtained from plants, animals, minerals, or marine sources. Products obtained from them remain the major foundation for the treatment of human diseases [1, 2]. A plethora of therapeutic substances have been stored in the womb of nature, among which botanicals are very unique and enormous. Initially, disease treatment was accomplished by using a crude or semi-pure fraction of botanicals, and after the twentieth century, the theory of drug action and receptor link was developed. The thought that drug effects on humans might be due to the interaction of drug substances with biological proteins, nucleic acids, or other macromolecules led scientists to conclude that individual constituents present in such drugs or extracts are responsible for the therapeutic activity of the drug. Eventually, this concept directed the separation of pure bioactive compounds from an extract or drug and the elucidation of their structure [3]. People started to switch over to natural botanicals due to their dissatisfaction with synthetic medicines for the treatment of chronic illnesses like cancer and diabetes. This interest in natural products led to the exploration of more chemical structures, which can be the basis for new drug development, proving that natural products were and will always remain important sources of new pharmaceuticals [4]. It is worth noting that more than half of existing drugs are naturally derived or modified forms of them, with 60% of them being used to treat cancer. This encourages the pharmaceutical industry and academia to focus on developing new drugs from botanicals [2, 5, 6]. Since the isolation of early phytoconstituents such as digitoxin, morphine, cocaine, and codeine, many of which are still in use for various purposes [7, 8], the concept of isolation or fractionation has persisted.

Cancer and Role of Botanicals - Historical Aspects

Cancer is considered a major cause of death worldwide, even after advances in chemotherapy and surgery [9]. In cancer, abnormal cell growth occurs in one place and can spread to other parts of the body, or we can say that it develops when normal cells start to grow abnormally or out of control. There are numerous types of cancer, including those of the blood, breast, lung, prostate, and uterus. Moreover, it is wise to prevent cancer before it requires treatment. Natural products are and will remain an important source of anticancer agents, especially botanicals. Moreover, because they possess a more structurally diverse nature [10] and are associated with less toxicity, it is wise to say that natural product research is a better approach for discovering new anticancer agents. Currently available cancer chemotherapeutics derived from botanicals are vincristine and vinblastine, taxol derivatives (paclitaxel and docetaxel), etoposide, irinotecan, and topotecan [11]. However, they suffer from poor solubility and the associated toxic effects. It leads to the synthesis of a few analogues and prodrugs of these medicines to overcome drugability issues. In the past many years, natural product drug discovery has gained momentum as researchers have tried to overcome the drugability issues of natural molecules, derive their semisynthetic analogues, and evaluate their efficacies *in vitro*, *in vivo*, and in clinics. Some of the most important anticancer agents are derived from plants, as well as their semisynthetic derivatives, which are widely used. According to Müller-Kuhrt [12], natural products complement synthetic drugs by exhibiting drug-like features. Newer combinatorial approaches for synthesis and computerised methods shifted pharmaceutical industries' interests toward synthetic chemicals for the discovery of new molecules, diminishing the importance of natural products in the drug discovery process. They fear carrying out research on natural products due to the ever-growing competition and time limit, but looking at the architect of natural products and past success utilising newer techniques with fresh strategies helps to overcome this aversion [3]. Table **1** represents some of the botanicals tested for anticancer activity utilising HTS screening techniques.

Table 1. Reported HTS Screening of Botanicals for Anticancer Potential

Sr. No.	Sample Screened by HTS	Biological Source	HTS Assay	HTS Method Adopted	Potent Anticancer Phyto-compounds Identified	Reference
1	Podophyllotoxin (S1, DP1, ET) & Tanshinone (TI, TIIA, TIIB)	*Podophyllum emodi* (Berberidaceae), *Salvia miltiorrhiza* (Lamiaceae)	DNA laddering assay on HeLa-C3 cells	Herrmann's method	DP1, TIIA	[13]
2	Subfraction (SF) 1 to 12	*Albuca setosa* (Asparagaceae)	HeLa cervical cancer cells	MTT viability assay.	C-glucosylflavonoidOglucoside	[14]
3	Approx. 2000 extract prepared from 1220 Brazilian plant	Plants grown in Amazon Rain Forest, Brazil	Breast, Prostate, Lung, Colon, Central nervous system and Leukemia cell lines	SRB colorimetric method	Topotecan, Irinotecan & Camptothecin (Terrestrialsources) and Bryostatin, Dolastatin-10 and Ecteinascidin 743 (Marine Source)	[15]
4	Ethyl acetate-soluble extract	*Ziziphus mauritiana* Lam. (Rhamnaceae)	Human melanoma cells (MEL-2)	Proteasome inhibition assay & Histone deacetylase (HDAC) inhibition assay	Betulinic acid	[16]
5	Chloroform-soluble extract	*Erythroxylum pervillei* Baill. (Erythroxylaceae)	Oral epidermoid cancer cell line (KB-V1)	Proteasome inhibition assay & Histone deacetylase (HDAC) inhibition assay	Pervilleine A	[17]
6	Chloroform-soluble extract	*Aglaia silvestris* (Meliaceae)	Lung, Prostate and Breast cancer cells as well as against Umbilical vein endothelial cells	Proteasome inhibition assay & Histone deacetylase (HDAC) inhibition assay	Silvestrol	[18]

(Table 1) cont.....

Sr. No.	Sample Screened by HTS	Biological Source	HTS Assay	HTS Method Adopted	Potent Anticancer Phyto-compounds Identified	Reference
7	Pet. Ether, Chloroform, Ethyl acetate & Aqueous Extract of weed plants	*Phytolacca Dodecandra, Cytisus Scoparius, Erigeron Karvinkianus, Cnicus wallichi, Solanum mauritianum, Cestrum aurantiacum*	VERO, A-549, MCF-7, HCT-116 Cell line	*In vitro* cytotoxic studies, Molecular docking studies, TLC based bio-autography studies.	Naringenin, Tetrahydro-2-(hydroxymethyl)-6-(octadecahydro-2,7,10a-trimethyl-1-propylchrysen-8-yloxy)-2H-Pyran-3,4,5-triol, 7-Methoxy Hesperetin & (1E)-1-hydroxyprop-1-en-2-yl (2E)--(4-hydroxy-3-methoxyphenyl)prop-2-enoate).	[19]
8	Aqueous extracts	897 commercially sold natural plant	MDA-MB-231 human breast cancer cells	Viable cell counter using a microplate fluorometer	Mayapple (*P. peltatum*), Truja Twigs (*T. occidentalis*), mistletoe (*P. flavescens*), Speranskia herb (*S. tuberculata*), Bunge root (*P. chinensis*) & Brucea fruit (*B. javanica*)	[20]
9	Formononetin	*AstragalusMembranaceus* (Fabaceae)	HeLa cells	MTT assay, Flow cytometry & ATP assay	Formononetin	[21]
10	Methanolic extract	*Plakortis quasiamphiaster, Crella spinulata*	V-C8 mutant cell line and the BRCA2-complemented BAC29 cell line	WST1 cell viability assay	Plakinidine A, Plakinidine B & Plakinidine C	[22]
11	Flavanoid rich fraction	*Dysoxylum binectariferum* Hook. (Meliaceae),	breast and lung carcinoma cell lines	MTT viability assay.	Rohitukine, Flavopiridol	[23]
12	Plant extract of different parts	65 Egyptian plants	HepG2 cells line	MTT viability assay.	Oleandrin, Polymethoxyflavones, Thaspine	[24]
13	Cotton seed extracts & Its derivatives	*Gossypium Spp.* (Malvaceae)	HeLa cells	MTT viability assay	Gossypol, Sabutoclax	[25]
14	622,079 compounds	Natural product library	Breast cancer (TNBC) cell line	Cell viability and cell-cycle assays	Curcumin, Garcinol, Anacardic acid	[26]
15	148,250 natural product extracts	Natural product library	GST-Bcl-2 proteins, FITC or Cy5-Bim BH3 peptide.	Fluorescence polarization assays (FPAs),	994 natural product extracts	[27]

Botanicals have demonstrated their effect on several cancers, like stomach, lung, breast, prostate, and endometrium cancer. Various mechanisms like antioxidant activity, alteration of enzyme activity, and antiviral or antibacterial effects are attributed to the presence of complex-natured constituents in botanicals [28]. Botanicals demonstrated mechanisms such as immune function alteration, inflammation reduction, hormone metabolism modulation, cell cycle progression arrest, and majority apoptosis stimulation for the arrest of cancer cell proliferation.(HTS) High-throughput screening (HTS) has gained wide popularity over the past few years as a tool of drug discovery, and the pharmaceutical and biotechnology industries prefer this technique for screening and assaying a large number of bioactives against specific targets [29, 30]. It provides a practical approach to screening a large number of compounds for the identification of bioactives through *in vitro* assay miniaturization, which is far more convenient in comparison to traditional drug discovery. The origin and evolution of HTS date back to 1984, when Pfizer, USA, started with a prototype of screening [31]. HTS is considered a segment of the drug discovery process, which can be described as the stage from target to lead [29]. It is employed by scientists and academic researchers for screening of different types of synthetic and natural product libraries, which include genomics, combinatorial chemistry, peptides, and protein libraries. Additionally, it is helpful to characterise the pharmacokinetic, metabolic, and toxicological profiles of a new drug under investigation. The key focus of the HTS is to speed up the drug discovery process by screening a large number of compound libraries, the rate of which may surpass a few thousand compounds per day or per week [32]. HTS involves different steps like identification of target, preparation of reagent, management of compound, development of assay, and screening of available high-throughput libraries [33]. The development of HTS techniques is attributed to combinatorial chemistry, where large numbers of compounds are produced for screening. Testing them within a short period of time is easily achievable by HTS, which has attracted the attention of so many researchers. However, the HTS technique almost never identifies a new drug candidate, but it is a reasonably chemical starting point where heat-to-lead discovery can be initiated. Lead is one of a series of compounds for which a chemical optimization plan can be carried out [34]. Currently, high-density arrays of microreaction wells are gaining popularity in the drug discovery process. Initially, 96-well plates were used for screening, which are now replaced by higher-density microplates with a capacity of up to 1586 wells per plate. The usual working volume for microplates is about 2.5–10 L total, where a standard volume is 5 L per well [35]. Moreover, there are still ongoing trends towards the miniaturisation of plates. Several reports were evident of the utilisation of 3456-well microplates with an assay volume of 1–2 L, but they were associated with technical hurdles [36]. Traditional HTS techniques can screen 10,000 compounds per day, but the advent of Ultra HTS allows screening of up to 100,000 compounds per day [32].

In HTS screening, if a compound gives the desired result in primary screening, it's called as "hit" then secondary screening is performed by adopting biological evaluation. Hence, HTS screening can be used for finding primary compounds with biological activity against the selected target called as hits and also for leads selection. However, there exists a perception that botanical extracts in comparison to pure compound create numerous artefacts As a result, it is preferable to carry out screening techniques using two different experimental detections when using various assay techniques. Here, the extracts or compounds that interfere with one recording system can be picked up because they are implausibly appearing as active in another detection system [37]. Different sample preparation methodologies can be found for HTS screening, as traditional manual sample preparation will be tedious and time-consuming. To solve this problem, the solid-phase extraction (SPE) procedure is employed in the majority of cases. This method generates high-quality samples from botanicals, allowing for rapidity in the process [31, 38]. For the general methodology to be followed, the heart of HTS screening is the microwell plates in which test samples and reagents are added, the plate is incubated, and their interactions are monitored in the form of signals that can be detected by different spectroscopy and chromatography methods. Spectroscopic methods like fluorescence spectroscopy, absorption and luminescence, nuclear magnetic resonance (NMR), Fourier transformed infrared (FTIR), and total internal reflection fluorescence (TIRF) are employed for detection. Liquid chromatography is widely used in HTS screening. Some microscopic techniques, like scanning and confocal microscopic techniques, and flow cytometry are sometimes employed for reaction detection or live imaging while HTS screening. After HTS screening, looking at the data complexity, it is needed to have an effective representation of the data obtained. One popular method is the utilisation of a "heat map," which is a simple data representation in the form of a map or diagram where data values are observed as different colours with different intensities [39].

Importance of HTS in Anticancer Drug Discovery

Cancer remains a major cause of death in the world, and so the majority of drug compounds in the pipeline of discovery are aimed at cancer treatment or elimination [40]. Although cancer drug development has a low success rate and high costs, HTS techniques have raised hopes for saving time and money while supporting anticancer drug discovery. Natural product research is revolutionised through computational and mathematical modelling by facilitating isolation, extraction, and structure characterization in a way that is less time-consuming and more precise. Also, it has greatly reduced the time and effort required for the generation of dereplicated phytocompound libraries. The design of target-focused libraries requires combinatorial and computational chemistry. Reports are available where researchers made attempts at designing phytochemical libraries for specific therapeutic targets. Flavonoids and alkaloids such as licorice are two examples. HTS techniques are best-suited for providing lead molecules with anticancer activity in order to complete the drug discovery process with the least amount of time and effort [39]. Fig. (**1**) depicts the general HTS screening steps for anticancer agents derived from botanicals.

HTS Techniques for Anticancer Agents

HTS involves mainly target identification steps, for which a large number of compound libraries can be tested. HTS assays are generally carried out in mainly two ways: cell-free and cell-based assays (Fig. **2**). Much advancement in robotics, system automization, assay miniaturization, sensible detection systems, data control and processing software, liquid handling devices, and the involvement of sophisticated instrumentation created a scope for botanical candidate screening that was accurate and faster. However, according to many researchers, botanical diversity, availability, chemical complexity, stability of compounds, nonreliability of the HTS assay system, and costs are among the many common problems for carrying out HTS screening of natural compounds. Also, many a time, such extracts are discontinued after HTS due to issues related to their availability and purity. Here, a more careful approach can be opted for to address the associated problems related to botanical drug discovery. It has been commonly found that cell-based assays are preferred for HTS screening of anticancer agents from botanicals because they do not involve target protein purification, reach intracellular sites, and give precise results.

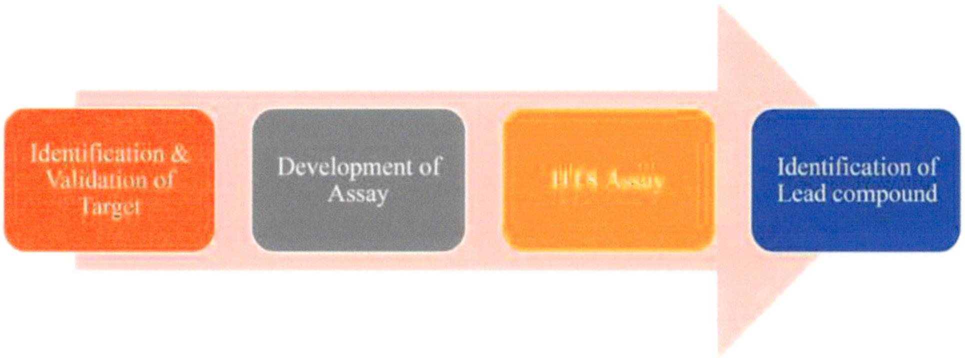

Fig. (1). HTS Screening of Anti-cancer Agents from Botanicals at Glance.

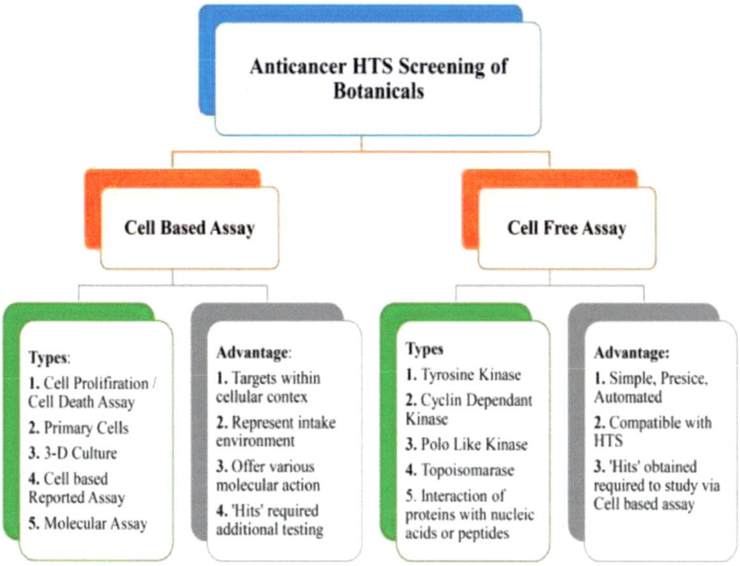

Fig. (2). Anticancer HTS Screening techniques of botanicals

Anticancer Drug Target Identification

The selection and validation of drug targets rely on the demonstration of a biological effect mediated by compound interaction with the target. Molecular targeting techniques should focus on the molecular essence of a target role to increase the possibility that the drug will not show a diverse range of effects. Kinases like Bcr-Abl kinase are currently viewed as best representing a molecular target in the modern era of anticancer drug development [41 - 43]. Other targets for therapy of solid tumours where Ras-mediated cell signalling caters to multiple potential points of target have been extensively studied by pharmaceutical industries [44]. A kinase inhibitor directed to the vascular endothelial cell growth receptor tyrosine kinase was used in this study to inhibit tumour angiogenesis [45]. Human genome projects combined with increased computerised approaches to exploit a large number of potential targets can be a good tool for drug discovery. Hundreds of kinases are coded in the human genome, which provides important information for regulating cancer signalling pathways [46].

Creating a Botanical Library for HTS Screening

Creating a botanical extract and compound library will aid in the systematic screening of a large number of compounds by HTS. As we are well aware of the potency of botanicals and other natural agents to provide novel anticancer agents, the US National Cancer Institute, known as the NCI, has already created a repository of natural products. It is considered one of the world's largest and most diverse collections, with over 30,000 extracts originating from different natural sources. These resources are readily available for researchers for HTS screening of extracts followed by bioactivity-guided isolation [47]. To make these extracts HTS-amenable, they have created a pre-fractioned library from over 1,25,000 natural product extracts. Computational tools provide varied means for assessing diversity in the botanical chemical library. Several early efforts were made to use selected molecular targets to develop focused libraries of compounds. The preliminary aim of this work is to define compound libraries that can be optimised against specific molecular targets [48]. HTS Screening Assay for Anticancer Agents Cell-Free HTS Assay For anticancer drug screening, simple cell-free assays evaluate the interaction of proteins with nucleic acids or peptides. These assays are simple to conduct in solution using fluorescence polarisation (FP) or any other detection technique. Also, it can be conducted in aqueous buffers as an ELISA with the target protein immobilised on an assay plate [49]. Conventional modes of FP detection are mostly useful for anticancer HTS assays from botanicals. However, due to the higher degree of intrinsic fluorescence of various kinds of botanical extracts, FP detection in an HTS assay can be problematic [29].

To combat this issue, the utilisation of europium-labelled reagents along with a time-resolved fluorescent detection approach can be adopted. HTS based on enzyme inhibitors, different receptor-linked tyrosine kinases, cyclin-dependent kinases, and Polo-like kinases were tested to avail agents for specific cancer treatment [50 - 52]. It is feasible to perform HTS screening against particular kinases as there are commercial suppliers and methods available [50, 53]. When hits are detected, their specificities can be confirmed against a broad panel of kinases [54]. 1200 compounds related to known kinase inhibitors were screened for PIM1 kinase, out of which 7 confirmed hits were reported. It is interesting to note that out of these 7 compounds, 6 were flavonoids [55]. 1,20,000 natural products were reported to be screened through a protein fragment complementation assay [56]. A natural compound called thymoquinone and a synthetic analogue, poloxin, were reported to inhibit polo-like kinase 1 [57]. Various botanicals are found to be active *via* assays for protein-protein interaction with Src kinases [58].

Another well-established enzyme, topoisomerases can be good target for anticancer drugs screening by HTS assays [59, 60]. Camptothecin and their derivatives irinotecan and camptothecan are active against topoisomerase I. Podophyllotoxin analogue, etoposide is active against topoisomerase II. Other enzymes like phosphatases, gamma-secretase, heparanase, histone deacetylases and leucine aminopeptidases are considered as active targets for HTS screening [61 - 65].

Cell Based HTS Assay

Cell-based assays can be one of the best ways to check drug effects on generalised pathways or specific targets. Many types of cell-based HTS assays for screening anticancer actives originated from botanicals have been reported, such as cell growth or cell death assays, molecular assays, cell-based reporter assays, and taking primary cells from tumours. A HTS homogeneous screening assay for detecting apoptosis in different human cancer cell lines has been reported [49].

Cell Proliferation/Cell Death Assay

Cancer cells are characterised by uncontrolled proliferation [66]. This property of cancer cells is a highly useful approach for testing the anticancer activity of compounds in HTS screening, where a reduction in the growth of cancer cells will be observed. The effects of compounds under testing can be evaluated on cell lines derived from a patient's tumor, and their effects on tumour cells can be compared to non-cancerous cells. Cell proliferation or cell death can be quantified using methods like trypan blue exclusion, radiolabelled thymidine, intracellular enzyme release, changes in ATP, and DNA staining dyes [67]. Methods are also reported for detecting apoptosis.

One of the widely used methods is the detection of caspases, a family of enzyme cysteine proteases. Caspase activation in the cell serves as a biochemical marker of cell death as it plays a central role in programmed cell death. Hence, their activation in the cells can easily be an indicator of the effect induced by the test substances. Also, DNA fragmentation, cytotoxicity and cell proliferation, membrane alterations, immunological detection and mitochondrial damage are employed for detection of cell apoptosis [68, 69].

These assays can be carried out even on 1536 well plates [70]. During detection, the test compound can create an interference with the measurement, so that no system is called an ideal detection method. The interference with fluorescent signals or visible light or reagent inhibition like luciferase is an example. Luciferases obtained from different organisms are widely used for HTS because of their bioluminescence property. Luciferase's active site binds to ATP and luciferin holding benzthiazole core proceeds *via* the formation of luciferyl-adenylate intermediate, which results in the generation of Adenosine monophosphate, oxyluciferin and light. The active cite environment affects the wavelength of the emitted light where single amino acid changes can shift the luminescence. Hence, the compounds which have a direct inhibition of enzyme can interfere with the detection and can be considered as potent luciferase inhibitors [71, 72].

To avoid such interferences, parallel screening, like for cell viability and cell death, can be helpful, and such assays can be performed on the same wells [73, 74] and can be multiplexed with cell assays for detection of caspase 3 and apoptotic markers [75]. Cell culture experiments are carried out in an artificial environment, where they grow faster than they would *in vivo*. In such conditions, major concerns arise related to the correlation of results and their ability to provoke the activity of drugs in patients [76]. To overcome this issue, trials have been reported using depleted medium and culture plates, which decrease the attachment and growth of cells, to construct a cellular environment like *in vivo* [77]. The MTT (3-(4,5-dimethylthiazol-2-yl)-2,5-diphenyl tetrazolium bromide) assay, in which this dye is taken up by viable cells and reduced by cell enzymes to blue formazan product and alamar blue, is used as a metabolic indicator of live cells. However, these metabolic indicators may produce false results because, during sampling, damaged cells are on the verge of dying, but their metabolism may be temporarily enhanced, potentially increasing the number of live cells. In this cell proliferation screening for cancer cells, the test compounds may be able to kill readily growing cells, but they may not be able to remove tumours due to cancer stem cells. Oppositely, the test compound may provoke the appearance of such stem cells, so the agents that are effective against these cells became a study of interest [78, 79].

The main challenge in cancer stem cells is their scarcity, which makes it difficult to develop a precise HTS assay. Stem cells can form colonies when plated at a lower density; such clonogenic assays are suitable for low-throughput screening. Thierbach and Steinberg published a soft agar method for HTS screening of test compounds against the colony-forming capacity of cells that relies on an automatic pipetting instrument [80]. Most cancer patients are treated with combinations of drugs for potential synergistic effects. Accordingly, screening methods have been developed for evaluating the synergistic potential of combinations of clinically used agents and have been tested on different human cancer cell lines [81]. Statistically, they are evaluated to check the synergism of the combination so that the possibility of an additive or antagonistic effect can be avoided. In a reported study, 50,000 compounds were tested for their capacity to kill prostate cancer cell line cells in a mixture with an anti-FAS antibody [82]. Booth *et al.* reported in their study that 16,480 synthetic and natural product substances could mimic the effects of the death receptor ligand TNF--related apoptosis-inducing ligand (TRAIL) on a renal cancer cell line [83]. In this study, 18 confirmed synergistic substances were detected, and 14 of these were natural products. The synergism of the test compounds at nanomolar concentrations was found to demonstrate their effectiveness *via* activation of caspase 8, mitochondrial membrane potential modulation, interference with DNA, or at any point of apoptosis.

Primary cells

Primary cell cultures derived from patient biopsies are more practical for use in cell-based assays than specific cell lines, which differ in their behavior. Glaysher *et al.*, in a pilot study, screened 5605 plant extracts against ovarian tumour primary cultures grown successfully in 384-well plates. They found 60 active extracts, out of which 47 were unknown previously and 13 had previously been reported with positive effects in ZR75 breast cancer cell lines [84]. Milroy *et al.* used chronic lymphocytic leukaemia cells for screening of natural product-based scaffolds, where they discovered effective apoptosis-inducing cytotoxic agents [85].

D Cultures

Actual solid tumours present in cancer patients are 3 dimensional (3-D), but when we grow cells in culture, they are in monolayer 2 dimensional. During cytotoxicity studies, cancer cells are cultured as a monolayer. In the monolayer cultures, microenvironment signals and cell to cell contacts are missing, so that they are not able to replicate the *in vivo* conditions. Therefore, it will be more accurate if we grow cancer cells in 3 dimensional systems. 3-D cultures are found to be promising system to bridge the gap between *in vivo* study and monolayer cell cultures. To facilitate anticancer drug discovery from 3-D cultures, it is highly required to develop new techniques which permit their use in HTS [86]. To overcome monolayer cultures related technical problems, 3-D cultures are being employed in different formats [87 - 89]. Here, co-cultures are coming out as a valuable methodology for predicting drug responses in different diseases *in vivo* [90 - 92]. Chitosan hydrogel co-culture, microfluidic devices, multi-well hanging drop, PDMS V-bottom microwells and 2-layer embryoid bodies are prominent reported methods for the generation of uniform spheroids to be utilized in 3-D culture [93, 94]. Howes *et al.* utilized the multi-well hanging drop method which was found to be the best HT amenable techniques due to less cross reactivity with test compound, cost and meeting liquid handling requirements [86].

Attempts have been reported to grow cells in small multicellular spheroids that were adapted for HTS [95, 96]. Documented evidence is available for the measurement of drug-induced apoptosis in cultured multicellular spheroids when grown from different human cancer cell lines [97]. However, reports are not available for anticancer HTS testing of natural products by spheroid culture. A 3-D matrix, like a network of electrospun collagen microfibers, was reported to support colony formation by providing a more real environment for cells to grow [98]. Automated imaging for tracking cancer cell movement through a matrix was developed. It was tested on A549 lung cancer cells grown in collagen, recommending the use of such methods for drug screening [99].

Cell-Based Reporter Assays

Simple proliferation and viability assays of cancer cells are highly convenient to carry out, but they will not be able to explain the probable mechanism of action of the compounds under screening. Cell engineering can be used to create mechanistic cell-based assays that demonstrate specific molecular targets. An assay for substances affecting the EGFR (epidermal growth factor receptor) was created by transfecting the receptor into a cell line for growth stimulation by EGF. Here, 9 compounds were documented as hits out of a total of 20,000 compounds under screening [100]. For the development of reporter assays to detect potential anticancer compounds, a luciferase-based system for autophagy was reported [101]. In the discovery of novel anticancer agents, many targets were identified and used for screening. Bortezomib, clinically used for multiple myeloma, was proven to be an inhibitor of the ubiquitin-proteosome pathway, which was one of the established targets identified for anticancer agents. Physalin B from the Physalis angulate plant was discovered as a novel proteasome function inhibitor *via* bioluminescence assay [102]. This assay was developed for use with natural product extracts [103].

Cell-based and molecular assays are being developed for hsp90 (heat shock protein 90). Natural products, radicol and geldanamycin, were found to inhibit hsp90 [104 - 106]. HTS assays of several natural products provided a few hits against the potential transcription factor target HIF-1, the hypoxia-inducible factor [107]. To overcome problems related to the utilisation of botanical extracts in protein interaction assays, the electrochemiluminescence method was developed and used for the screening of 1,44,000 extracts [108]. Sempervirine, an indole alkaloid derived from a shrub, was discovered to inhibit MDM2-mediated p53 degradation, auto-ubiquitination, and apoptosis in cells. In such cases, detected hits must be validated to ensure that they are not interfering with the reporter system and tested against the predefined target to demonstrate their action *via* the desired mechanism.

Molecular Assays

With the advent of targeted anticancer agents, the trend moved toward the utilization assays which are based on molecular targets [109]. Molecular assays are highly advantageous compared to cell based assays. Molecular assays require fewer test substances, are less laborious and faster. They are more feasible with ultra-HTS. Hits, arising from molecular assays, are needed to be tested for the selectivity of targets and for retaining their integrity.

The success of Taxanes, which stabilise microtubules and vinca alkaloids like vincristine and vinblastine, which disrupt microtubules, have paved a pillar of utilization of tubulin and microtubule as targeted agents. They along with related proteins like kinesins are considered as screening criterion for HTS and novel inhibitors have been found from botanicals [110].

Analysis of Botanicals for Characterization of Identified Compounds

Fluorescent techniques are widely employed for botanicals analysis in HTS screening. Botanicals comprise complexnatured compounds and and sometimes fluorescent techniques cannot be applied screening. When there is a requirement for structural characterization of compounds or products, a technique like MS (mass spectrometry) is used due to its sensitivity, selectivity, resolution and structural elucidation capability. Further, MS is providing easy and selective separation of interested molecules from a complex mixture which does not require a complicated sample preparation process. FIA MS (flow injection analysis MS) associated with 8 probe autosampler makes it possible to characterize combinatorial library compounds in a 96 well plate in 5 min [111]. Tutko *et al.* reported that an automated version of MALDI-FT-MS (matrix-assisted laser desorption/ionization Fourier transform MS) can analyse 20 samples in an hour [112]. Liquid chromatography MS (LC-MS) and nuclear magnetic resonance (NMR) spectroscopy are other analytical techniques employed. LC-MS is employed for metabolic identification in HTS assays. High-performance LC (HPLC) is utilized for the purity determination of compounds [113, 114].

HPLC linked with MS is the most preferable for botanicals. The Anticancer Drug Discovery process from botanicals involving HT screening and compound identification is represented in Fig. (**3**).

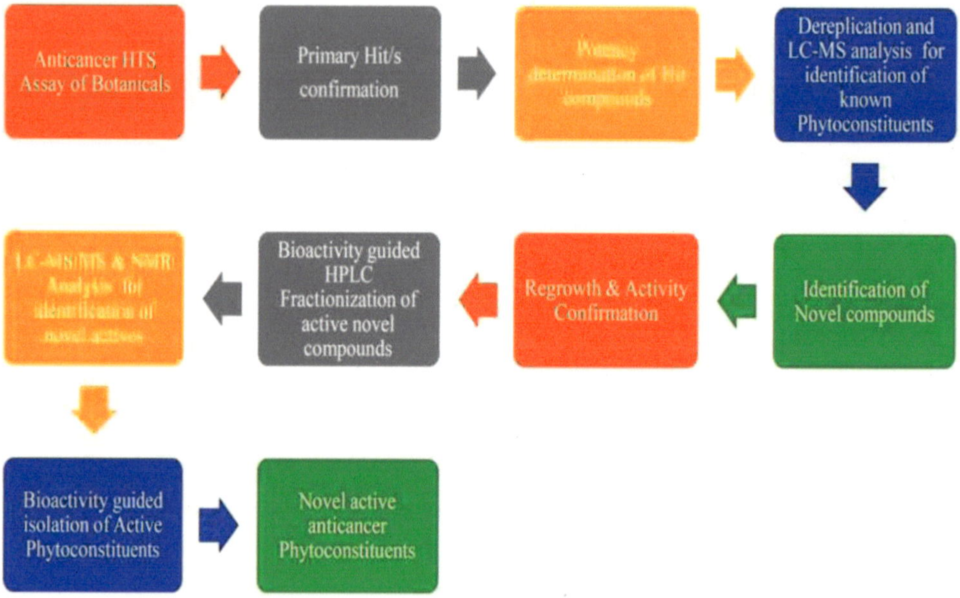

Fig. (3). Anticancer drug discovery process from botanicals using HTS

Assay Miniaturization and Advancement in HTS

The advancement of technology causes changes in the HTS screening strategy. related to liquid handling automation, the design of novel platforms, and a quantitative data analysis tool that facilitates fast drug screening Thus, HTS's functioning is commendable. Miniaturization with automation reduces the analysis's labour, time, and costs. Through HTS miniaturization, it is now possible to test the toxicity of compounds in quantities ranging from 1-3 mg. This method of cytotoxicity research saves money and shortens the study period [30]. Ultra

HTS was performed on nearly 150,000 natural product extracts for the identification of proapoptotic inhibitors of Bcl-2 family proteins using fluorescence-conjugated peptide ligands in 1536 well plates. Confirmed HTS extracts were further tested for caspase-3/7 activation in tumour cells. Active extracts were carried forward to bioactivity guided fractionation. The study depicts the feasibility of ultra HTS in the screening of natural products [115]. Molecular modification of a natural product containing lead can establish a structure-activity relationship. Pharmacomodulation is one of the methods used to search for new compounds and involves taking a chemical substance with an established structure and known bioactivity and preparing and testing its structural analogues. Pharmacomodulation techniques are mainly aimed at establishing a correlation between pharmacology and structure. In this case, the obtained drugs may be better than prototypes. In the study of natural products, pharmacomodulation has provided notable achievements and important improvements in biological activity and the drug's pharmacokinetics [116]. HTS assays in primary tumour cultures can identify actives with high potential for clinical trials. Quantitative HTS (qHTS) of clinically approved agents is important, and such reproducible assays can be utilised for identifying actives for cancer therapy and for other diseases as well [117].

Dereplication Techniques: Assistance in Drug Discovery from Botanicals

Botanicals have the most chemical diversity and have proven to be a significant source of therapeutic substances. Drug discovery based on such a diverse library requires a method of bioassay-guided isolation and structure characterization, which can be a herculean task. When a confirmed hit was obtained from botanicals in the HTS screen, the investigators want to find out what may be the active compound, whether it is known/ already established or it is novel and if so, how to catch more amount of it. For this purpose, recollection and dereplication are requirements. Recollection means we must be able to get more sources for follow on studies [3].

Dereplication against the increasing number of known bio-actives is becoming highly important for drug discovery screening. Dereplication techniques, for the identification and elimination of known compounds from the discovery process, demand skill and utilization of chemical informatics. The advancement of sensitive equipment like LC-MS facilitated this process. In many cases, this process along with different spectral data provides a fast identity of already known compounds and permits investigators to move on to novel lead compounds. National Cancer Institute (NCI) created a library of aqueous and organic extracts from diverse nature of natural sources like plants, and marine and microbial cultures [118]. Many intra and extramural investigators have utilized this library for isolation of novel molecules possessing anticancer property and other property [119]. NCI compound library can be found on the web of NCI. Many investigators have reported separation and characterization of anticancer leads from NCI library [120].

Merits And Demerits of HTS Screening for Anticancer Agents

Anticancer agents' drug discovery from botanicals through HTS provides a high degree of efficiency in lead identification. HTS automation and high-density plates make the screening task fast after target identification if compound libraries for screening are available. HTS for anticancer screening is associated with advantages such as high sensitivity, high speed, minimization of reagents and samples, and sensitive detection techniques. Such techniques will send a clear message about the status of compound activity. It will aid in the enhancement of anticancer discoveries from botanicals. Despite its many benefits, HTS screening suffers from high investment costs in automated assay detection techniques. Also, precise sample preparation with modern techniques are required. Such facilities are not available to every investigator, which hampers the process of finding novel anticancer agents.

CONCLUSION

In the beginning, HTS screening was developed for screening large compound libraries generated from combinatorial synthesis, where automation and robotics provided a fast process of drug discovery. Initially, botanicals remained unnoticed for HTS screening because there was no availability of natural products with duplicated libraries. Various computational tools and modelling facilitated the isolation and identification of bioactive phytochemicals with utmost speed and precision, resulting in phytocompound libraries. The phytocompound libraries offered by the US National Cancer Institute and other commercial producers allowed researchers and academia to carry out research on botanicals and other natural products *via* the HTS process.

It is unopposed truth that plants are the most perfect laboratories where various simple to high complexity molecules are synthesized. These phytochemicals are highly superior in their therapeutic activity. If we have to move forward with drug discovery from botanicals, we need to utilize bioactivity-guided isolation and identification of some important drugs including anticancer agents. Botanical drug discovery starts with the attempts to find out phytochemicals responsible for the specific biological effect. In the current competitive era of pharmaceutical research, botanicals provide uniqueness in terms of biological activity and molecular diversity which is a bit difficult to obtain manually. To combat with the current scenario, botanicals drug discovery also needs to improve continuously for the screening speed, identification and isolation of actives, structural characterization and large-scale phytocompounds supply. There is a tremendous scope for countries who have rich biodiversity and can take up the correct measures for the supply of medicinal plants in a scientific way, so that plant material quality will be promising. With the utilization of good and rapid extraction technologies, HTS screening methodologies, automization, and robotics involvement in finding lead compounds may lead to the generation of potent anticancer agents form botanicals.

However, it is not easy to discover novel anticancer agents from botanicals, but HTS and combinatorial approach made it possible to establish potent anticancer drugs and or their semisynthetic derivatives in the market. With the advancement in various HTS techniques an assay miniaturization, HTS field becomes dynamic and competitive. In this competitive environment, several pharmaceutical companies are joining hands to accelerate drug discovery process. High density micro well plates and nanoscale capillaries will certainly change the scenario and provide positive outcome for such dreadful disease, although these techniques are still few years away for routine screening of compounds.

REFERENCES

[1] Patwardhan B, Vaidya AD, Chorghade M. Ayurveda and natural products drug discovery. Curr Sci 2004; 789-99.

[2] Newman DJ, Cragg GM. Natural products as sources of new drugs over the last 25 years. J Nat Prod 2007; 70(3): 461-77.
[http://dx.doi.org/10.1021/np068054v] [PMID: 17309302]

[3] Lahlou M. The success of natural products in drug discovery. Pharmacol Pharm 2013; 4(3): 17-31.
[http://dx.doi.org/10.4236/pp.2013.43A003]

[4] Lahlou M. Screening of natural products for drug discovery. Expert Opin Drug Discov 2007; 2(5): 697-705.
[http://dx.doi.org/10.1517/17460441.2.5.697] [PMID: 23488959]

[5] Wilson RM, Danishefsky SJ. Small molecule natural products in the discovery of therapeutic agents: the synthesis connection. J Org Chem 2006; 71(22): 8329-51.
[http://dx.doi.org/10.1021/jo0610053] [PMID: 17064003]

[6] Wilson RM, Danishefsky SJ. Applications of total synthesis toward the discovery of clinically useful anticancer agents. Chem Soc Rev 2007; 36(8): 1207-26.
[http://dx.doi.org/10.1039/b611967k] [PMID: 17619682]

[7] Butler MS. The role of natural product chemistry in drug discovery. J Nat Prod 2004; 67(12): 2141-53.
[http://dx.doi.org/10.1021/np040106y] [PMID: 15620274]

[8] Newman DJ, Cragg GM, Snader KM. The influence of natural products upon drug discovery (Antiquity to late 1999). Nat Prod Rep 2000; 17(3): 215-34.
[http://dx.doi.org/10.1039/a902202c] [PMID: 10888010]

[9] Cragg GM, Pezzuto JM. Natural products as a vital source for the discovery of cancer chemotherapeutic and chemopreventive agents. Med Princ Pract 2016; 25(Suppl 2) (Suppl. 2): 41-59.
[http://dx.doi.org/10.1159/000443404] [PMID: 26679767]

[10] Clardy J, Walsh C. Lessons from natural molecules. Nature 2004; 432(7019): 829-37. [http://dx.doi.org/10.1038/nature03194] [PMID: 15602548]

[11] Cragg GM, Kingston DG, Newman DJ, Eds. Anticancer agents from natural products. Boca Raton: Taylor & Francis 2005. [http://dx.doi.org/10.1201/9781420039658]

[12] Müller-Kuhrt L. Putting nature back into drug discovery. Nat Biotechnol 2003; 21(6): 602-4. [http://dx.doi.org/10.1038/nbt0603-602] [PMID: 12776140]

[13] Tian H, Ip L, Luo H, Chang DC, Luo KQ. A high throughput drug screen based on fluorescence resonance energy transfer (FRET) for anticancer activity of compounds from herbal medicine. Br J Pharmacol 2007; 150(3): 321-34. [http://dx.doi.org/10.1038/sj.bjp.0706988] [PMID: 17179946]

[14] Nyambe MN, van de Venter M, Beukes DR, Swanepoel B, Smith N, Hlangothi B. Anticancer Activity of a Novel Flavonoid Capioglucoside from Albuca setosa Jacq.(Asparagaceae). FEBS Open Bio 2018; 8: 336-6.

[15] Younes RN, Varella AD, Suffredini IB. Discovery of new antitumoral and antibacterial drugs from brazilian plant extracts using high throughput screening. Clinics (São Paulo) 2007; 62(6): 763-8. [http://dx.doi.org/10.1590/S1807-59322007000600017] [PMID: 18318049]

[16] Pisha E, Chai H, Lee IS, *et al.* Discovery of betulinic acid as a selective inhibitor of human melanoma that functions by induction of apoptosis. Nat Med 1995; 1(10): 1046-51. [http://dx.doi.org/10.1038/nm1095-1046] [PMID: 7489361]

[17] Silva GL, Cui B, Chávez D, *et al.* Modulation of the multidrug-resistance phenotype by new tropane alkaloid aromatic esters from Erythroxylum pervillei. J Nat Prod 2001; 64(12): 1514-20. [http://dx.doi.org/10.1021/np010295+] [PMID: 11754602]

[18] Hwang BY, Su BN, Chai H, *et al.* Silvestrol and episilvestrol, potential anticancer rocaglate derivatives from Aglaia silvestris. J Org Chem 2004; 69(10): 3350-8. [http://dx.doi.org/10.1021/jo040120f] [PMID: 15132542]

[19] Chaitanya MVNL. Drug Discovery of Anticancer Agents from the Weeds of the Niligiris Using High Throughput Screening Techniques. Broadway Edmond, OK: MedCrave Group LLC 2016.

[20] Mazzio E, Badisa R, Mack N, Deiab S, Soliman KFA. High throughput screening of natural products for anti-mitotic effects in MDA-MB-231 human breast carcinoma cells. Phytother Res 2014; 28(6): 856-67. [http://dx.doi.org/10.1002/ptr.5065] [PMID: 24105850]

[21] Jin Y, Xu T, Zhao Y, Wang Y, Cui M. *In vitro* and *in vivo* anti-cancer activity of formononetin on human cervical cancer cell line HeLa. Tumour Biol 2014; 35(3): 2279-84. [http://dx.doi.org/10.1007/s13277-013-1302-1] [PMID: 24272199]

[22] Bugni TS, Richards B, Bhoite L, Cimbora D, Harper MK, Ireland CM. Marine natural product libraries for high-throughput screening and rapid drug discovery. J Nat Prod 2008; 71(6): 1095-8. [http://dx.doi.org/10.1021/np800184g] [PMID: 18505284]

[23] Sausville EA, Zaharevitz D, Gussio R, *et al.* Cyclin-dependent kinases: initial approaches to exploit a novel therapeutic target. Pharmacol Ther 1999; 82(2-3): 285-92. [http://dx.doi.org/10.1016/S0163-7258(98)00062-X] [PMID: 10454206]

[24] El-Menshawi BS, Fayad W, Mahmoud K, *et al.* Screening of natural products for therapeutic activity against solid tumors. Indian J Exp Biol 2010; 48(3): 258-64. [PMID: 21046978]

[25] Hedvat M, Emdad L, K, Das S, *et al.* Selected approaches for rational drug design and high throughput screening to identify anti-cancer molecules. Anti-Cancer Agents in Medicinal Chemistry 2012; 12(9): 1143-55.

[http://dx.doi.org/10.2174/187152012803529709]

[26] Yang H, Pinello CE, Luo J, *et al.* Small-molecule inhibitors of acetyltransferase p300 identified by high-throughput screening are potent anticancer agents. Mol Cancer Ther 2013; 12(5): 610-20. [http://dx.doi.org/10.1158/1535-7163.MCT-12-0930] [PMID: 23625935]

[27] Hassig CA, Zeng FY, Kung P, *et al.* Ultra-high-throughput screening of natural product extracts to identify proapoptotic inhibitors of Bcl-2 family proteins. SLAS Discov 2014; 19(8): 1201-11. [http://dx.doi.org/10.1177/1087057114536227] [PMID: 24870016]

[28] Lampe JW. Spicing up a vegetarian diet: chemopreventive effects of phytochemicals. Am J Clin Nutr 2003; 78(3) (Suppl.): 579S-83S. [http://dx.doi.org/10.1093/ajcn/78.3.579S] [PMID: 12936952]

[29] Mishra KP, Ganju L, Sairam M, Banerjee PK, Sawhney RC. A review of high throughput technology for the screening of natural products. Biomed Pharmacother 2008; 62(2): 94-8. [http://dx.doi.org/10.1016/j.biopha.2007.06.012] [PMID: 17692498]

[30] Szymański P, Markowicz M, Mikiciuk-Olasik E. Adaptation of high-throughput screening in drug discovery-toxicological screening tests. Int J Mol Sci 2011; 13(1): 427-52. [http://dx.doi.org/10.3390/ijms13010427] [PMID: 22312262]

[31] Pereira DA, Williams JA. Origin and evolution of high throughput screening. Br J Pharmacol 2007; 152(1): 53-61. [http://dx.doi.org/10.1038/sj.bjp.0707373] [PMID: 17603542]

[32] Martis EA, Radhakrishnan R, Badve RR. High-throughput screening: the hits and leads of drug discovery-an overview. J Appl Pharm Sci 2011; 1(1): 2-10.

[33] Armstrong JW. A review of high-throughput screening approaches for drug discovery. Am Biotechnol Lab 1999; 17(1): 26-8.

[34] Wildey MJ, Haunso A, Tudor M, Webb M, Connick JH. High-Throughput Screening. Annu Rep Med Chem 2017; 50: 149-95. [http://dx.doi.org/10.1016/bs.armc.2017.08.004]

[35] Mayr LM, Fuerst P. The future of high-throughput screening. SLAS Discov 2008; 13(6): 443-8. [http://dx.doi.org/10.1177/1087057108319644] [PMID: 18660458]

[36] Brandish PE, Chiu CS, Schneeweis J, *et al.* A cell-based ultra-high-throughput screening assay for identifying inhibitors of D-amino acid oxidase. SLAS Discov 2006; 11(5): 481-7. [http://dx.doi.org/10.1177/1087057106288181] [PMID: 16760370]

[37] Harvey A, Cree I. High-throughput screening of natural products for cancer therapy. Planta Med 2010; 76(11): 1080-6. [http://dx.doi.org/10.1055/s-0030-1250162] [PMID: 20635309]

[38] Schmid I, Sattler I, Grabley S, Thiericke R. Natural products in high throughput screening: automated high-quality sample preparation. SLAS Discov 1999; 4(1): 15-25. [http://dx.doi.org/10.1177/108705719900400104] [PMID: 10838408]

[39] Ismail FM, Nahar L, Sarker SD. High-Throughput Screening of Phytochemicals: Application of Computational Methods. Computational Phytochemistry 2018; 165-92.

[40] Maziasz T, Kadambi VJ, Silverman L, Fedyk E, Alden CL. Predictive toxicology approaches for small molecule oncology drugs. Toxicol Pathol 2010; 38(1): 148-64. [http://dx.doi.org/10.1177/0192623309356448] [PMID: 20075108]

[41] Buchdunger E, Zimmermann J, Mett H, *et al.* Inhibition of the Abl protein-tyrosine kinase *in vitro* and *in vivo* by a 2-phenylaminopyrimidine derivative. Cancer Res 1996; 56(1): 100-4. [PMID: 8548747]

[42] Carroll M, Ohno-Jones S, Tamura S, *et al.* CGP 57148, a tyrosine kinase inhibitor, inhibits the growth of cells expressing BCR-ABL, TEL-ABL, and TEL-PDGFR fusion proteins. Blood 1997; 90(12):

4947-52.
[http://dx.doi.org/10.1182/blood.V90.12.4947] [PMID: 9389713]

[43] Deininger MWN, Goldman JM, Lydon N, Melo JV. The tyrosine kinase inhibitor CGP57148B selectively inhibits the growth of BCR-ABL-positive cells. Blood 1997; 90(9): 3691-8.
[http://dx.doi.org/10.1182/blood.V90.9.3691] [PMID: 9345054]

[44] End DW. Farnesyl protein transferase inhibitors and other therapies targeting the Ras signal transduction pathway. Invest New Drugs 1999; 17(3): 241-58.
[http://dx.doi.org/10.1023/A:1006380320290] [PMID: 10665477]

[45] Sun L, Tran N, Liang C, *et al.* Identification of substituted 3-[(4,5,6, 7-tetrahydro-1H-indl-2-yl)methylene]-1,3-dihydroindol-2-ones as growth factor receptor inhibitors for VEGF-R2 (Flk-1/KDR), FGF-R1, and PDGF-Rbeta tyrosine kinases. J Med Chem 2000; 43(14): 2655-63.
[http://dx.doi.org/10.1021/jm9906116] [PMID: 10893303]

[46] Robinson DR, Wu YM, Lin SF. The protein tyrosine kinase family of the human genome. Oncogene 2000; 19(49): 5548-57.
[http://dx.doi.org/10.1038/sj.onc.1203957] [PMID: 11114734]

[47] Thornburg CC, Britt JR, Evans JR, *et al.* NCI program for natural product discovery: a publicly-accessible library of natural product fractions for high-throughput screening. ACS Chem Biol 2018; 13(9): 2484-97.
[http://dx.doi.org/10.1021/acschembio.8b00389] [PMID: 29812901]

[48] Becker RA, Chambers JMS. A language and system for data analysis bell laboratories computer information service. Murray Hill, New Jersey 1981.

[49] Shoemaker R, Scudiero D, Melillo G, *et al.* Application of high-throughput, molecular-targeted screening to anticancer drug discovery. Curr Top Med Chem 2002; 2(3): 229-46.
[http://dx.doi.org/10.2174/1568026023394317] [PMID: 11944818]

[50] Eglen RM, Reisine T. The current status of drug discovery against the human kinome. Assay Drug Dev Technol 2009; 7(1): 22-43.
[http://dx.doi.org/10.1089/adt.2008.164] [PMID: 19382888]

[51] Hartmann J, Haap M, Kopp HG, Lipp HP. Tyrosine kinase inhibitors - a review on pharmacology, metabolism and side effects. Curr Drug Metab 2009; 10(5): 470-81.
[http://dx.doi.org/10.2174/138920009788897975] [PMID: 19689244]

[52] Gautschi O, Heighway J, Mack PC, Purnell PR, Lara PN Jr, Gandara DR. Aurora kinases as anticancer drug targets. Clin Cancer Res 2008; 14(6): 1639-48.
[http://dx.doi.org/10.1158/1078-0432.CCR-07-2179] [PMID: 18347165]

[53] Ma H, Deacon S, Horiuchi K. The challenge of selecting protein kinase assays for lead discovery optimization. Expert Opin Drug Discov 2008; 3(6): 607-21.
[http://dx.doi.org/10.1517/17460441.3.6.607] [PMID: 19662101]

[54] Karaman MW, Herrgard S, Treiber DK, *et al.* A quantitative analysis of kinase inhibitor selectivity. Nat Biotechnol 2008; 26(1): 127-32.
[http://dx.doi.org/10.1038/nbt1358] [PMID: 18183025]

[55] Holder S, Zemskova M, Zhang C, *et al.* Characterization of a potent and selective small-molecule inhibitor of the PIM1 kinase. Mol Cancer Ther 2007; 6(1): 163-72.
[http://dx.doi.org/10.1158/1535-7163.MCT-06-0397] [PMID: 17218638]

[56] Hashimoto J, Watanabe T, Seki T, *et al.* Novel *in vitro* protein fragment complementation assay applicable to high-throughput screening in a 1536-well format. SLAS Discov 2009; 14(8): 970-9.
[http://dx.doi.org/10.1177/1087057109341406] [PMID: 19641222]

[57] Reindl W, Yuan J, Krämer A, Strebhardt K, Berg T. Inhibition of polo-like kinase 1 by blocking polo-box domain-dependent protein-protein interactions. Chem Biol 2008; 15(5): 459-66.
[http://dx.doi.org/10.1016/j.chembiol.2008.03.013] [PMID: 18482698]

[58] Sperl B, Seifert MHJ, Berg T. Natural product inhibitors of protein–protein interactions mediated by Src-family SH2 domains. Bioorg Med Chem Lett 2009; 19(12): 3305-9. [http://dx.doi.org/10.1016/j.bmcl.2009.04.083] [PMID: 19427202]

[59] Pommier Y. DNA topoisomerase I inhibitors: chemistry, biology, and interfacial inhibition. Chem Rev 2009; 109(7): 2894-902. [http://dx.doi.org/10.1021/cr900097c] [PMID: 19476377]

[60] Nitiss JL. Targeting DNA topoisomerase II in cancer chemotherapy. Nat Rev Cancer 2009; 9(5): 338-50. [http://dx.doi.org/10.1038/nrc2607] [PMID: 19377506]

[61] Johnston PA, Foster CA, Tierno MB, *et al.* Cdc25B dual-specificity phosphatase inhibitors identified in a high-throughput screen of the NIH compound library. Assay Drug Dev Technol 2009; 7(3): 250-65. [http://dx.doi.org/10.1089/adt.2008.186] [PMID: 19530895]

[62] Hammond E, Li CP, Ferro V. Development of a colorimetric assay for heparanase activity suitable for kinetic analysis and inhibitor screening. Anal Biochem 2010; 396(1): 112-6. [http://dx.doi.org/10.1016/j.ab.2009.09.007] [PMID: 19748475]

[63] Shelton CC, Tian Y, Shum D, Radu C, Djaballah H, Li YM. A miniaturized 1536-well format γ-secretase assay. Assay Drug Dev Technol 2009; 7(5): 461-70. [http://dx.doi.org/10.1089/adt.2009.0202] [PMID: 19715456]

[64] Huang H, Tanaka H, Hammock BD, Morisseau C. Novel and highly sensitive fluorescent assay for leucine aminopeptidases. Anal Biochem 2009; 391(1): 11-6. [http://dx.doi.org/10.1016/j.ab.2009.05.004] [PMID: 19433052]

[65] Hauser AT, Jung M, Jung M. Assays for histone deacetylases. Curr Top Med Chem 2009; 9(3): 227-34. [http://dx.doi.org/10.2174/156802609788085269] [PMID: 19355987]

[66] Hanahan D, Weinberg RA. The hallmarks of cancer. Cell 2000; 100(1): 57-70. [http://dx.doi.org/10.1016/S0092-8674(00)81683-9] [PMID: 10647931]

[67] Galluzzi L, Aaronson SA, Abrams J, *et al.* Guidelines for the use and interpretation of assays for monitoring cell death in higher eukaryotes. Cell Death Differ 2009; 16(8): 1093-107. [http://dx.doi.org/10.1038/cdd.2009.44] [PMID: 19373242]

[68] Hägg M, Bivén K, Ueno T, *et al.* A novel high-through-put assay for screening of pro-apoptotic drugs. Invest New Drugs 2002; 20(3): 253-9. [http://dx.doi.org/10.1023/A:1016249728664] [PMID: 12201488]

[69] Antczak C, Takagi T, Ramirez CN, Radu C, Djaballah H. Live-cell imaging of caspase activation for high-content screening. SLAS Discov 2009; 14(8): 956-69. [http://dx.doi.org/10.1177/1087057109343207] [PMID: 19726787]

[70] Shum D, Radu C, Kim E, *et al.* A high density assay format for the detection of novel cytotoxic agents in large chemical libraries. J Enzyme Inhib Med Chem 2008; 23(6): 931-45. [http://dx.doi.org/10.1080/14756360701810082] [PMID: 18608772]

[71] Auld DS, Southall NT, Jadhav A, *et al.* Characterization of chemical libraries for luciferase inhibitory activity. J Med Chem 2008; 51(8): 2372-86. [http://dx.doi.org/10.1021/jm701302v] [PMID: 18363348]

[72] Shoichet BK. Screening in a spirit haunted world. Drug Discov Today 2006; 11(13-14): 607-15. [http://dx.doi.org/10.1016/j.drudis.2006.05.014] [PMID: 16793529]

[73] Riss TL, Moravec RA. Use of multiple assay endpoints to investigate the effects of incubation time, dose of toxin, and plating density in cell-based cytotoxicity assays. Assay Drug Dev Technol 2004; 2(1): 51-62.

[http://dx.doi.org/10.1089/15406580432296631 5] [PMID: 15090210]

[74] Niles AL, Moravec RA, Riss TL. Multiplex caspase activity and cytotoxicity assays. Apoptosis and Cancer. 2008; pp. 151-62.

[75] Cen H, Mao F, Aronchik I, Fuentes RJ, Firestone GL. DEVD–NucView488: a novel class of enzyme substrates for real–time detection of caspase–3 activity in live cells. FASEB J 2008; 22(7): 2243-52. [http://dx.doi.org/10.1096/fj.07-099234] [PMID: 18263700]

[76] Halliwell B. Oxidative stress in cell culture: an under-appreciated problem? FEBS Lett 2003; 540(1-3): 3-6. [http://dx.doi.org/10.1016/S0014-5793(03)00235-7] [PMID: 12681474]

[77] Fernando A, Glaysher S, Conroy M, *et al.* Effect of culture conditions on the chemosensitivity of ovarian cancer cell lines. Anticancer Drugs 2006; 17(8): 913-9. [http://dx.doi.org/10.1097/01.cad.0000224445.23953.d9] [PMID: 16940801]

[78] Kawasaki BT, Hurt EM, Mistree T, Farrar WL. Targeting cancer stem cells with phytochemicals. Mol Interv 2008; 8(4): 174-84. [http://dx.doi.org/10.1124/mi.8.4.9] [PMID: 18829843]

[79] Desbordes SC, Placantonakis DG, Ciro A, *et al.* High-throughput screening assay for the identification of compounds regulating self-renewal and differentiation in human embryonic stem cells. Cell Stem Cell 2008; 2(6): 602-12. [http://dx.doi.org/10.1016/j.stem.2008.05.010] [PMID: 18522853]

[80] Thierbach R, Steinberg P. Automated soft agar assay for the high-throughput screening of anticancer compounds. Anal Biochem 2009; 387(2): 318-20. [http://dx.doi.org/10.1016/j.ab.2009.01.029] [PMID: 19454240]

[81] Budman DR, Calabro A, Kreis W. Synergistic and antagonistic combinations of drugs in human prostate cancer cell lines *in vitro.* Anticancer Drugs 2002; 13(10): 1011-6. [http://dx.doi.org/10.1097/00001813-200211000-00005] [PMID: 12439335]

[82] Larsson DE, Hassan S, Larsson R, Öberg K, Granberg D. Combination analyses of anti-cancer drugs on human neuroendocrine tumor cell lines. Cancer Chemother Pharmacol 2009; 65(1): 5-12. [http://dx.doi.org/10.1007/s00280-009-0997-6] [PMID: 19381631]

[83] Booth NL, Sayers TJ, Brooks AD, *et al.* A cell-based high-throughput screen to identify synergistic TRAIL sensitizers. Cancer Immunol Immunother 2009; 58(8): 1229-44. [http://dx.doi.org/10.1007/s00262-008-0637-8] [PMID: 19089423]

[84] Glaysher S, Clements C, Harvey AL, Cree IA. High throughput screening of potential anti-cancer agents in primary cell culture using an ATP based luminescence assay AACR 101st Annual meeting. Washington, DC. 2010.

[85] Milroy LG, Zinzalla G, Loiseau F, *et al.* Natural-product-like spiroketals and fused bicyclic acetals as potential therapeutic agents for B-cell chronic lymphocytic leukaemia. ChemMedChem 2008; 3(12): 1922-35. [http://dx.doi.org/10.1002/cmdc.200800265] [PMID: 19025736]

[86] Howes AL, Richardson RD, Finlay D, Vuori K. 3-Dimensional culture systems for anti-cancer compound profiling and high-throughput screening reveal increases in EGFR inhibitor-mediated cytotoxicity compared to monolayer culture systems. PLoS One 2014; 9(9): e108283. [http://dx.doi.org/10.1371/journal.pone.0108283] [PMID: 25247711]

[87] Tung YC, Hsiao AY, Allen SG, Torisawa Y, Ho M, Takayama S. High-throughput 3D spheroid culture and drug testing using a 384 hanging drop array. Analyst (Lond) 2011; 136(3): 473-8. [http://dx.doi.org/10.1039/C0AN00609B] [PMID: 20967331]

[88] Vinci M, Gowan S, Boxall F, *et al.* Advances in establishment and analysis of three-dimensional tumor spheroid-based functional assays for target validation and drug evaluation. BMC Biol 2012; 10(1): 29.

[http://dx.doi.org/10.1186/1741-7007-10-29] [PMID: 22439642]

[89] Mikhail AS, Eetezadi S, Allen C. Multicellular tumor spheroids for evaluation of cytotoxicity and tumor growth inhibitory effects of nanomedicines *in vitro*: a comparison of docetaxel-loaded block copolymer micelles and Taxotere®. PLoS One 2013; 8(4): e62630. [http://dx.doi.org/10.1371/journal.pone.0062630] [PMID: 23626842]

[90] Costa EC, Gaspar VM, Marques JG, Coutinho P, Correia IJ. Evaluation of nanoparticle uptake in co-culture cancer models. PLoS One 2013; 8(7): e70072. [http://dx.doi.org/10.1371/journal.pone.0070072] [PMID: 23922909]

[91] Burguera EF, Bitar M, Bruinink A. Novel *in vitro* co-culture methodology to investigate heterotypic cell-cell interactions. Eur Cell Mater 2010; 19(166): 166-79. [http://dx.doi.org/10.22203/eCM.v019a17] [PMID: 20419629]

[92] Duell BL, Cripps AW, Schembri MA, Ulett GC. Epithelial cell coculture models for studying infectious diseases: benefits and limitations. J Biomed Biotechnol 2011; 2011: 1-9. [http://dx.doi.org/10.1155/2011/852419] [PMID: 22007147]

[93] Hirschhaeuser F, Menne H, Dittfeld C, West J, Mueller-Klieser W, Kunz-Schughart LA. Multicellular tumor spheroids: An underestimated tool is catching up again. J Biotechnol 2010; 148(1): 3-15. [http://dx.doi.org/10.1016/j.jbiotec.2010.01.012] [PMID: 20097238]

[94] Fennema E, Rivron N, Rouwkema J, van Blitterswijk C, de Boer J. Spheroid culture as a tool for creating 3D complex tissues. Trends Biotechnol 2013; 31(2): 108-15. [http://dx.doi.org/10.1016/j.tibtech.2012.12.003] [PMID: 23336996]

[95] Kunz-Schughart LA, Freyer JP, Hofstaedter F, Ebner R. The use of 3-D cultures for high-throughput screening: the multicellular spheroid model. SLAS Discov 2004; 9(4): 273-85. [http://dx.doi.org/10.1177/1087057104265040] [PMID: 15191644]

[96] Friedrich J, Seidel C, Ebner R, Kunz-Schughart LA. Spheroid-based drug screen: considerations and practical approach. Nat Protoc 2009; 4(3): 309-24. [http://dx.doi.org/10.1038/nprot.2008.226] [PMID: 19214182]

[97] Herrmann R, Fayad W, Schwarz S, Berndtsson M, Linder S. Screening for compounds that induce apoptosis of cancer cells grown as multicellular spheroids. SLAS Discov 2008; 13(1): 1-8. [http://dx.doi.org/10.1177/1087057107310442] [PMID: 18040052]

[98] Hartman O, Zhang C, Adams EL, *et al.* Microfabricated electrospun collagen membranes for 3-D cancer models and drug screening applications. Biomacromolecules 2009; 10(8): 2019-32. [http://dx.doi.org/10.1021/bm8012764] [PMID: 19624098]

[99] Adanja I, Debeir O, Mégalizzi V, Kiss R, Warzée N, Decaestecker C. Automated tracking of unmarked cells migrating in three-dimensional matrices applied to anti-cancer drug screening. Exp Cell Res 2010; 316(2): 181-93. [http://dx.doi.org/10.1016/j.yexcr.2009.10.004] [PMID: 19835872]

[100] Lin WH, Song JS, Chang TY, *et al.* A cell-based high-throughput screen for epidermal growth factor receptor pathway inhibitors. Anal Biochem 2008; 377(1): 89-94. [http://dx.doi.org/10.1016/j.ab.2008.02.027] [PMID: 18358823]

[101] Farkas T, Høyer-Hansen M, Jäättelä M. Identification of novel autophagy regulators by a luciferase-based assay for the kinetics of autophagic flux. Autophagy 2009; 5(7): 1018-25. [http://dx.doi.org/10.4161/auto.5.7.9443] [PMID: 19652534]

[102] Vandenberghe I, Créancier L, Vispé S, *et al.* Physalin B, a novel inhibitor of the ubiquitin-proteasome pathway, triggers NOXA-associated apoptosis. Biochem Pharmacol 2008; 76(4): 453-62. [http://dx.doi.org/10.1016/j.bcp.2008.05.031] [PMID: 18577376]

[103] Ausseil F, Samson A, Aussagues Y, *et al.* High-throughput bioluminescence screening of ubiquitin-proteasome pathway inhibitors from chemical and natural sources. SLAS Discov 2007; 12(1): 106-16. [http://dx.doi.org/10.1177/1087057106296494] [PMID: 17175525]

[104] Taldone T, Sun W, Chiosis G. Discovery and development of heat shock protein 90 inhibitors. Bioorg Med Chem 2009; 17(6): 2225-35. [http://dx.doi.org/10.1016/j.bmc.2008.10.087] [PMID: 19017562]

[105] Galam L, Hadden MK, Ma Z, *et al.* High-throughput assay for the identification of Hsp90 inhibitors based on Hsp90-dependent refolding of firefly luciferase. Bioorg Med Chem 2007; 15(5): 1939-46. [http://dx.doi.org/10.1016/j.bmc.2007.01.004] [PMID: 17223347]

[106] Amolins M, Blagg B. Natural product inhibitors of Hsp90: potential leads for drug discovery. Mini Rev Med Chem 2009; 9(2): 140-52. [http://dx.doi.org/10.2174/138955709787316056] [PMID: 19200020]

[107] Nagle D, Zhou YD. Natural product-based inhibitors of hypoxia-inducible factor-1 (HIF-1). Curr Drug Targets 2006; 7(3): 355-69. [http://dx.doi.org/10.2174/138945006776054979] [PMID: 16515532]

[108] Sasiela CA, Stewart DH, Kitagaki J, *et al.* Identification of inhibitors for MDM2 ubiquitin ligase activity from natural product extracts by a novel high-throughput electrochemiluminescent screen. SLAS Discov 2008; 13(3): 229-37. [http://dx.doi.org/10.1177/1087057108315038] [PMID: 18270365]

[109] Goldstein DM, Gray NS, Zarrinkar PP. High-throughput kinase profiling as a platform for drug discovery. Nat Rev Drug Discov 2008; 7(5): 391-7. [http://dx.doi.org/10.1038/nrd2541] [PMID: 18404149]

[110] Kozielski F, DeBonis S, Skoufias DA. Screening for inhibitors of microtubule-associated motor proteins.Microtubule Protocols. Humana Press 2007; pp. 189-207. [http://dx.doi.org/10.1007/978-1-59745-442-1_14]

[111] Wang T, Zeng L, Strader T, Burton L, Kassel DB. A new ultra-high throughput method for characterizing combinatorial libraries incorporating a multiple probe autosampler coupled with flow injection mass spectrometry analysis. Rapid Commun Mass Spectrom 1998; 12(16): 1123-9. [http://dx.doi.org/10.1002/(SICI)1097-0231(19980831)12:16<1123::AID-RCM293>3.0.CO;2-W]

[112] Tutko DC, Henry KD, Winger BE, Stout H, Hemling M. Sequential mass spectrometry and MSn analyses of combinatorial libraries by using automated matrix-assisted laser desorption/ionization Fourier transform mass spectrometry. Rapid Commun Mass Spectrom 1998; 12(6): 335-8. [http://dx.doi.org/10.1002/(SICI)1097-0231(19980331)12:6<335::AID-RCM160>3.0.CO;2-T]

[113] Hajduk PJ, Burns DJ. Integration of NMR and high-throughput screening. Comb Chem High Throughput Screen 2002; 5(8): 613-21. [http://dx.doi.org/10.2174/1386207023329996] [PMID: 12470258]

[114] Ermer J, Vogel M. Applications of hyphenated LC-MS techniques in pharmaceutical analysis. Biomed Chromatogr 2000; 14(6): 373-83. [http://dx.doi.org/10.1002/1099-0801(200010)14:6<373::AID-BMC29>3.0.CO;2-S] [PMID: 11002275]

[115] Hassig CA, Zeng FY, Kung P, *et al.* Ultra-high-throughput screening of natural product extracts to identify proapoptotic inhibitors of Bcl-2 family proteins. SLAS Discov 2014; 19(8): 1201-11. [http://dx.doi.org/10.1177/1087057114536227] [PMID: 24870016]

[116] Gordaliza M. Natural products as leads to anticancer drugs. Clin Transl Oncol 2007; 9(12): 767-76. [http://dx.doi.org/10.1007/s12094-007-0138-9] [PMID: 18158980]

[117] Zhang L, He M, Zhang Y, Nilubol N, Shen M, Kebebew E. Quantitative high-throughput drug screening identifies novel classes of drugs with anticancer activity in thyroid cancer cells: opportunities for repurposing. J Clin Endocrinol Metab 2012; 97(3): E319-28. [http://dx.doi.org/10.1210/jc.2011-2671] [PMID: 22170715]

[118] Cragg GM, Newman DJ, Weiss RB. Coral reefs, forests, and thermal vents: The worldwide exploration of nature for novel antitumor agents. Seminars in oncology 24(2): 156-63.1997;

[119] Cragg GM, Newman DJ. Antineoplastic agents from natural sources: achievements and future directions. Expert Opin Investig Drugs 2000; 9(12): 2783-97.
[http://dx.doi.org/10.1517/13543784.9.12.2783] [PMID: 11093353]

[120] Roberge M, Cinel B, Anderson HJ, *et al.* Cell-based screen for antimitotic agents and identification of analogues of rhizoxin, eleutherobin, and paclitaxel in natural extracts. Cancer Res 2000; 60(18): 5052-8.
[PMID: 11016628]

CHAPTER 6

Anticancer Phytochemicals of 21st Century: A Multitargeted Approach and Role of Humanism in Oncology

Jubie Selvaraj[1,*], **Motamarri Venkata Naga Lalitha Chaitanya**[2], **Akey Krishna Swaroop**[1], **Prabha Thangavelu**[3] and **Rashmi Saxena Pal**[4]

[1] *Department of Pharmaceutical Chemistry, JSS College of Pharmacy, JSS Academy of Higher Education & Research, Ooty, The Nilgiris, Tamil Nadu, India*

[2] *School of Pharmacy, Lovely Professional University Phagwara, 144402 Punjab, India*

[3] *Department of Pharmaceutical Chemistry, Nandha College of Pharmacy, Affiliated to The Tamil Nadu Dr. MGR Medical University, Erode-638052, Tamil Nadu, India*

[4] *Department of Pharmacognosy, School of Pharmaceutical Sciences, Lovely Professional University, Phagwara, India*

Abstract: Unfortunately, we are living in a century where cancer has become an epidemic that is uncontrollable. Although the plant kingdom has been explored for cancer therapeutics due to its antimutagenic, antioxidant, antiproliferative, and alteration of the human immune system potential; these efforts are still underway due to inadequate knowledge of their biochemical mechanisms and molecular pathways. Phytochemicals exert anticancer activity due to their agonistic and antagonistic potentials on different proteins and enzymes involved in the molecular pathways of cancer. This classical phytotherapy treatment has various pitfalls, such as resistance, side effects, and a lack of target specificity. Because of the target-specificity effects, traditional phytotherapy does not distinguish tumour cells from normal cells. A multitargeted approach, in which a single phytochemical act on different points of the same signalling cascade, plays an important role in this regard. Polypharmacology, system biology, and networking pharmacology are the different terminologies to use to explain in detail the multitargeting approach. Classical phytotherapy is replaced with this multitargeted approach where different "omics" such as genomics, epigenomics, transcriptomics, proteomics, metabolomics, and various cytogenic technologies are involved. In this chapter, the various multitargeted approaches involved in cancer therapy and the phytochemicals that were prominent in cancer prevention in the 21st century have been explained. At the end of the chapter, the holistic approach to the treatment of oncology has also been emphasized.

* **Corresponding author Jubie Selvaraj:** Department of Pharmaceutical Chemistry, JSS College of Pharmacy, JSS Academy of Higher Education & Research, Ooty, The Nilgiris, Tamil Nadu, India; E-mail: jubie@jssuni.edu.in

Motamarri Venkata Naga Lalitha Chaitanya, Galvina Pereira, & Heyam Saad Ali (Eds.)

Keywords: Cancer, Cytogenic technologies, Genomics, Holistic approach, Humanism, Multi targeting, Networking pharmacology, Oncology, Omics, Pathways, Phytochemicals, Polypharmacology, Phytotherapy, System biology, Targets.

INTRODUCTION

In today's world, maybe they are on the path to success, but in fact, there is so much that is out of our control today, and one thing is cancer [1]. Cancer is a community of diseases that alter and spread because of the physiological and metabolic imbalance of cells in the human body. Most cancer cell types eventually form a lump or mass known as a tumor, which is named after the body part where the tumour is located. One of the most multidimensional and complex diseases in the world is cancer, which is a non-communicable disease. Until 2018, the death rate was 9.6 million, and new cases were 18.1 million. According to the WHO, this global disease will be doubled by 2040 (10.108). The primary causes of cancer are environmental (90–95%) and genetic (5–10%), as well as some other lifestyle factors such as the consumption of alcohol, smoking, and junk food. More than 277 cancer types (including prostate, breast, lung, colon, rectum, bronchus, and urinary bladder cancer, *etc.*) have been identified and diagnosed until now. The subtyping of cancer (Fig. **1**) is essential for an enhanced understanding of this complex disease, its diagnosis, and treatment. Cancer disrupts cell connectivity and signaling, which leads to critical gene malfunction. It is a multi-stage process in humans that mimics genetic changes responsible for cancer progression and malignancy [2].

Cancer is now recognised as a multifactorial disorder rather than a single-factor disease [3]. While cancer cells have a complex cellular machinery, the most significant barriers to cancer treatment are cancer tissue regeneration and chemical resistance. This allows researchers to study the widespread use of current drugs in complementary and safe treatment methods to resolve problems in chemotherapy. A multidisciplinary approach with multiple ways of addressing multiple changes in cell signalling machinery that controls expansion, motility, and survival is a viable option [4]. The use of complementary medicines, particularly herbal supplements, is common in cancer patients [5]. Many patients believe that the use of "natural" medicine is efficient and safe.

Since there are many negative effects of anticancer drugs of synthetic origin, it is urgently important to develop safe compounds. In recent years, secondary plant metabolites have become more significant because they may have fewer harmful effects. For many years, oncologists have understood that today's conventional cancer treatment has taken a more individual approach using multiple modalities

[5]. Cancer-friendly agents are more effective in cancer control with multiple targets than agents targeting individual pathways [2]. It is incorrect to say that cancer is incurable, but breast cancer patients also have a very high mortality rate.

Most breast cancers start in the breast tissue of the milk-producing gland, called lobules, or in the conduits connecting the lobules with the nipple. There are fatty, connective, and lymphatic tissues in the majority of the breast [6]. According to the WHO, breast cancer is the most common cancer in women, affecting millions of women worldwide. It is also an advertisement factor. However, because of screening, early detection, sensitivity, and constantly improving care, the death rate has steadily declined since 1990. Age, sex, prosperity, family history, breast disorders, alcohol intake, and obesity are some of the main risk factors for breast cancer [7].

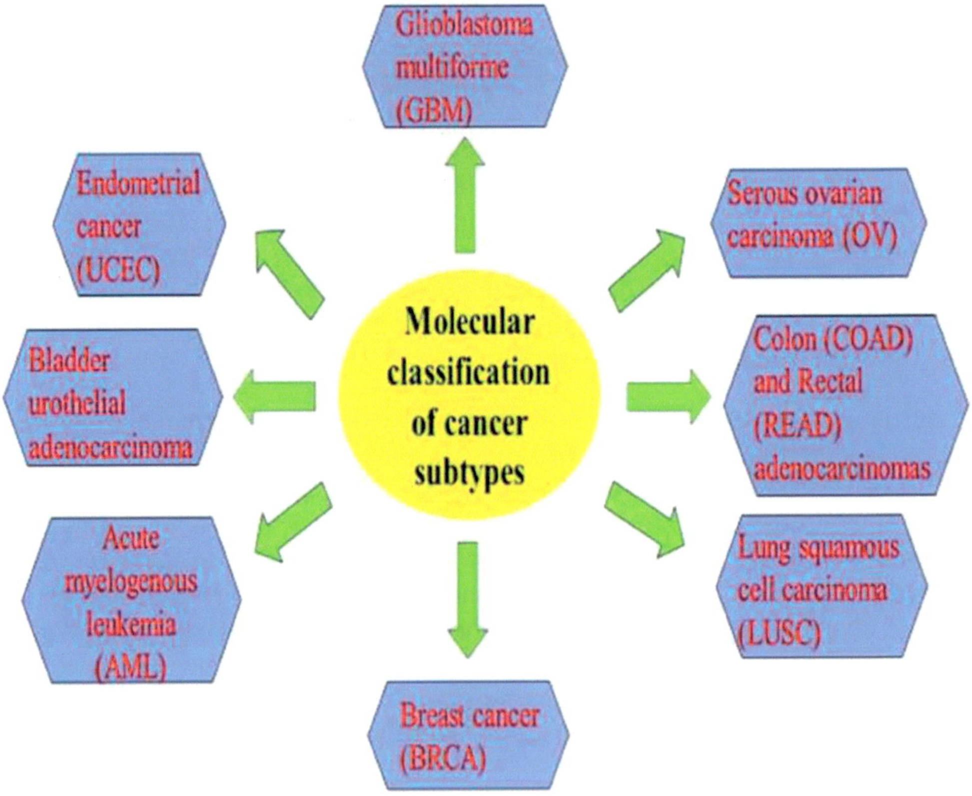

Fig. (1). Molecular Classification of Cancer Subtypes.

The primary cause of cancer was thought to be a variety of mutations throughout various cancer genes, mainly classified as tumour suppressor genes, oncogenes, and stability genes. These genes communicate with various characteristics of cancer advancement, including receptor tyrosine kinases (RTKs), serine/threonine kinases (STKs), tumour suppressor protein (p53), base excision repair (BER), chromosomal instability (CIN), DNA mismatch repair (MMR), nucleotide excision repair (NER), adenomatous polyposis coli (APC), apoptosis (APOP), zinc, finger protein (GLI), hypoxia-inducible factor 1 (HIF1), phosphoinositide 3-kinase (PI3K), and retinoblastoma tumour suppressor gene (RB) [4]. There are various smart reporting network signalling types that can be targeted therapeutically to promote tumorigenesis and tumour progression (Fig. **2**).

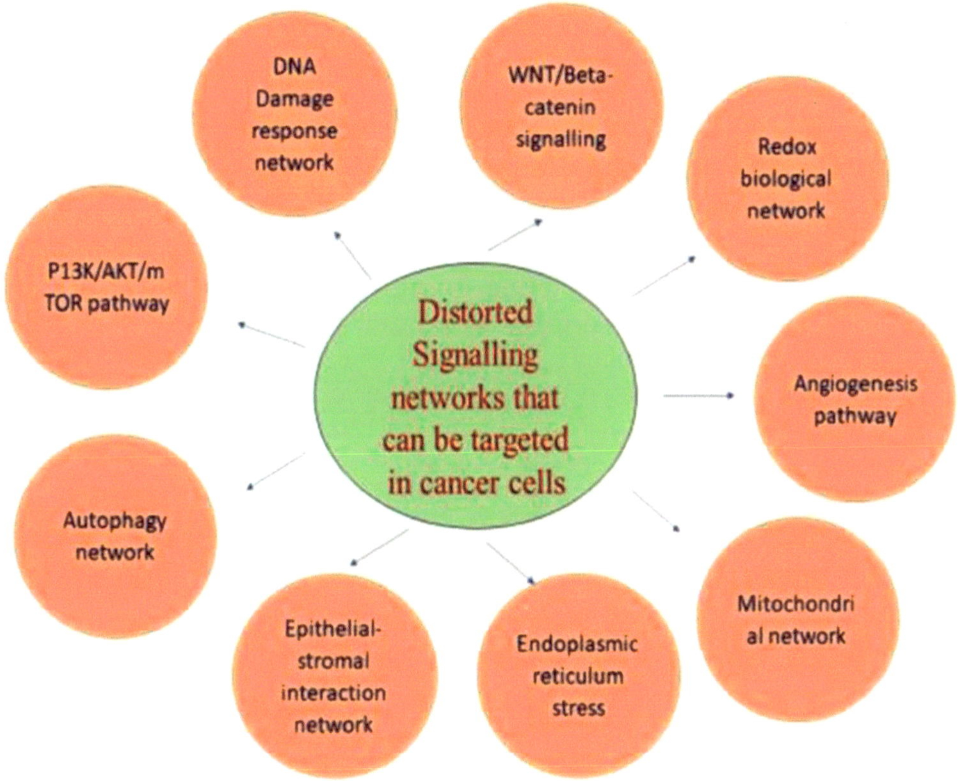

Fig. (2). Altered signalling networks aimed at cells of cancer

APPROACH TO MULTI-DRUG TARGETING

Multi-target lead discovery is one of the newly developed combination therapeutics to identify unexpected new drug combination effects. Besides, traditional drugs and remedies often contain multi-component natural product extracts [8]. Many strategies for drug production are designed to complement multiple targets. Combined therapy for many diseases, such as AIDS, atherosclerosis, cancer, and depression, are some of the most popular multitarget approaches. Ideally, the effect or expression of several proteins contributing to illness is re-balanced with a multi-target epidrug instead of abolishing a single protein that dramatically affects cell pathways or network functions [3].

An approach that is multi-targeted requires either partial inhibition or reduction of chosen goals in the direction it is targeted. Interference in the natural direction of a signalling pathway can increase the effectiveness of its inherent effects, reinforcing multi-target strategies. Tumor cells resist pharmacological treatment. When cancer occurs, the tumour begins to grow again, and the patient is called relapsed. On the other hand, stromal cells, which are standard, seldom undergo genomic mutations and have a significant reduction in the chances of being resistant to medicines when compared to cancer cells. Therefore, the repetition problem should be reduced by multi-target agents directed against host cells [9]. The mixture of two and more molecules unique to various enzymes results in most of the multi-target epi medications. Merging could be achieved by connecting atoms to a linker that is closed in physiological (pro-drug) conditions or to a secure linker to allow the single aspect of the medication to interfere with its particular intent without interfering in principle with the interaction of its counterpart. Multitargeted epi-drugs may contain molecules influencing one or more epigenetic enzymes, or they may control one cancer-related epi-enzyme and its targets. The compounds of a multi-target epi-medicine may influence symphonic on the same or various routes and thus increase their therapeutic impact in diseases where therapeutic resistance is achieved, at least on a conceptual level.

The creation of a multi-target drug may yield a medication that interacts with a lower affinity target than a single-target drug because it is impossible that a small drug molecule can similarly bind to several other objectives. In multi-target medicines, a smaller prevalence and reduced number occur compared to the greater affinity of single-target medicines [3]. LCS-101 is a botanical multitargeted formula for cancer treatment. LCS-101 is composed of 14 biologically active constituents. It affects the immune system, has anticancer effects, and enhances the symptoms and quality of life associated with chemotherapy [5]. Natural pleiotropic products are one of the most successful and promising strategies because they target multiple targets and have fewer side effects. Some of them are shown in Table **1**.

Table 1. Plant constituents with multi-targeting effects in cancer

Plant Name	Constituents	Multi-Target molecules	References
Tinospora cardifolia	Berberine	JNK, P38, Wnt, Beta-catenin	[1]
Centella asiatica	Asiaticoside	MAP Kinase, apoptosis, P38	[2]
Ziziphus nummularia	Betulin, betulinic acid	MAP kinase, P53, CD95	[3]
Curcuma longa	Curcumin	EGFR, HER2, Tyrosine kinase, serine/threonine kinase	[4]
Phyllanthus amarus	Phyllanthin, nirtetralin, phyltetralin	MAP Kinase, Wnt, P13k/AKT	[5]
Annona squamosa	Acetogenin	Downregulation of Antiapoptotic, caspase 3 activity	[6]
Eclipta prostrata	Terthiophenes	Apoptotic, autophagic cell death	[7]
Abrus precatorius	Abrin	P53, p21, apoptosis through the mitochondrial pathway	[8]
Tephrosia sinapou	Tephrosin	Mainly used in skin cancer and hepatocellular cancer	[9]
Uncaria guianensis	Oxindole alkaloids	Apoptosis, immunomodulatory, cytotoxic effects.	[10]
Mappia foetida	Camptothecin	DNA topoisomerase 1	[11]
Withania somnifera	Withaferin-A, Withanlide-A	Apoptosis, VEGF, stress response	[12]
Cedrus deodara	Methairesinol, Dibenzyl butylrolactol	Apoptosis, inhibits cell proliferation	[13]
Boswellia serrata	Beta boswellic acid, acetyl-1--keto-beta-boswellic acid.	Caspase leading to PARP cleavage, loss of mitochondrial membrane, oxidative stress	[14]
Brassica sp	Sulphoraphane	Inhibits tumour growth in breast cancer, antiproliferative effects.	[15]
Taxus brevefolia	Paclitaxel	Disruption of spindle formation, block mitosis, microtubule polymerization	[16]
Podophyllum peltatum	Epipodophyllotoxin	Proapoptotic effects, cell cycle interference	[17]
Catharanthus roseus	Vincristine, Vinblastine	Hodgkin's leukaemia, Beta-tubulin, microtubule inhibitors.	[18]
Maclura pomifera	Pomiferin	DNA fragmentation, oxidative damage of DNA, inhibits histone deacetylases.	[19]
Catechin	Epigallocatechin-3-gallate	Kinases, oxidative stress	[20]

(Table 1) cont.....

Plant Name	Constituents	Multi-Target molecules	References
Combretum caffrum	Combretastatin A-4 phosphate	The vascular shutdown of tumours, angiogenesis	[21]
Rafphanus sativus	Roscovitine	Inhibition of cyclin kinase-dependent kinases	[22]
Dysoxylum binectariferum	Flavoperidol	Immunomodulator effect, Tyrosine kinase activity	[23]
Papaver somniferum	Noscapine	Microtubule interfering, antiproliferative property	[24]
Artemisinin annuna	Dihydroartemisinin	MAP kinases, cell division protein kinases, Janus kinases.	[25]
Boerhaavia diffusa	Boeravinone b, punarnavin	Inhibits S phase of the cell cycle, antioxidant	[26]
Andrographis panuculate	andrographolide	Tumor suppressor proteins P53, P21, cell cycle arrest G2/M phase.	[15]
Azadirachta indica	Azadirachtin	P53, pTEN genes, angiogenesis, VEGF	[16]
Acacia catechu	Catechin	Apoptosis, caspase activity	[16]
Aloe barbadensis	Aloin, barbaloin	P53, Bcl-2, apoptosis	[16]

NETWORK PHARMACOLOGY APPROACHES

The pharmacological network has become a powerful instrument for revealing complicated biological relations. The created data group of parameters helps establish networks between genomics and metabolomics to identify molecular activities in ailments. A single target intervention has been proven ineffective to fight complex systemic conditions that harbour solid biological networks, such as cancer.

In such instances, pharmacological network approaches are highly useful because of their ability to target a large number of protective networks or networks involved in the disease, which is different from conventional drug discovery [10]. The multi-target consequences of the active drug and the conceptual evaluation of biological network properties established a new paradigm called poly-pharmacology [11]. Some of the approaches and suggestions in network pharmacology were shown in Fig. (**3**).

One of the most evidence-based network approaches to recommending targeted cancer therapies is the CDG network (cancer-drug-gene network). CDGnet is a user-friendly computer interface that extends the spectrum of treatment options tailored for cancer patients who receive molecular profiling by presenting pathway information in the biological sense. CDGnet explicitly considers biological pathway data from targets or biomarkers downstream of oncogenes and is tailored to individual patients based on user feedback, molecular changes, and cancer type.

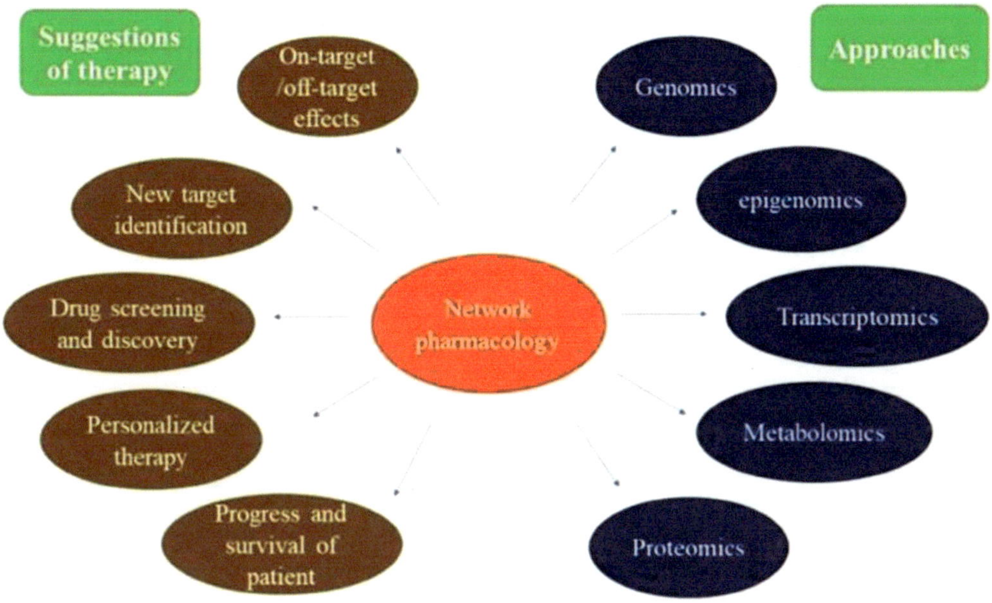

Fig. (3). Approaches and suggestions of network pharmacology

It integrates a variety of different knowledge sources: patient-specific input, the US Food and Drug Administration's (DailyMed) approved therapies, pathways for a specific type of cancer (the Kyoto Encyclopedia of Genomics and Genomes (KEGG)), gene-drug links (the Drug Bank) and oncological information (KEG). It combines knowledge from various sources (including KEGG). CDGnet offers a collection of readily accessible and useful findings that separate the categories of targeted cancer treatments into evidence-based categories that integrate knowledge about biological pathways [12].

CANCER THERAPY THROUGH MULTITARGETING

As a consequence of the participation of adverse sites in target-specific treatment, several multitasking drugs have been documented for their unwanted properties. In 2015–2017, 21 percent of the multitargeted drugs were licenced as primarily anti-infectious and antineoplastic agents for use in the classification of anatomical therapeutic chemicals (ATC) [22]. Multi-targeted drugs not only show multiple pathways of cancer but also exhibit one pathway related to cancer and another pathway that may have anti-inflammatory, anti-oxidant, anti-mitotic, or antibiotic effects. This chapter discusses natural compounds that have antioxidant, immune-boosting, antimitotic, anti-inflammatory, antibiotic, and anti-carcinogenic properties. The researchers focused on treating cancer with infection, inflammation, and a high degree of free radicals. In cancer treatment, which is primarily responsible for the role of the genes in this underlying pathology and can be viewed as multitasking cancer treatment targets, multi-target encounters with anti-inflammatory, antioxidant, and antibiotics, and anti-mitotic effects. This work is aimed at treating cancer with infection, inflammation, and a high degree of free radicals [4].

CORRELATION OF ANTICANCER COMPOUNDS WITH ANTI-INFLAMMATORY, ANTIOXIDANT, ANTIBIOTIC AND ANTIMITOTIC DRUGS

The role of the primary responsible genes in the underlying pathways is attempted to be understood, which can be thought of as multi-target therapies in cancer, anti-inflammatory antioxidants, antibiotics, and anti-mitotics. We first investigated the function and usage of the mechanisms of anti-inflammatory, antioxidant, antibiotic, and antimitotic drugs in alleviating cancer [4]. They are mainly used to explore the role of cancer with anti-inflammatory, anti-oxidant, antibiotic, and anti-mitotic activity by using a multitargeting drug approach. Here we explain four categories, which are shown in Fig. (**4**). The inflammatory cytokines are mainly IL-6, IL-8, IL-10, TNF-alpha, interferon-gamma, STAT-3 (signal transducer and activator of transcription), macrophage inflammatory protein (MIP), macrophage colony-stimulating factor (M-CSF), and vascular endothelial growth factor (VEGF). For the role of cancer and inflammation, the mainly used multi-target drugs are salicin, gingerol, prostaglandin, celecoxib, and valdecoxib [23]. The second category is of anti-oxidants, which are used to prevent the generation of free radicals like superoxide ions, hydrogen peroxide (H2O2), and hydroxyl ions (OH-). For the role of cancer and antioxidants, the drugs that are mainly used are quercetin, kaempferol, myricetin, selenium, and vitamin E [24]. The next category are antibiotics, which are azithromycin, methotrexate, doxycycline, and tigecycline, which block protein synthesis in the cell wall [25]. And the final category is anti-mitotic, which are mainly stabilising and destabilising agents of the microtubule. For the roles of anti-mitotic and cancer, drugs mainly used for multi-targeting are taxol, taxanes, vinblastine, and epothilones [26].

Role of Antioxidants in Cancer Therapy

The protection of our body against free radicals produced by endogenous and exogenous stimuli like medication, radiation, pollutants, and cigarette smoking is essential and is majorly done by antioxidant compounds. Because cancer cells multiply quickly, they have a high metabolic rate, which increases the intracellular cell environment of reactive oxygen species (ROS) [27]. Combination therapy with radiation and other synthetic cancer compounds has also been investigated with antioxidants. Research by Albanes *et al.* has shown that antioxidants can prevent excess ROS, suppress tumours, selectively destroy cancer cells, and stop cancer cell line progression [28]. Studies have also demonstrated the use of natural agents to target ROS accumulation, which can destroy cancer cells selectively and keep normal cells healthy *via* apoptosis and cell death. They are said to work by chelating ROS and maintaining the body's redox balance [24]. Cell organelles are preserved against chronic oxidative stress by antioxidants including superoxide dismutase, glutathione, and catalase [29].

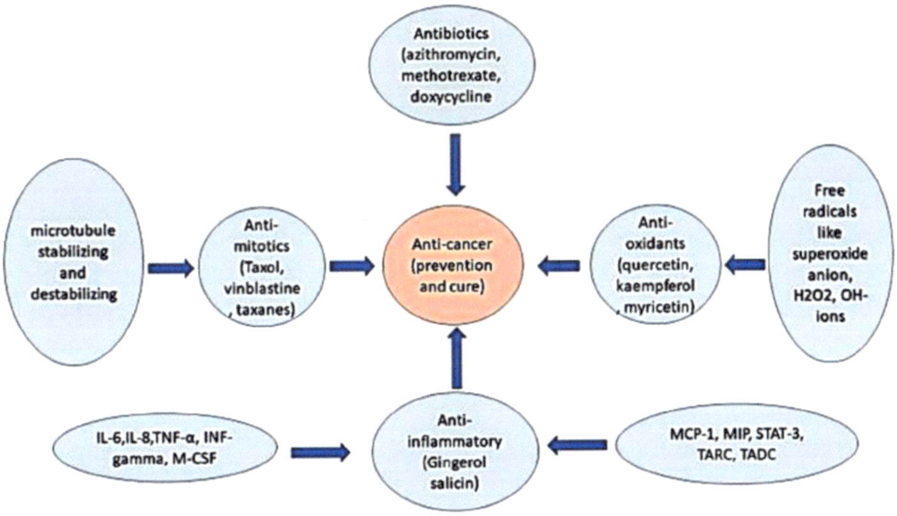

Fig. (4). A multidisciplinary strategy for preventing and treating cancer by the application of anti-inflammatory, antioxidants, antimitotic and antibiotics.

Role of Anti-inflammatory Agents in Cancer

The role of pro-inflammatory mediators in understanding the connection between inflammation and cancer is included in the mechanics of tissue wounds and their repair. Chemicals, biologics, and irritants that cause inflammation of the tissue can lead to cancer. Chronic inflammation is the first site for the growth of cancer, according to Virchow's hypothesis. The inflammatory process involves the aggregation of platelets at the tissue injury stage, plug formation, platelet release, and vasoactive amines [30]. This causes an accumulation of serum fibrinogenic factors as well as chemotactic factors such as platelets. These factors play a major role in the initiation of granular tissue and pathways for repair. Carcinogens recruit inflammatory mediators directly or indirectly and increase ROS generation. ROS changes DNA irreversibly, resulting in cancer promotion [31]. Cancer is caused by signalling pathways and inflammatory intermediate products. Cytokines can restore normal inflammation. The weakened DNA cannot regulate chronic inflammation, however. The cell loses control over cellular activity, directly leading to cancer initiation [30]. The combination of both COX and EGFR inhibitors resulted in lower doses of cancer reduction than in previous trials and literature reviews. Indole, isoquinoline, quinazoline, and piperidine are naturally occurring alkaloids with COX-2 inhibitory activity, which is important in tumour development [4].

Antibiotics and Anticancer Compounds

The mechanism of antibiotic activity depends on the chemical structure, its affinity for cell organelles, and its site concentration. They are the primary medications used in the treatment of cancer. Mitochondria are the leading cell organelles involved in inflammation and apoptosis control during bacterial infection [32, 33].

Antibiotics that specifically affect mitochondria can effectively eradicate infectious diseases such as cancer [4]. Bacterial mitochondria are affected by aminoglycosides, tetracyclines, and erythromycin, and researchers have tested them for their anti-cancer action. Azithromycin, an erythromycin group derivative, binds to the mitochondrial ribosome subunit 50S and obstructs mRNA transmission in protein synthesis. In 2015, Lamb used this tool to control its cancer activity on cell lines MCF7 and T47D. At 50 mM concentration, azithromycin inhibited mammosphere formation in MCF7 cells. Lung, pancreas, breast, melanoma, and ovarian lines of cancer cells with concentrations of 250mm were also inhibited [25].

Antimitotics and Anticancer Compounds

Drug-class antibiotics can be used at some cell cycle levels. In cancer chemotherapy, bioactive compounds used as antimitotics are also unique to cells, such as vinflunine, vinorelbine, and eribulin [34]. These medications primarily inhibit microtubular polymerizations, which are a component of mitosis spindle proteins. This causes mitosis to be blocked by activating spindle control points from the metaphase to the anaphase stage [27, 35]. The microtubule stabilisation agents work by activating polymerization and preventing the depolymerization of the compounds taxanes and eribulin caused by cold or calcium [36]. Antimitosis targets four steps, including the target cell cycle, spindle mounting, apoptosis, and autophagy. Also reported as drug targets for antimitotics during mitosis are checkpoint kinases (Chk) and cyclin-dependent kinases (Cdk1) [37]. The damage to DNA results in the activation of control point kinases, resulting in cell cycle arrest and the remedial repair of the damage. Centrosome maturation and spindle formation during mitosis are involved in Cdk1/cyclin B, which is activated by Ser/Thr polo-like kinases [38].

CADD IN MULTITARGETED APPROACH

The polypharmacology approach is a concept in drug discovery where a drug with multiple targets and off-target effects may offer multiple mechanisms of action [39]. The molecular docking approach plays a crucial role in structural-based virtual screening based on the free binding energies, predicts ligand binding, and estimates how the molecules can inhibit the target protein [40].

DHA is an antimalarial drug synthesised by artemisinin, an active agent found in the Artemisia annua plant in China. It's among the first-line antimalarial drugs on the World Health Organization's (WHO) recommendations. Previous studies have demonstrated that DHA possesses remarkable and selective anticancer activity with minimal or no cytotoxic effect on normal cells. Numerous studies have shown that DHA inhibits the growth and metastasis of numerous human cancers, including hepatocellular carcinoma, laryngeal carcinoma, breast, ovarian, bladder, gastric, head and neck squamous, cervical, prostate, esophageal, colon, lung, and leukemia. A sesquiterpene lactone molecule (Fig. **5**) that has interesting features contains a three-cyclic ring system with an oxepane bridge [21].

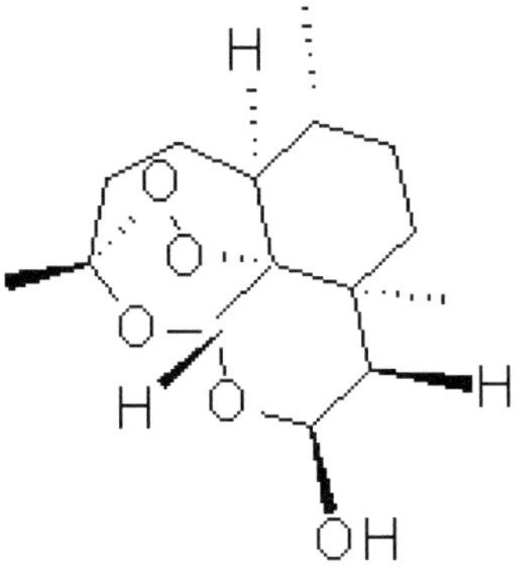

Fig. (5). Structure of DHA

DHA binds human protein kinases to ATP binding sites like mitogen-activated protein kinases; molecular docking studies on human MAPK1, MAPK8, MAPK10, MAPK14, and MAPKAPK2 confirmed the predictions in the presence of DHA. The MAP kinases were then predicted to bind DHA [41]. The molecular docking of DHA at the CDK2 ATP-binding sites was estimated at the lowest concentration of 5.82 mM at 7.14 kcal. Mol-1 binds free energy [21]. c) Janus kinase (JAKs), JAK2, and JAK3 are essential to the survival of cancer cells; among the members of the Janus kinase family, DHA was estimated at 1.52 kcal mol1 (1.52 mM) and 2.42 kcal mol1 (2.41 mM), respectively, to bind to JAK2 and JAK3 [42]. DHA was estimated to bind at the ATP site of c-Scr at 6.95 kcal mol1 in proto-oncogene tyrosine protein kinases [43].e) Heat shock protein 90, or HS90, is a molecular chaperone that contributes to the development and survival of cancer and is thus targeted for carcinogenic therapy; the affinity of Hsp90 for DHA has been measured at 6.81 kcal/mol [44]. The structural-based virtual studies indicate potential antitumor properties of DHA as a whole [21].

ROLE OF HUMANISM IN ONCOLOGY

Novel holistic approaches for upcoming therapy resistance in cancers involve the design of a computational multi-targeted drug. One of the novel approaches is network pharmacology which offers new solutions for a holistic approach. The holistic computational analysis involves certain pathways which are genetic and epigenetic that support the resistance. Network biology and polypharmacology holistic approaches can qualify pharmacology as an appropriate drug development tool for complex diseases, for example, cancer. Thus, the pharmacology network consolidates its position in the medicine of cancer.

The holistic approach of herbal medicine can often not be satisfactorily explored using western medicine and reductionist scientific methods [10]. The team offers a holistic needs assessment (HNA) in the role of humanism in oncology for all newly-referred patients. Worry, anxiety, fear, memory and concentration problems, difficulty making plans, anger or a sense of guilt, sadness, and depression, sexual concerns, housing or financial concerns, caring responsibilities, feelings of hopelessness, loneliness, and isolation, and regrets about the past are some of the holistic needs [45].

Holistic cancer care is an integral part of inclusive care [46]. The holistic care of cancer patients requires extensive screening for supportive care needs [47]. People need to live with and beyond cancer to meet their individual needs in a holistic and patient-centered way [48]. A critical unmet need is a holistic care that incorporates physical needs, such as recovery from treatment effects and response to recurrence risk factors, as well as other needs of the body and spirit [49, 50]. The next phases of your cancer journey are often not known to patients and survivors, and holistic care becomes an increasingly important approach [50]. Evidence to support holistic care shows that there is a lack of evidence for post-treatment services in empirical research [51]. Bloomhill Cancer Care (BCC) is a holistic, comprehensive treatment model [50]. A team strategy takes a holistic approach to the child's treatment, creating resilience through the child's family support system [52]. It offers much-needed results on the provision of care in an integrated comprehensive cancer system, guarantees the service is delivered to patients as evidence-based treatments, and helps obtain grants and assistance outside the government.

REFERENCES

[1] Dubey AK, Gupta U, Jain S. Breast cancer statistics and prediction methodology: a systematic review and analysis. Asian Pac J Cancer Prev 2015; 16(10): 4237-45. [http://dx.doi.org/10.7314/APJCP.2015.16.10.4237] [PMID: 26028079]

[2] Ikram N, Mirza MU, Vanmeert M, *et al.* Inhibition of oncogenic kinases: An *in vitro* validated computational approach identified potential multi-target anticancer compounds. Biomolecules 2019; 9(4): 124. [http://dx.doi.org/10.3390/biom9040124] [PMID: 30925835]

[3] Benedetti R, Conte M, Iside C, Altucci L. Epigenetic-based therapy: From single- to multi-target approaches. Int J Biochem Cell Biol 2015; 69: 121-31. [http://dx.doi.org/10.1016/j.biocel.2015.10.016] [PMID: 26494003]

[4] Kumar MS, Adki KM. Marine natural products for multi-targeted cancer treatment: A future insight. Biomed Pharmacother 2018; 105(May): 233-45. [http://dx.doi.org/10.1016/j.biopha.2018.05.142] [PMID: 29859466]

[5] Maimon Y, Samuels N, Cohen Z, Berger R, Rosenthal DS. Botanical Formula LCS101: A Multi-Targeted Approach to Cancer Care. Integr Cancer Ther 2018; 17(4): 1020-6. [http://dx.doi.org/10.1177/1534735418801528] [PMID: 30303021]

[6] Facts BC. Cancer 2000; 8(2): 55-7.

[7] Singletary SE. Rating the risk factors for breast cancer. Ann Surg 2003; 237(4): 474-82. [http://dx.doi.org/10.1097/01.SLA.0000059969.64262.87] [PMID: 12677142]

[8] Korcsmáros T, Szalay MS, Böde C, Kovács IA, Csermely P. Multitarget Drug Are Often Low Affinity Binderspdf. Expert Opin Drug Discov 2007; 2: 1-10.

[9] Petrelli A, Valabrega G. Multitarget drugs: the present and the future of cancer therapy. Expert Opin Pharmacother 2009; 10(4): 589-600. [http://dx.doi.org/10.1517/14656560902781907] [PMID: 19284362]

[10] Poornima P, Kumar JD, Zhao Q, Blunder M, Efferth T. Network pharmacology of cancer: From understanding of complex interactomes to the design of multi-target specific therapeutics from nature. Pharmacol Res 2016; 111: 290-302. [http://dx.doi.org/10.1016/j.phrs.2016.06.018] [PMID: 27329331]

[11] Hopkins AL. Network pharmacology: the next paradigm in drug discovery. Nat Chem Biol 2008; 4(11): 682-90. [http://dx.doi.org/10.1038/nchembio.118] [PMID: 18936753]

[12] Kancherla J, Rao S, Bhuvaneshwar K, *et al.* Evidence-Based Network Approach to Recommending Targeted Cancer Therapies. JCO Clin Cancer Inform 2020; 4(4): 71-88. [http://dx.doi.org/10.1200/CCI.19.00097] [PMID: 31990579]

[13] Palmieri A, Scapoli L, Iapichino A, *et al.* Berberine and *Tinospora cordifolia* exert a potential anticancer effect on colon cancer cells by acting on specific pathways. Int J Immunopathol Pharmacol 2019; 33 [http://dx.doi.org/10.1177/2058738419855567] [PMID: 31663444]

[14] Liu YT, Chuang YC, Lo YS, *et al.* Asiatic acid, extracted from centella asiatica and induces apoptosis pathway through the phosphorylation p38 mitogen-activated protein kinase in cisplatin-resistant nasopharyngeal carcinoma cells. Biomolecules 2020; 10(2): 184.
[http://dx.doi.org/10.3390/biom10020184] [PMID: 31991751]

[15] Desai A, Qazi G, Ganju R, *et al.* Medicinal plants and cancer chemoprevention. Curr Drug Metab 2008; 9(7): 581-91
[http://dx.doi.org/10.2174/138920008785821657] [PMID: 18781909]

[16] Padmaharish V, Lakshmi T. Anticancer activities of medicinal plants –An update. Journal of Pharmaceutical Sciences and Research 2017; 9(4): 432-40.

[17] Harikrishnan H, Jantan I, Alagan A, Haque MA. Modulation of cell signaling pathways by Phyllanthus amarus and its major constituents: potential role in the prevention and treatment of inflammation and cancer. Inflammopharmacology 2020; 28(1): 1-18.
[http://dx.doi.org/10.1007/s10787-019-00671-9] [PMID: 31792765]

[18] Mans RA. Anticancer activity of uncommon medicinal plants from the republic of suriname: Traditional claims, preclinical findings, and potential clinical applicability against cancer.Pharmacognosy - Medicinal Plants. 2019.

[19] Sultana S, Asif HM. Review: Medicinal plants combating against hypertension: A green antihypertensive approach. Pak J Pharm Sci 2017; 30(6): 2311-9.
[PMID: 29175804]

[20] Greenwell M, Rahman PKSM. Medicinal Plants: Their Use in Anticancer Treatment. Int J Pharm Sci Res 2015; 6(10): 4103-12.
[PMID: 26594645]

[21] Malami I, Bunza AM, Alhassan AM, Muhammad A, Abubakar IB, Yunusa A, *et al.* Dihydroartemisinin as a potential drug candidate for cancer therapy: a structural-based virtual screening for multitarget profiling. J Biomol Struct Dyn 2020; 0(0): 1-16.
[PMID: 32964804]

[22] Ramsay RR, Popovic-Nikolic MR, Nikolic K, Uliassi E, Bolognesi ML. A perspective on multi□target drug discovery and design for complex diseases. Clin Transl Med 2018; 7(1): 3.
[http://dx.doi.org/10.1186/s40169-017-0181-2] [PMID: 29340951]

[23] Medzhitov R. Origin and physiological roles of inflammation. Nature 2008; 454(7203): 428-35.
[http://dx.doi.org/10.1038/nature07201] [PMID: 18650913]

[24] Sharma N. Free radicals, antioxidants and disease. Biol Med (Aligarh) 2014; 6(3): 1-6.
[http://dx.doi.org/10.4172/0974-8369.1000214]

[25] Lamb R, Ozsvari B, Lisanti CL, *et al.* Antibiotics that target mitochondria effectively eradicate cancer stem cells, across multiple tumor types: Treating cancer like an infectious disease. Oncotarget 2015; 6(7): 4569-84.
[http://dx.doi.org/10.18632/oncotarget.3174] [PMID: 25625193]

[26] van Vuuren RJ, Visagie MH, Theron AE, Joubert AM. Antimitotic drugs in the treatment of cancer. Cancer Chemother Pharmacol 2015; 76(6): 1101-12.
[http://dx.doi.org/10.1007/s00280-015-2903-8] [PMID: 26563258]

[27] Ames BN, Gold LS. Endogenous mutagens and the causes of aging and cancer. Mutat Res 1991; 250(1-2): 3-16.
[http://dx.doi.org/10.1016/0027-5107(91)90157-J] [PMID: 1944345]

[28] Taylor R. Effects of alpha-tocopherol and beta-carotene supplements on cancer incidence in the Alpha-Tocopherol Beta-Carotene Cancer Prevention Study. Am J Clin Nutr 1995; 62: 1427S-30S.

[29] Le Corre L, Chalabi N, Delort L, Bignon YJ, Bernard-Gallon DJ. Resveratrol and breast cancer chemoprevention: Molecular mechanisms. Mol Nutr Food Res 2005; 49(5): 462-71.

[http://dx.doi.org/10.1002/mnfr.200400094] [PMID: 15786518]

[30] Balkwill F, Mantovani A. Inflammation and cancer: back to Virchow? Lancet 2001; 357(9255): 539-45.
[http://dx.doi.org/10.1016/S0140-6736(00)04046-0] [PMID: 11229684]

[31] Strowig T, Henao-Mejia J, Elinav E, Flavell R. Inflammasomes in health and disease. Nature 2012; 481(7381): 278-86.
[http://dx.doi.org/10.1038/nature10759] [PMID: 22258606]

[32] Martinou JC, Youle RJ. Mitochondria in apoptosis: Bcl-2 family members and mitochondrial dynamics. Dev Cell 2011; 21(1): 92-101.
[http://dx.doi.org/10.1016/j.devcel.2011.06.017] [PMID: 21763611]

[33] Baltrusch S. Mitochondrial network regulation and its potential interference with inflammatory signals in pancreatic beta cells. Diabetologia 2016; 59(4): 683-7.
[http://dx.doi.org/10.1007/s00125-016-3891-x] [PMID: 26873508]

[34] Overmoyer B. Options for the treatment of patients with taxane-refractory metastatic breast cancer. Clin Breast Cancer 2008; 8 (Suppl. 2): S61-70.
[http://dx.doi.org/10.3816/CBC.2008.s.002] [PMID: 18637401]

[35] Bennett LL, Rojas S, Seefeldt T. Role of Antioxidants in the Prevention of Cancer. J Exp Clin Med 2012; 4(4): 215-22.
[http://dx.doi.org/10.1016/j.jecm.2012.06.001]

[36] Vogelstein B, Kinzler KW. Cancer genes and the pathways they control. Nat Med 2004; 10(8): 789-99.
[http://dx.doi.org/10.1038/nm1087] [PMID: 15286780]

[37] Zhou BBS, Elledge SJ. The DNA damage response: putting checkpoints in perspective. Nature 2000; 408(6811): 433-9.
[http://dx.doi.org/10.1038/35044005] [PMID: 11100718]

[38] da Rocha A, Lopes RM, Schwartsmann G. Natural products in anticancer therapy. Curr Opin Pharmacol 2001; 1(4): 364-9.
[http://dx.doi.org/10.1016/S1471-4892(01)00063-7] [PMID: 11710734]

[39] Nowak-Sliwinska P, Scapozza L, Ruiz i Altaba A. Drug repurposing in oncology: Compounds, pathways, phenotypes and computational approaches for colorectal cancer. Biochim Biophys Acta Rev Cancer 2019; 1871(2): 434-54.
[http://dx.doi.org/10.1016/j.bbcan.2019.04.005] [PMID: 31034926]

[40] Mishra A, Dey S. Molecular docking studies of a cyclic octapeptide-cyclosaplin from sandalwood. Biomolecules 2019; 9(11): 740.
[http://dx.doi.org/10.3390/biom9110740] [PMID: 31731771]

[41] Giri H, Cai X, Panicker SR, Biswas I, Rezaie AR. Thrombomodulin regulation of mitogen-activated protein kinases. Int J Mol Sci 2019; 20(8): 1851.
[http://dx.doi.org/10.3390/ijms20081851] [PMID: 30991642]

[42] Cioccio J, Claxton D. Therapy of acute myeloid leukemia: therapeutic targeting of tyrosine kinases. Expert Opin Investig Drugs 2019; 28(4): 337-49.
[http://dx.doi.org/10.1080/13543784.2019.1584610] [PMID: 30775933]

[43] Anguita E, Villalobo A. Src-family tyrosine kinases and the Ca^{2+} signal. Biochim Biophys Acta Mol Cell Res 2017; 1864(6): 915-32.
[http://dx.doi.org/10.1016/j.bbamcr.2016.10.022] [PMID: 27818271]

[44] Bickel D, Gohlke H. C-terminal modulators of heat shock protein of 90 kDa (HSP90): State of development and modes of action. Bioorg Med Chem 2019; 27(21): 115080.
[http://dx.doi.org/10.1016/j.bmc.2019.115080] [PMID: 31519378]

[45] Muls AC, Lalji A, Marshall C, *et al.* The holistic management of consequences of cancer treatment by a gastrointestinal and nutrition team: a financially viable approach to an enormous problem? Clin Med (Lond) 2016; 16(3): 240-6.
[http://dx.doi.org/10.7861/clinmedicine.16-3-240] [PMID: 27251913]

[46] Cramer H, Cohen L, Dobos G, Witt CM. Integrative oncology: Best of both worlds - Theoretical, practical, and research issues. Evidence-based Complementary and Alternative Medicine 2013.

[47] Rushton M, Morash R, Larocque G, *et al.* Wellness Beyond Cancer Program: building an effective survivorship program. Curr Oncol 2015; 22(6): 419-34.
[http://dx.doi.org/10.3747/co.22.2786] [PMID: 26715879]

[48] Bower WF, Vlantis AC, Chung TML, Van Hasselt CA. Mode of treatment affects quality of life in head and neck cancer survivors: Implications for holistic care. Acta Otolaryngol 2010; 130(10): 1185-92.
[http://dx.doi.org/10.3109/00016481003667366] [PMID: 20331408]

[49] Schloss J, Steel A. Thriving after cancer: The role of integrative medicine (IM) in cancer survivorship and wellbeing programs. Adv Integr Med 2015; 2(3): 123-4.
[http://dx.doi.org/10.1016/j.aimed.2016.02.002]

[50] Cadet T, Davis C, Elks J, Wilson P. A Holistic Model of Care to Support Those Living with and beyond Cancer. Healthcare (Basel) 2016; 4(4): 88.
[http://dx.doi.org/10.3390/healthcare4040088] [PMID: 27869728]

[51] Davies NJ, Batehup L. Towards a personalised approach to aftercare: a review of cancer follow-up in the UK. J Cancer Surviv 2011; 5(2): 142-51.
[http://dx.doi.org/10.1007/s11764-010-0165-3] [PMID: 21253881]

[52] Kazak AE, Rourke MT, Alderfer MA, Pai A, Reilly AF, Meadows AT. Evidence-based assessment, intervention and psychosocial care in pediatric oncology: a blueprint for comprehensive services across treatment. J Pediatr Psychol 2007; 32(9): 1099-110.
[http://dx.doi.org/10.1093/jpepsy/jsm031] [PMID: 17626069]

CHAPTER 7

Importance of *In silico* Tools in Anticancer Drug Discovery from Nature

Gnana Ruba Priya Muthaiah[1,*], Motamarri Venkata Naga Lalitha Chaitanya[2], Seema Sajjan Singh Rathore[1], Maida Engels S.E.[4] and **Vishnu Nayak Badavath[3]**

[1] *College of Pharmaceutical Sciences, Department of Pharmaceutical Chemistry, Dayananda Sagar University, Bangalore, Karnataka, India*

[2] *School of Pharmacy, Lovely Professional University Phagwara, 144402 Punjab, India*

[3] *Department of Pharmaceutical Chemistry, College of Pharmacy, Chitkara University, Chitkara, Panjab, India*

[4] *PSG College of Pharamacy,Coimbatore,Tamil Nadu, India*

Abstract: Currently, cancer has become one of the most dreadful diseases threatening human health. Natural plant sources play a vital role in the development of several anti-cancer drugs such as vincristine, vinblastine, vinorelbine, docetaxel, paclitaxel, camptothecin, etoposide, teniposide, *etc.* Various chemotherapies fail due to adverse reactions, target specificity, and drug resistance of some types of drugs. Researchers are attentive to developing drugs that overcome the problems stated above by using natural compounds that may affect multiple targets with reduced adverse effects and that are effective against several cancer types. The development of a new drug is a highly complex, expensive, and time-consuming endeavour. In the traditional drug discovery process, ending with a new medicine ready for the market can take up to 15 years and cost more than one billion dollars. Fortunately, this situation has changed with the arrival of novel approaches recently. Many new technologies and methodologies have been developed to increase the efficiency of the drug discovery process, and computational methodologies utilise the existing data to generate knowledge that affords valuable understanding for addressing current complications and guiding the further research and development of new naturally derived drugs. Consequently, the application of *in silico* techniques and optimization algorithms in drug discovery ventures can provide versatile solutions to understand the molecular-level interactions of chemical constituents and identify the hits. Lead optimization techniques such as ligand-based or structure-based drug design are widely used in many discovery efforts. In this chapter, we first introduce the concepts of CADD, *in silico* tools, *etc.* we then describe how this virtual screening has been successfully applied. Furthermore, we review the concept of natural product anticancer therapies

* **Corresponding author Gnana Ruba Priya Muthaiah:** College of Pharmaceutical Sciences, Department of pharmaceutical chemistry, Dayananda Sagar University, Bangalore, Karnataka, India; E-mail: gnana-sps@dsu.edu.in

Motamarri Venkata Naga Lalitha Chaitanya, Galvina Pereira, & Heyam Saad Ali (Eds.)

and present some of the most representative examples of molecules identified through this method.

Keywords: Anticancer, ADME Tool, Bioinformatics, Cancer, CADD, Drug discovery, Drug likeness, *In silico* tools, Ligand, Lead optimization. Phytochemical properties, Molecular docking, Natural anticancer molecule, Molecular dynamics, Pass Tool, Targets, Virtual screening.

INTRODUCTION

Historically, over the years, many natural products from earthly sources have gained popularity for their role in providing better health care and disease prevention. During the early 19th century, Friedrich Serturner, a scientist, performed research on numerous medicinal plants and isolated morphine as an active constituent. This investigation led to the screening of terrestrial natural products for medicinal activity. Over 100 anticancer agents were developed between the end of the nineteenth and the beginning of the twentieth centuries. Out of this, 25 are from natural sources: 9 are purely natural products, 18 are derivatives of natural products, and 11 are derivatives of natural product pharmacophores [1]. The advancement of knowledge and research regarding the prevention and treatment of disease using drugs from plant or animal sources has been observed for years.

Unlike food, cloth, and shelter, medicines are a basic need to fight against illness and to amend mood and consciousness. Natural substances are extremely valued because of their advantageous activities, but modern medicines used nowadays are the advancement of natural products. Hence, a drug used for treatment can be defined as a constituent obtained from either a natural or synthetic origin that is used for the purpose of diagnosing, curing, treating, relieving, or preventing any disease or that is intended to affect the body's function and structure. Thus, a drug is a chemical moiety or compound that affects the body along with its processes. In recent times, a tremendous increase in research on natural products from plant sources has been observed, and they have gained popularity because of their pharmaceutical applications. The phytochemical substances from natural sources produce various molecules with distinctive structures. These molecules tend to produce biological effects through chemical variety and structural complexity.

Nature is the best source of drugs, and it is not very well explored by researchers in the fields of pharmaceuticals, cosmetics, functional foods, and nutritional supplements. Around 25 natural products, like vincristine, vinblastine, docetaxel, paclitaxel, etoposide, teniposide, *etc.*, have been developed for the treatment of cancer and are in various phases of clinical trials. Tools like bioinformatics and chemoinformatics aid in providing leads and targets. They help in discovering leads against individual targets by using pharmacophores, molecular docking, machine learning, and quantitative and qualitative structure-activity relationship methods. With the aid of molecular docking, quantitative or qualitative structural activity relationships (QSAR), pharmacophores, and machine learning methods, leads can be discovered for targeting.

Most of these approaches have the potential to ease the process of lead discovery against individual targets by using molecular docking, QSAR, pharmacophores, and machine learning methods. Combinatorial approaches, as well as simultaneous interaction with multiple targets, can be used to explore an individual target. 3D target-based methods have their own disadvantages, and 2D structures are better and more reasonable to enable leads for multiple targets. Phytoconstituents obtained from plant extracts are discovered based on their random screening and bioactivity-guided fractionation. The bioactive principle from traditional activities acts as a base for the discovery of drugs with known bioactivities by using molecular docking, and hence, the other natural constituents whose activities are not known are largely unexplored. The activity of those constituents can be determined by using multi-targeted in silico models. Along with chemoinformatics, bioinformatics and system biology approaches are gaining popularity as ways to know the therapeutic activity of medicinally active plants. These methods are used in docking to select the target and identify the relationship between the activity of a phytoconstituent and its therapeutic activity. (Fig. **1**). However, the traditional approach to drug discovery is really time-consuming and cost-intensive. Thus, the new approach to drug discovery exceeds the limitations of traditional research. After studying about 5,000 to 10,000 compounds, only one drug comes to market. Each drug costs about $156 million in the discovery phase. Food and Drug Administration (FDA) processes I, II, and III cost another $75 million. This brings the total to about $231 million for each drug placed on the market for consumers. Then, to gain FDA approval, a long and expensive procedure also needs to be followed.

In recent times, drug design has been carried out with the help of software. Taking into account the fine structure of the target molecule, a whole new ligand is constructed (Fig. **2**). The figure given below is the de novo finding of a lead substance. It has been a powerful tool to build a lead compound.

Drug discovery method: The most important stages of the process of drug discovery in the identification of biologic targets involve the following:

1. Hit identification: Many compounds are screened and analysed at this stage in order to identify the biological target. "Hit" here is referred to as the compound that reacts with the target protein [2].

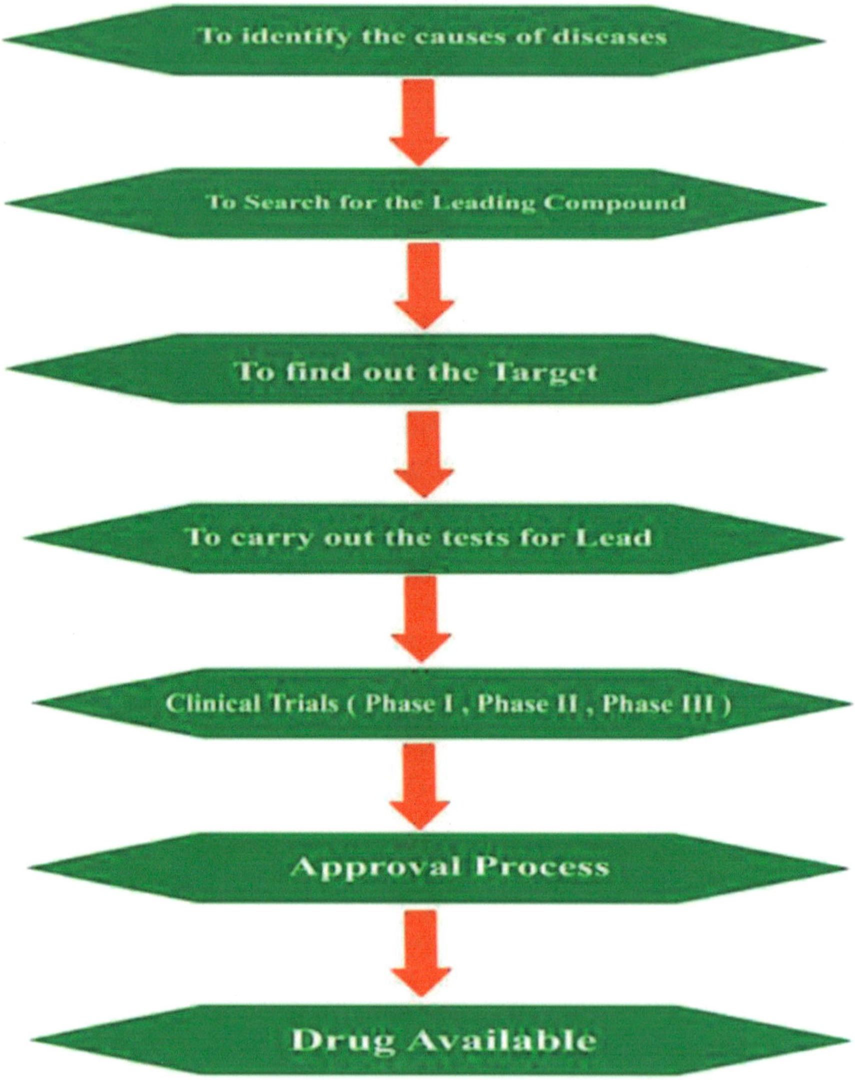

Fig. (1). Rational drug design.

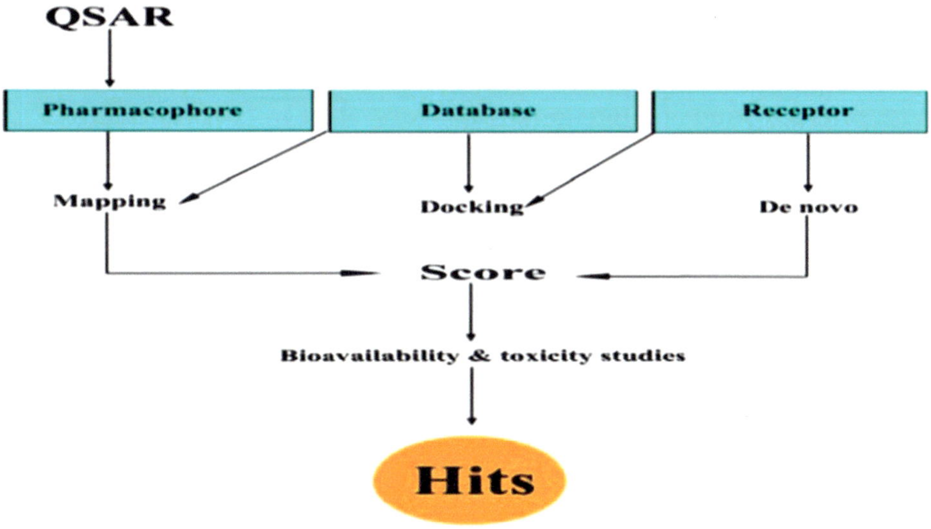

Fig. (2). Flow chart for drug design.

Role of Computers in Drug Design

During the 1990s, a new technique called CADD was introduced, which was believed to replace the traditional method of drug discovery and development. Computers were procured by the pharmaceutical industries to apply CADD in the development of drugs and to estimate ligand-receptor complementarities.

Researchers were able to produce chemical structure and modify them using vector models. It was believed by the computational chemists that by using computers, the time and effort for synthesizing a drug and testing its activity can be reduced. The design by which a lead molecule was developed through computer model was named as de novo design. This design was a big disappointment and had no effect in discovering lead compounds due to its computing power restrictions and unavailability of software.

To run the computers for a limited period of time, shortcuts are required, and this could not be fulfilled with the use of computing techniques. The most challenging scenario with de novo design is no association of the computed chemical structure with that of reality or the formation of chemical structures that are useful. The usage of computers is gaining popularity and is growing very fast, but the accuracy in predicting the binding of ligand, which is obtained by the de novo method, to its receptor needs substantial estimates. It has been observed that researchers are making an effort to dock a ligand that is produced from scratch within the receptors. An attempt was made to overcome the problems associated with de novo design by using RACHEL, which was an advancement in technology.

This technique gained recognition in the design of a lead molecule as it was useful in mass screening and combinatorial chemistry. Researchers discovered that this was an important step in discovering lead compounds because it took much less time and was more effective. This advancement proved that to optimise the lead compounds to their potent moieties, computational tools are required. When de novo ligand generation design is compared with drug optimization, it can be observed that de novo design creates the complete structure from the base, whereas in the case of drug optimization, the process begins with the lead molecule binding with the receptors, which is characterised by the x-ray crystallographic method. Computers are widely used in generating potential molecules, predicting the binding of the molecules to the receptors, and choosing the best one. Hence, by using CADD software, a lead compound that is weakly bound to the receptors can be modified to show the best effects (Fig. **3**).

Advancement in Drug discovery with Natural Products and CADD

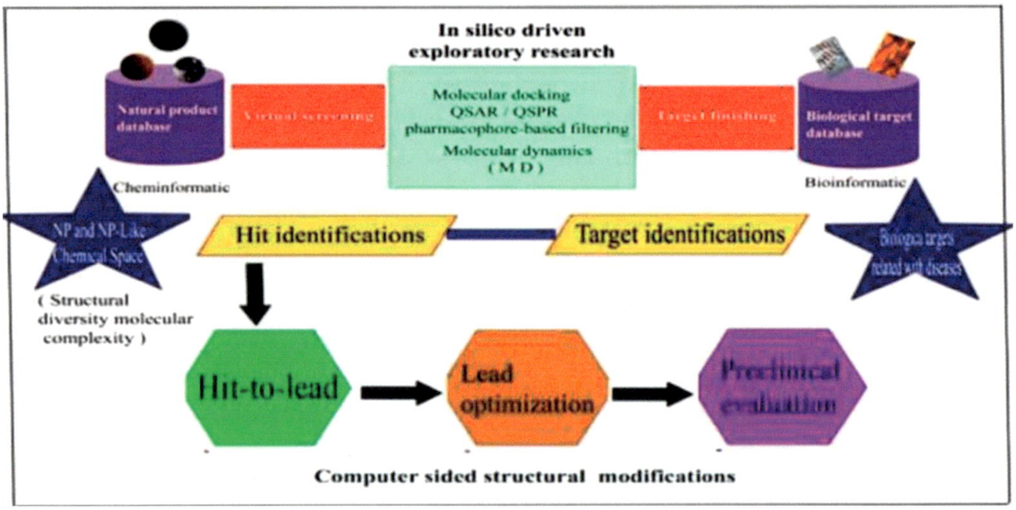

Fig. (3). Innovative *in silico* strategies have contributed valuably to the NP research in drug discovery processes as reviewed herein.

Many scholars have worked in the area of drug discovery by using various in silico methods or CADD to determine the lead compounds from natural products [3]. They implemented computer-generated screening on 329 types of flavonoid derivatives from natural sources. The screening was performed by using the naturally available plant-based anticancer compound activity target (NPACT) database to recognise the poly ADP-ribose polymerase (PARP) inhibitors. The screening was performed by using various *in silico* methods, like the prediction of the drug's likeness, molecular docking, and *in silico* toxicity studies. The results obtained were compared with Rucaparib, which is an FDA-approved agent for the inhibition of PARP, and it was found that out of 329 compounds, 15 showed better docking. The 15 flavonoids were termed as "hits" and were again evaluated for their accurate mode of docking and drug similitude properties.

The docking method's accuracy was determined with the help of the re-docking method. Two flavonoids, *i.e.*, NPACT00280 and NPACT00183, with docking scores of -129.36 and -139.237, respectively, were recognised as potential agents in inhibiting PARP, and when predicted with ADMET SAR, they didn't show any AMES toxicity nor carcinogenicity. Hence, these 2 flavonoids can be used as potential agents, and further research can be carried out [4]. and stated that different plants contain pharmacologically active substances which can be effective in the treatment and prevention of disease. WHO has identified 252 drugs, considered to be basic and essential drugs. According to the researcher 11% of the above-mentioned drugs are obtained from flowering plant origin. Most of the compounds like Paclitaxel from *Taxus Brevifolia* are derived, developed and marketed for the treatment of ovarian and breast cancer. When compared with chemical compounds, the phytoconstituents have advantages like less cost, fewer side effects, high bioavailability, *etc.*

The computational methods can be used to determine the pharmacokinetic and pharmacodynamic parameters. As the researchers are exploring nature and its products, an increase in medicines from plant sources has been observed due to their pharmacological properties. In modern times, CADD is reported to be a widely used tool for the progression of drug discovery. In the drug invention field, many other technologies like ligand-based drug discovery (LBDD), structure-based drug design (SBDD), and virtual library screening (VLS), as well as commercially available free tools like Auto Dock, Schrodinger Suite, Discovery Studio, and Flex, are being used. Other than these, the molecular modelling method, a medicinal chemistry tool, is gaining popularity among researchers because of its use in studying SARs. It has been stated by various researchers that natural products are grown as an intuition for drug discovery, and these have led to the discovery of drugs and supplements in modern medicine. CADD, along with experimental validation techniques, had a major role in recognising and intending new drug moieties.

The structure of natural products has been crucial in identifying novel anti-disease compounds. Structure-based methods and ligand-based methods find are used in CADD. By using the structure-based method, a 3D model can be created if the site of target binding is known, and this can be used for docking molecules, generating pharmacophores, or screening molecular dynamics simulations as described in a study [5]. A ligand-based method is used to identify the structure of the compound that is responsible for producing the biological activity by taking active and inactive molecules into consideration.

Virtual Screening

The development of lead compounds in drug discovery led to increased usage of computational resources and molecular databases. Due to the increased usage of computational techniques like CADD and chemical bio informatics, many virtual screening technologies like homology search, high-throughput docking, and pharmacophore search in the database are observed. Virtual screening has found its way to be a significant part of CADD methods. Virtual screening has established as a successful and economical technique in the identification of lead molecules.

Molecular Docking

In the rational drug design method, molecular docking follows a structure-based protocol. The docking is done by learning and envisaging the binding pattern and interaction affinity between the ligand and the receptors [6]. Molecular docking is classified into rigid and flexible molecular docking based on the flexibility of the ligand during the computational process [7, 8]. In a rigid method, the binding model overlooks flexibility and induced fit theory but considers the static chemical, physical, and geometrical complementarity between the target and ligand proteins [9]. This method is quick, efficient, and useful for the virtual screening of large small molecule databases. In case of flexible docking, more comprehensive and precise information is required. Docking *via* flexible methods is becoming increasingly easy with advancement in computational methods. Various software like AutoDock, Discovery Studio, DOCK, FlexX, Glide, Sybyl, *etc.* are available.

The molecular docking process occurs in 3 steps

1. In advance, the structure of small molecules and the target proteins must be prepared. By using the PDB database, many structures solved experimentally can be obtained. This can help in understanding the physiological process based on the crystal structure, and if the molecule's docking structure is of interest, then a homologous template can be used.

2. It is a search engine that can be used to know the orientations, conformations, and positional space of the binding site of a ligand [10]. The abiding of binary complexes using conformational search algorithms can be performed using systemic and stochastic search methods. The different methods for systematic search include conformational ensemble search, fragmentation search, exhaustive search, and stochastic search methods including evolutionary algorithms' Monte Carlo methods, swarm optimization methods, and Tabu search methods. During the molecular docking process, the aforementioned programmes aid in determining the compound with the highest affinity for the target [11].

3. Various types of scoring functions for docking purposes have been developed, including force-field-based scoring functions, empirical scoring functions, consensus scoring functions, knowledge-based scoring functions [12], interactive fingerprints, machine learning technologies, and quantum mechanical scores [13].

Structure Based Pharmacophore Mapping

During the process of drug discovery and development, pharmacophore mapping has been considered the best and the most useful tool. In the de novo design, virtual screening, and lead optimization, structure-based approaches have been performed. This is done to improve the modelling of pharmacophores [14, 15]. Another useful technique is structure-based pharmacophore (SBP) mapping, which is classified into two types based on ligand structure availability. Target-ligand complex and target-binding site-based methods (without ligand) are the two types of SBP modelling methods [16]. In case of the target ligand complex method, the ligand binding pocket of a protein can be easily located and the main ligand-protein interactions can be evaluated. This approach is clearly explained by considering an example from Ligand Scout [17 - 19]. But this method has its own limitations and is useless if the ligand is not known. To overcome this limitation, a macromolecule-based (without ligand) method was instigated in Discovery Studio [20]. This can be considered one of the best examples where the ligand and receptor-ligand interactions are not observed. The interaction occurring within the binding sites is explained by the LUDI programme [21]. This process has the benefit of defining the complete interaction ability of the binding pocket and the associated restriction on the production of maps with unrequired interface features.

Ligand-Based Drug Discovery

Molecular resemblance works on the principle of molecules producing similar pharmacological effects, due to their structural similarities. This approach acts as a base for ligand-based approaches in the field of drug discovery [22].

The structure of an active ligand that interacts with a target protein serves as the foundation for ligand-based drug discovery. These compounds with remarkable pharmacological properties can be used as query templates, which will help in recognising and envisaging newer chemical moieties with comparable properties. In this method, only the structure of the small molecule is important and can be used if the 3D target protein structure is not available or predicted. This method can be used for the screening of ligands with good pharmacological activities and the optimization of the same to improve the pharmacokinetic parameters, including toxicity. To signify the reference compounds, physicochemical properties like the weight of the molecule, the logP value, the energy of the highest occupied and lowest unoccupied orbitals, charges, 2D fingerprints, and 3D shape resemblance searches can be added. In virtual screening for molecular representation, methods like extended-connectivity fingerprints (ECFP), 2D fingerprints (Molprint2D and Unity 2D), 3D shape similarity (MACCS), phase shapes, and rapid overlay of chemical structures (ROCS) are used [23].

An investigator [24] found a novel agonist of the estradiol receptor family receptor GPR30 by applying 2D fingerprint and 3D shape-similarity methods. Both the methods were applied in virtual screenings with respect to scalability and time, and were seen to exhibit better activity against many targets when compared with that of docking methods. The major problem associated with both methods is the difficulty in choosing the structure of the input molecule.

Advantages of 3D Molecular Docking Studies

Over the past few decades, QSAR (quantitative structure-activity relationship) techniques have advanced at a rapid pace. The QSAR method has long been crucial in the optimization of lead structures, and with the advent of big data methods and increased computing power, it is now able to deal with the vast amounts of information related to combinatorial chemistry as well.

The 3D QSAR is a relatively new advancement in the field of QSAR. Successful applications of 3D-OSAR to numerous datasets, most notably those containing enzyme and receptor ligands, have been made over the past two decades. Protein-ligand docking studies and 3D QSAR analyses generally go hand in hand because they complement one another. Here, we provide an overview of the most up-t--date developments in 3D QSAR, protein-ligand docking, and hybrid methods for both traditional organic molecules and nanostructured materials including fullerenes and carbon nanotubes.

Ligand-based Pharmacophore

Mapping by considering a set of active moieties, a pharmacophore (PH4) is developed in contrast with molecular descriptors. According to IUPAC, "a pharmacophore is a collection of spatial and electronic characteristics necessary to ensure optimal supramolecular interactions with specific biological targets and to trigger or block their biological reactions" [25]. Hence, to signify the most feasible chemical characteristic, structural overlap from active constituents can act as the main feature of a molecule. Newly identified and developed molecules can be the best candidates for performing future investigations if they are active against the target protein. If macromolecular structures are not available, this computational method can be used to improve, encourage, and monitor the drug discovery process [26]. The summarization for pharmacophore modelling is done as follows: (i) Choosing a ligand training set that includes both active and inactive compounds (ii) The molecular preparation (low energy conformations)(iii) Ligand alignment or superimposition and pharmacophore model generation (iv) pharmacophore model validation [27].

Quantitative Structure-Activity Relationship Modeling

QSAR, an additional ligand-based method, can be used to determine the biological and pharmacological activities of drug molecules using molecular descriptors (MDs) or fingerprints (FPs). This model can be used to mathematically study the response produced by activities to the target in accordance with ligand structural characteristics. Various approaches like Deep learning (DL) and material learning (ML) have been applied for the development of QSAR models, QSAR is calculated by associating the properties of the ligand binding agent with the biological activity [27]. Other than ML and DL, other approaches are used, such as artificial neural networks (ANN), multi-linear regression (MLR),

Polynomial Regression (PR), Random Forest (RF), and Support Vector Machine (SVM) QSAR models which are used to determine quantitative biological activity as well as positive and negative effects on molecule activity. Other than the activities mentioned above, QSAR can be applied for many other purposes in drug discovery, like predicting the activity of a new molecule analogue, analysing the optimising lead, and predicting the new lead molecule. The 2D-QSAR method has its own approaches to the physical and chemical nature of drugs, and the relationships can be obtained as a mathematical equation [28]. The 3D-QSAR method is more advanced when compared to 2D-QSAR and has comparative molecular field analysis [29] and molecular similarity indexes [30], which are created using force field calculations. A 3D method can be used to obtain 3D contour maps, which are helpful in the visualisation and interpretation of the structure of the molecule.

Multiscale De Novo Drug Design

Quantum Chemical Approaches to Structure-Based and Ligand-Based QSAR Models

Proteochemometrics (PCM) is a newer approach in the area of drug discovery. QSAR models can be used in this field as a powerful tool because of their virtual screening activity, but for calculating the enthalpy of contributors of protein-ligand interactions, the QM method can be preferred because it uses descriptors in ligand-based QSARs. The energies of the contributing fragments the molecular orbital calculation from structure-based QSARs, which produces a clear enthalpy and a model, but changes the binding energy and calculates the contribution of free energy to ligand-target complex formation in both structure- and ligand-based QSAR models. Optimization steps can be used to predict and interpret the change in binding affinity.

The QSAR models and QM approaches can be used to describe the molecule accurately and to provide enhanced information and understanding of the molecular and structural characteristics of drugs and ligands, respectively. Many QSAR models have been developed, each with a different computational precision. Several QSAR studies involve small and large molecules and refer to structure description. In case of microscales, mesoscales, and macroscales, different approaches for molecules will be used. Atom based QSAR is one such microscale method for precisely calculating the QM approaches; fragment-based QSAR is used as a mesoscopic scale simulation for a molecular force field; and macromolecule-based QSAR and cell-based QSAR are macroscopic scales studied on a coarse-grained scale. Other than these, multiscale can be used in QSAR, as these scales can replicate at different dimensions. Skeleton transition and substitution of R- groups to obtain various structures of a new drug can be done by CoMFA, which is a 3D fragment-based QSAR method. When compared to the 3D QSAR approach, 2.5D kino chemometrics (KCM), which is derived from PCM, can increase the proficiency and precision using 3D descriptors and 2D fingerprints for protein kinase and ligands use respectively. The precise predictions for drug discovery are obtained by multiscale QSAR. This incorporates QSAR systematically and effectively applies all QSAR models. An amalgamation of QM calculations, QSAR models, and fragment-based drug discovery is observed in multiscale de novo drug design. Taking molecular structure into consideration in QM calculations, the significance of explicit molecular descriptors can be studied. The primary goal of drug design is to create a novel molecule with maximum biological activity, favourable pharmacokinetic parameters, and a low toxic level in a variety of environmental conditions. The amount of data from clinical and biochemical sources can be easily handled by using a multiscale de novo drug design, and chemical characteristics can be attained that can enhance the properties of the drug. Hence, it is known to be more efficacious and safer for the discovery of new drugs.

Using Molecular Dynamics Simulation to Find New Drug Binding Sites

A computer simulation method used for analysing the movements of atoms and molecules is known as molecular dynamics (MD). The majority of critical biological events are dependent on information about protein-ligand complex interactions. Coupled receptors are the foremost group of membrane receptors in our body, and they play a major role in studying various physiological processes [31]. Ligands have been found to bind the allosteric sites other than their orthosteric sites [32 - 34], which are far from their target binding pockets. The location of these allosteric sites is not known, but evidence can be obtained from the experimental structures, and the prediction of such sites can help in the advancement of new drug discovery [35]. Many computational tools are being used for the estimation of functional sites like 3DLigandSite (http:// www.sbg.bio.ic.ac.uk/3dligandsite/), COACHD (http:// yanglab. nankai.edu.cn/COACH-D/), Site Map (https:// www. schrodinger.com/sitemap), *etc.* These above-mentioned tools have their own limitations; they create many ligand binding sites where it becomes difficult to predict the active pocket to which the compound binds, and this can be overcome by MD. Precise identification and characterization of ligand binding sites [36, 37] and application of a new drug binding site are done using the MD approach [38]. An reported in his study regarding the presence of sodium ions, located in the orthosteric site, which was found by MD simulations. This method can also be used to identify the allosteric sites, which are intricate in protein kinases [39, 40] and Staphylococcus aureus [41]. These data can be used to advance drug discovery prospects using MD models.

Artificial Intelligence in Anticancer Drug Discovery

Over the years, computational drug design has gained too much popularity and is widely used in discovering new anticancer agents like Abiraterone [42], Gefitinib [43], Erlotinib [44], Lapatinib [45], Sorafenib [46], and Crizotinib [47], which are breakthroughs in this era. By using computational and artificial intelligence (AI) methods, the research on anticancer drugs is speedily developing. By using the PH4 design, the molecule SR13668 is optimised from indole-3-carbinol and has revealed a resilient effect on different types of cancer in phase I trials [47]. The

ML method was used to identify and develop a potent inhibitor of 5-lipoxygenase based on physicochemical and pharmacophore features [48]. AI has found its own advantages over other models in drug discovery, and it has been widely used in discovering anticancer drugs by using in silico models [49]. The first anti-cancer compound was developed by executing variational autoencoders using ML models [50], and the product's activity for types of cancer was demonstrated [51].

Successful Stories of Computational Drug Discovery

In the modern era, computational methods have a vibrant role in drug discovery. The use of computational methods in the field of drug discovery has gained too much popularity with respect to investment, resources, and time. In the development of anticancer drugs, computational methods play a major role. Some anticancer agents have found positive effects through computational methods. Crizotinib is one such agent that has found application in computational structure-based drug design. It is a cMet/ALK dual inhibitor approved by the USFDA. c-Met, along with its natural ligand, hepatocyte growth factor, plays a dangerous role in cell activities, and overexpression of c-Met is seen in human cancer [52 - 55]. Its irregular function is seen in solid and blood tumour cancers; hence, it is the best objective for oncology. The indolin-2-one derivatives were studied for the inhibition of c-MET, and the sequence was assessed by 3-substituted indolin---ones, an effective class of kinase inhibitors. A strong effect against the c-MET autophosphorylation process was observed by compound 1 with the code PHA-665752, Schemndolin-2-one derivatives, and it also showed *in vivo* and *in vitro* biological activities, but this compound had some untoward effects, which led to the suspension of further research. The key inhibitor binding site was identified by the co-crystal structure of compound 1, which had a kinase domain of c-MET, which encouraged researchers to work more in this area. The redesign of compound 1's central ring was performed and led to the discovery of the 5-substituted 3-benzyloxy-2-aminopyridine series; compound 2 showed a considerably good response in inhibition of c-MET among the lately designed derivatives. The development in optimization can be screened by employing lipophilic efficiency for binding purposes. To improve the effect of compound 2, a docked structure of the same was developed along with the c-MET kinase domain. Most of the drugs showed better effects in inhibiting the growth of tumours through the optimization process or examination of the chiral centre. The functional group 3-benzyloxy group at position 5 is optimised in 2-aminopyridine, and the chiral centre is examined in crizotinib (see Scheme 1A), and as such it has activity against esophageal, lung, and lymphoma cancer [56 - 58].A new treatment using Axitinib (AG-013736) for renal cell carcinoma was approved by the USFDA [59]. Axitinib was created using structure-based drug design and functions as an inhibitor by binding to the vascular endothelial growth factor

(VEGF) kinase domain in the DFG-out conformation [60]. VEGF are signalling regulators involved in angiogenesis; they have been found in tumour cells, and their signalling plays a critical role in the progression of malignant disease. The VEGF receptors act as ligands for the network of signaling, and these receptors belong to the class of tyrosine kinases along with VEGFR-1, VEGFR-2, and VEGFR-3. These VEGFR-1, 2, and 3 can be inhibited with a pan kinase inhibitor, which has been used to develop anti-angiogenic agents.

The phosphorylated crystal structure was developed for p-VEGFR2D50, and the structure of the unphosphorylated kinase inhibitor VEGFR2D50 was resolved. The structural activity relationship aids him in the design of drugs. Few compounds have been evaluated by conjoining the information from complex structures; for example, pyrazoles 3 and benzamide 4 are used as a prototypes for drug design design.

Pyrazole 3 was modelled into a ligand-free p-VEGFR2D50 structure, resulting in the formation of an indazole substance, a novel kinase inhibitor. The 5th derivative at the 3rd position had the styryl functional group of the indazole ring with increased levels of LipE and LE, which produced an inhibitory effect when compared to the other derivatives. Compound 5 with the crystal structure of VEGFR2D50 showed the detailed enzyme-ligand mode, and the basic indazole core was bound to open DFG in the endorsement of VEGFR2D50. Two co-crystal structures of VEGFR2D50–inhibitors are overlaid to obtain a more detailed 3D structure; this edifice helps in knowing the important binding sites for initiation of the DFG-out conformation. To capture the inhibition interactions as mentioned above, a chimera design protocol was used by taking overlapping or superimposing into consideration, and access was provided to the sulfur-linked indazole compound 6 and the corresponding amide analogs. In the presence of an extra amide group on the orthosteric site of the S-phenyl group, superimposing in the VEGFR2D50-bound co-crystal structures of benzamide 4 and indazole 6 revealed the formation of two hydrogen bonds, which were important for hydrogen binding. The hydrogen bonding was formed by Glu885 and Asp1046 of VEGFR2D50 and was caused by highly potent inhibitors. Notable improvements were observed on the cellular potency and desired physicochemical and pharmacokinetic properties of axitinb (AG-013736) (Scheme 1B), which were generated by applying a truncation strategy. Many drugs in combination are widely approved and used for the treatment of renal cell carcinoma (RCC). The combination of axitinib (Inlyta®) and pembrolizumab (Keytruda®) is one such approved treatment for RCC. Some exact and vital effects on protein performance are observed due to heat shock protein (HSP90). The effects of HSP90 are observed in cancer development and are associated with their activation, conformation, stabilization, and localization functions; hence, this is used as a favourable target for cancer therapy [61, 62].

The HSP90 has a crystal structure, and it has four domains that are functionally active. The domains present are the ATP/ADP binding domain, the C-term dimerization domain, the middle domain, and the N-term domain. A high screening performance was conducted to obtain the active drug inhibitor, compound 7 (CCT018159), based on the information obtained from the structure of HSP90 [63 - 65]. When the co-crystal structure of HSP90-compound 7 (CCT018159) is modified by adding or substituting specific functional groups, they tend to upgrade the pharmacokinetic property. If the methyl group is replaced by an amide group, the pyrazolyl ring is transformed into an isoxazole aromatic ring, which has a strong effect on animal cancer models. Luminespib (NVP-AUY922) is a HSP90 inhibitor that is currently in clinical trials. When patients with ALK disarray took the Phase I clinical trial drug Luminespib, a decisive outcome was observed [66]. This drug has also been used in combination with other drugs for anticancer therapy, and the combinations are at various stages of clinical trials (Table **3**) [67, 68].

To represent how computational drug discovery facilitates in the development of anticancer drugs, some FDA-approved anticancer agents in recent 3 years which are obtained from National Cancer Institute database [76] are listed in Table **4**.

Abbreviations: NSCLC: non- small cell lung cancer, EGFR: Epidermal growth factor receptor, VEGFR: Vascular epidermal growth factor receptor, ERBB2: erb-b2 receptor tyrosine kinase 2 (also known as NEU, NGL, HER2, TKR1, CD340, HER-2, MLN 19, HER-2/neu), ALK: Anaplastic lymphoma kinase.

Table 3. FDA Approved anticancer drugs

Name	Chemical structure	Therapeutic area	Target and Function	Year of Approval
Ribociclib	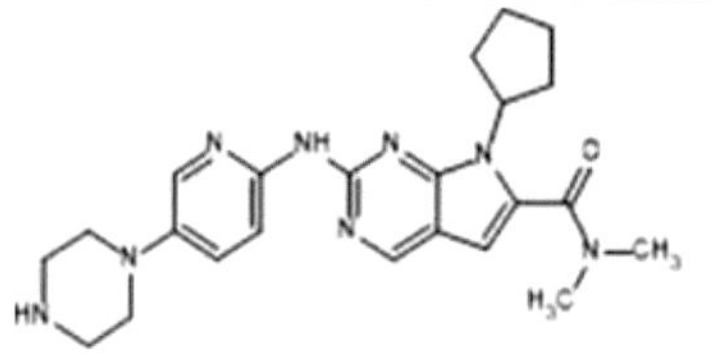	Breast cancer	Cyclin-Dependent Kinase (CDK) inhibitor	Syed *et al.*,2017 [69]
Niraparib Tosylate Monohydrate	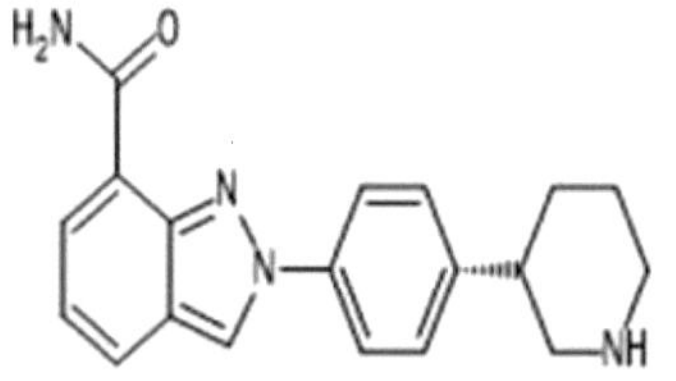	Recurrent epithelial ovarian, Fallopian tube and primary peritoneal cancer	Poly (ADP-ribose) polymerase (PARP)inhibitor	Mittica *et al.*,2017 [70]

(Table 3) cont.....

Name	Chemical structure	Therapeutic area	Target and Function	Year of Approval
Neratinib Maleate	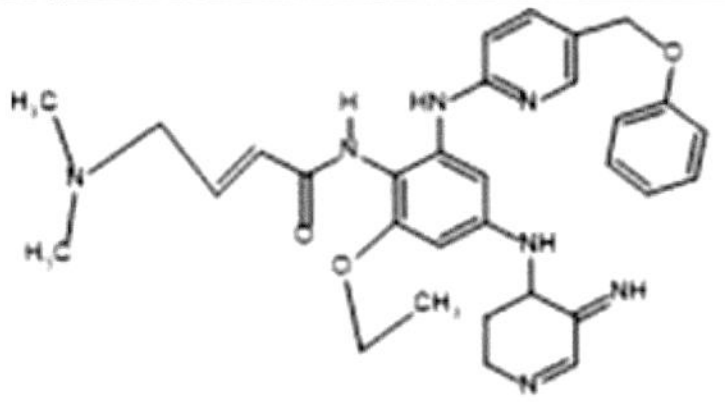	Breast cancer	Receptor tyrosine kinase (RTKs),Human epidermal growth factor receptor (EGFR)inibitor	Kotecki *et al.*,2017 [71]
Enasidenib Mesylate	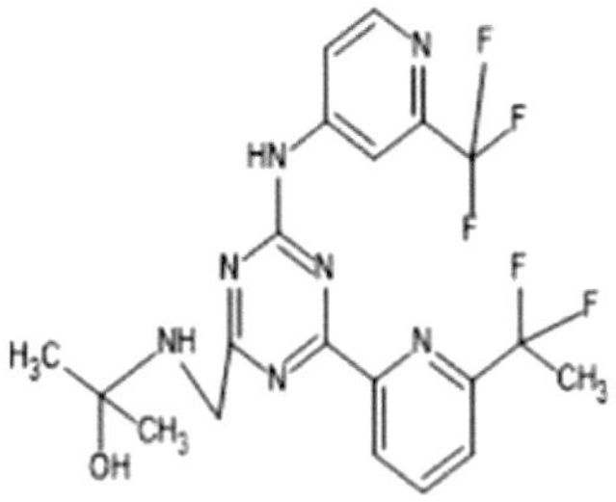	Acute myeloid leukemia	Isocitrate dehydrogenase-2inhibitor	Gras *et al.*,2017 [72]
Copanisib hydrochloride		Follicular lymphoma	Phosphonositide-3-kinase (P13K) inhibitor	Markham *et al.*,2017 [73]
	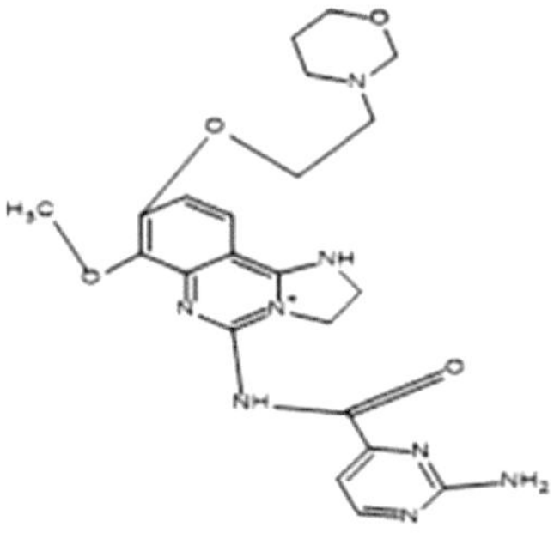			
Brigatinib	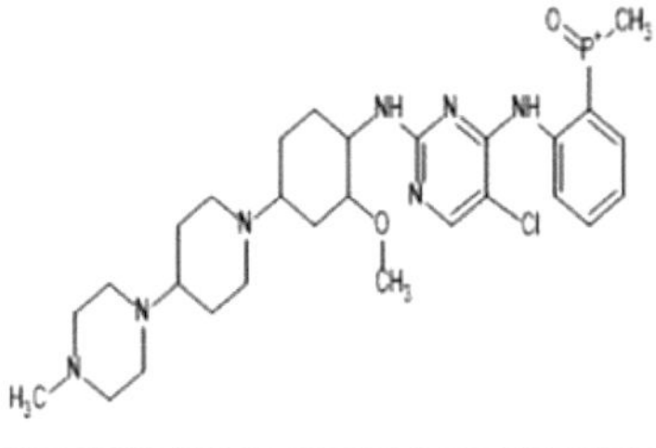	NSCLC	Anaplastic lymphoma kinase (ALK) and epidermal growth factor receptor (EGFR)kinase inhibitor	Markham *et al.*,2017 [73]

(Table 3) cont.....

Name	Chemical structure	Therapeutic area	Target and Function	Year of Approval
TolazoparibTosylate	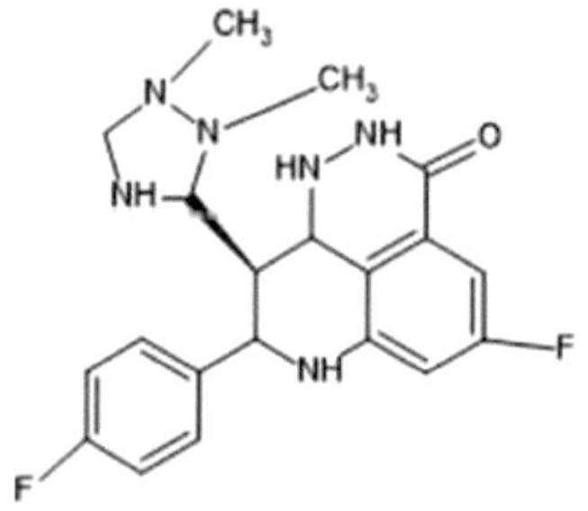	Breast cancer	Poly (ADP-ribose)polymerase (PARP)inhibitor	Esialer *et al.*,2017 [74]
Duvelisib	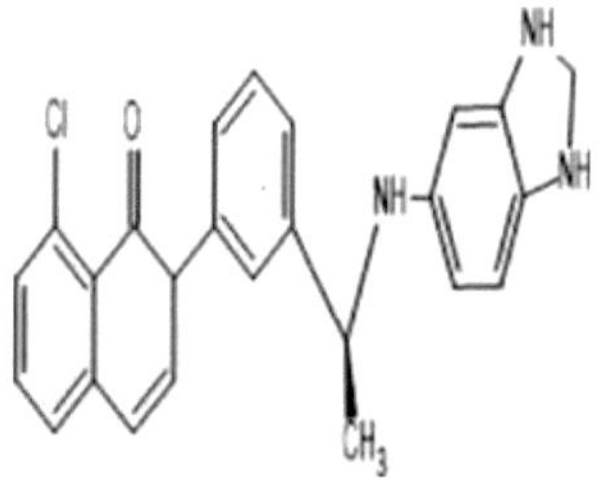	Chronic lymphocytic leukemiaand follicular lymphoma	P13K Kinase inhibitor	Blain *et al.*, 2018 [75]

Table 4. Compounds Developed with Computational Chemistry And Rational Drug Design Statistics

Name of the compound	Therapeutic area	Function	Approvals	References
Erlotinib	NSCLC	EGFR kinase inhibitor	2005	Pollack *et al.* (1999) [77] Bulgaru *et al.* (2003) [78]
Gefitinib	NSCLC	EGFR kinase inhibitor	2003	Baselga *et al.* (2000) [79] Sirotnak *et al.* (2002) [80]
Abiraterone	Metastatic castration-resistant prostate cancer or Hormone refractory prostate cancer	Androgen synthesis inhibitor	2011	Jarman *et al.* (1998) [81] Jagusch *et al.* (2008) [82]
Sorafenib	Renal, liver and thyroid cancer	VEGFR kinase inhibitor	2005	Heim *et al.* (2003) [83] Ahmad and Eisen (2004) [84]
Lapatinib	ERBB2-positive breast cancer	EGFR/ERBB2 inhibitor	2007	Xia *et al.* (2004) [85] Wood *et al.* (2004) [86]

(Table 4) cont.....

Name of the compound	Therapeutic area	Function	Approvals	References
Crizotinib	NSCLC	ALK inhibitor	2011	Butrynski *et al.* (2010) [87] Rodig *et al.* (2010) [88]
Imatinib	Chronic myeloid leukaemia	Tyrosine kinase inhibitor	1990	Buchnger *et al.* (1996) [89] Drunker *et al.* (1996) [90]

Cancer Modeling & Network

According to the WHO, cancer is one of the most dreadful diseases in the world. The treatment line is very complicated, and the therapy given should act on the multiple intracellular pathways, as it is known that cancer is a multifactorial disease. The analysis of anticancer agents is complex as the data available are large. There are numerous databases available to store massive amounts of data. Heterogeneous preclinical assay data are stored in the ChEMBL database. This Channel database has many models; one such model is PTML-LDA, which is used for preclinical discrimination of anticancer agents. To resolve similar issues, the PTML model is preferred, which is a combination of perturbation theory (PT) and ML methods. A comparison was made between the combinational model and the PTML model, and it was found that the combinational model had an advanced method to determine the activity of drugs against multiple cancers. A multi-task chemical information model was developed by uniting Broto Moreau with ANN, and a dataset carrying 1933 peptides was derived [91]. The model developed is used to virtually design and screen the peptide molecules and also to study the anti-cancer activity of peptides on cancer cell lines. The model showed more than 92% precision in both actual and predicted values, and the various healthy mammalian cells showed lower cytotoxicity. The tumours are constitutively complex, and hence their growth at different stages and scales must be studied carefully, from the tissues to the molecular length. The development of cancer cells is complicated, and it is studied at 3 different scales, such as micro, meso, and macroscale, which are the mathematical models. Many studies have been conducted to identify and combine drug targets for therapy using the multiscale models mentioned above by Wang *et al.* The evaluation of this method is based on an analysis of intracellular epidermal growth factor receptor [EGFR] signalling kinetics, lung cancer extracellular EGFR stimulation, and multicellular growth. A practically potent drug can be formed when the multi-scale model for tumours is cumulated with systemic pharmacology; by doing so, a broad system-level approach is developed, which can be further used to determine the effective form of currently available and new drug moieties used for preclinical studies, model organisms, and specific patients. Many factors affecting the drug effect can be interpreted by using computational and mathematical models. As a result, these can be used to comprehend advanced methods of disease prevention through therapy.

Summary

Cancer is one of the most dreadful diseases affecting mankind and has become hazardous for human health. According to reports, more than 9.5 million people are dying every year due to different forms of cancer. When a new type of cancer comes into existence, researchers start finding out the best therapy by developing various drugs, but in the case of cancer, the process of drug discovery is difficult as the pharmacology is not well known, and developing a new drug moiety takes more than 12 years and costs more than 2.7 billion US dollars. To overcome these issues, various tools, as discussed above, can be used to design a drug of our choice. The drug designed can be used to predict drug targets, perform network analysis of protein interaction, binding site prediction, and much more.

CONCLUSION

The advanced methods discussed above can be used to improve and increase drug discovery for anti-cancer therapy. The progression of artificial intelligence—mapping, docking, the de novo method, various models, *etc.*—can be very well used in the field of drug discovery. The computational models can be pooled with experimental validation, and this would increase the process of drug development.

REFERENCES

[1] Surh YJ. Reverse pharmacology applicable for botanical drug development - inspiration from the legacy of traditional wisdom. J Tradit Complement Med 2011; 1(1): 5-7. [http://dx.doi.org/10.1016/S2225-4110(16)30051-7] [PMID: 24716100]

[2] Foye WO. Foye's principles of medicinal chemistry. Lippincott williams & wilkins 2008.

[3] Suleria HA, Barrow C, Eds. Bioactive Compounds from Plant Origin: Extraction, Applications, and Potential Health Benefits. Principles of Medicinal chemistry. 3rd ed., CRC Press 2019.

[4] Veeresham C, Rama Rao A, Asres K. Aldose reductase inhibitors of plant origin. Phytother Res 2014; 28(3): 317-33. [http://dx.doi.org/10.1002/ptr.5000] [PMID: 23674239]

[5] Ntie-Kang F, Nwodo JN, Ibezim A, *et al.* Molecular modeling of potential anticancer agents from African medicinal plants. J Chem Inf Model 2014; 54(9): 2433-50. [http://dx.doi.org/10.1021/ci5003697] [PMID: 25116740]

[6] Ferreira L, dos Santos R, Oliva G, Andricopulo A. Molecular docking and structure-based drug design strategies. Molecules 2015; 20(7): 13384-421. [http://dx.doi.org/10.3390/molecules200713384] [PMID: 26205061]

[7] Halperin I, Ma B, Wolfson H, Nussinov R. Principles of docking: An overview of search algorithms

and a guide to scoring functions. Proteins 2002; 47(4): 409-43.
[http://dx.doi.org/10.1002/prot.10115] [PMID: 12001221]

[8] Rincones J, Scarpari LM, Carazzolle MF, *et al.* Differential gene expression between the biotrophic-like and saprotrophic mycelia of the witches' broom pathogen Moniliophthora perniciosa. Mol Plant Microbe Interact 2008; 21(7): 891-908.
[http://dx.doi.org/10.1094/MPMI-21-7-0891] [PMID: 18533830]

[9] Salmaso V, Moro S. Bridging molecular docking to molecular dynamics in exploring ligand-protein recognition process: an overview. Front Pharmacol 2018; 9: 923.
[http://dx.doi.org/10.3389/fphar.2018.00923] [PMID: 30186166]

[10] Mathi P, Prasad MV, Botlagunta M, Ravi M, Ramachandran D. De novo design of selective Sortase-A inhibitors: Synthesis, structural and *in vitro* characterization. Chemical Data Collections 2018; 15: 126-33.

[11] Huang SY, Grinter SZ, Zou X. Scoring functions and their evaluation methods for protein–ligand docking: recent advances and future directions. Phys Chem Chem Phys 2010; 12(40): 12899-908.
[http://dx.doi.org/10.1039/c0cp00151a] [PMID: 20730182]

[12] Kortagere S, Krasowski MD, Reschly EJ, Venkatesh M, Mani S, Ekins S. Evaluation of computational docking to identify pregnane X receptor agonists in the ToxCast database. Environ Health Perspect 2010; 118(10): 1412-7.
[http://dx.doi.org/10.1289/ehp.1001930] [PMID: 20558333]

[13] Yuriev E, Holien J, Ramsland PA. Improvements, trends, and new ideas in molecular docking: 2012-2013 in review. J Mol Recognit 2015; 28(10): 581-604.
[http://dx.doi.org/10.1002/jmr.2471] [PMID: 25808539]

[14] Yang W, Lu J, Weng J, *et al.* Prevalence of diabetes among men and women in China. N Engl J Med 2010; 362(12): 1090-101.
[http://dx.doi.org/10.1056/NEJMoa0908292] [PMID: 20335585]

[15] Sanchez-Vega F, Mina M, Armenia J, *et al.* Oncogenic signaling pathways in the cancer genome atlas. Cell 2018; 173(2): 321-337.e10.
[http://dx.doi.org/10.1016/j.cell.2018.03.035] [PMID: 29625050]

[16] Pirhadi S, Shiri F, Ghasemi JB. Methods and applications of structure based pharmacophores in drug discovery. Curr Top Med Chem 2013; 13(9): 1036-47.
[http://dx.doi.org/10.2174/1568026611313090006] [PMID: 23651482]

[17] Wolber G, Dornhofer AA, Langer T. Efficient overlay of small organic molecules using 3D pharmacophores. J Comput Aided Mol Des 2007; 20(12): 773-88.
[http://dx.doi.org/10.1007/s10822-006-9078-7] [PMID: 17051340]

[18] Liu X, Gu X, Li Z, *et al.* Neuregulin-1/erbB-activation improves cardiac function and survival in models of ischemic, dilated, and viral cardiomyopathy. J Am Coll Cardiol 2006; 48(7): 1438-47.
[http://dx.doi.org/10.1016/j.jacc.2006.05.057] [PMID: 17010808]

[19] Chimenti F, Cottiglia F, Bonsignore L, *et al.* Quercetin as the active principle of Hypericum hircinum exerts a selective inhibitory activity against MAO-A: extraction, biological analysis, and computational study. J Nat Prod 2006; 69(6): 945-9.
[http://dx.doi.org/10.1021/np060015w] [PMID: 16792415]

[20] Sanchez-Vega F, Mina M, Armenia J, *et al.* Oncogenic signaling pathways in the cancer genome atlas. Cell 2018; 173(2): 321-337.e10.
[http://dx.doi.org/10.1016/j.cell.2018.03.035] [PMID: 29625050]

[21] Böhm G, Muhr R, Jaenicke R. Quantitative analysis of protein far UV circular dichroism spectra by neural networks. Protein Eng Des Sel 1992; 5(3): 191-5.
[http://dx.doi.org/10.1093/protein/5.3.191] [PMID: 1409538]

[22] Zhavoronkov A, Ivanenkov YA, Aliper A, *et al.* Deep learning enables rapid identification of potent

DDR1 kinase inhibitors. Nat Biotechnol 2019; 37(9): 1038-40.
[http://dx.doi.org/10.1038/s41587-019-0224-x] [PMID: 31477924]

[23] Rush TS III, Grant JA, Mosyak L, Nicholls A. A shape-based 3-D scaffold hopping method and its application to a bacterial protein-protein interaction. J Med Chem 2005; 48(5): 1489-95.
[http://dx.doi.org/10.1021/jm040163o] [PMID: 15743191]

[24] Bologa CG, Revankar CM, Young SM, *et al.* Virtual and biomolecular screening converge on a selective agonist for GPR30. Nat Chem Biol 2006; 2(4): 207-12.
[http://dx.doi.org/10.1038/nchembio775] [PMID: 16520733]

[25] Murray CJL, Barber RM, Foreman KJ, *et al.* Global, regional, and national disability-adjusted life years (DALYs) for 306 diseases and injuries and healthy life expectancy (HALE) for 188 countries, 1990–2013: quantifying the epidemiological transition. Lancet 2015; 386(10009): 2145-91.
[http://dx.doi.org/10.1016/S0140-6736(15)61340-X] [PMID: 26321261]

[26] Hoshida Y, Nijman SMB, Kobayashi M, *et al.* Integrative transcriptome analysis reveals common molecular subclasses of human hepatocellular carcinoma. Cancer Res 2009; 69(18): 7385-92.
[http://dx.doi.org/10.1158/0008-5472.CAN-09-1089] [PMID: 19723656]

[27] Mendenhall J, Meiler J. Improving quantitative structure–activity relationship models using Artificial Neural Networks trained with dropout. J Comput Aided Mol Des 2016; 30(2): 177-89.
[http://dx.doi.org/10.1007/s10822-016-9895-2] [PMID: 26830599]

[28] Hansch C, Fujita T. p-σ-π Analysis. A method for the correlation of biological activity and chemical structure. J Am Chem Soc 1964; 86(8): 1616-26.
[http://dx.doi.org/10.1021/ja01062a035]

[29] Cramer RD, Patterson DE, Bunce JD. Comparative molecular field analysis (CoMFA). 1. Effect of shape on binding of steroids to carrier proteins. J Am Chem Soc 1988; 110(18): 5959-67.
[http://dx.doi.org/10.1021/ja00226a005] [PMID: 22148765]

[30] Klebe G, Abraham U, Mietzner T. Molecular similarity indices in a comparative analysis (CoMSIA) of drug molecules to correlate and predict their biological activity. J Med Chem 1994; 37(24): 4130-46.
[http://dx.doi.org/10.1021/jm00050a010] [PMID: 7990113]

[31] Conn VS, Hafdahl AR, Cooper PS, Brown LM, Lusk SL. Meta-analysis of workplace physical activity interventions. Am J Prev Med 2009; 37(4): 330-9.
[http://dx.doi.org/10.1016/j.amepre.2009.06.008] [PMID: 19765506]

[32] Tautermann CS. GPCR structures in drug design, emerging opportunities with new structures. Bioorg Med Chem Lett 2014; 24(17): 4073-9.
[http://dx.doi.org/10.1016/j.bmcl.2014.07.009] [PMID: 25086683]

[33] Cheng J, Bernstein MS. Flock: Hybrid crowd-machine learning classifiers. Proceedings of the 18th ACM conference on computer supported cooperative work & social computing. 600-11.

[34] DeVree BT, Mahoney JP, Vélez-Ruiz GA, *et al.* Allosteric coupling from G protein to the agonist-binding pocket in GPCRs. Nature 2016; 535(7610): 182-6.
[http://dx.doi.org/10.1038/nature18324] [PMID: 27362234]

[35] Tautermann CS. GPCR structures in drug design, emerging opportunities with new structures. Bioorg Med Chem Lett 2014; 24(17): 4073-9.
[http://dx.doi.org/10.1016/j.bmcl.2014.07.009] [PMID: 25086683]

[36] Sabbadin D, Moro S. Supervised molecular dynamics (SuMD) as a helpful tool to depict GPCR-ligand recognition pathway in a nanosecond time scale. J Chem Inf Model 2014; 54(2): 372-6.
[http://dx.doi.org/10.1021/ci400766b] [PMID: 24456045]

[37] Saha S, Singh G, Sapienza M, Torr PH, Cuzzolin F. Deep learning for detecting multiple space-time action tubes in videos. arXiv 2016.
[http://dx.doi.org/10.5244/C.30.58]

[38] Forde PM, Chaft JE, Smith KN, *et al.* Neoadjuvant PD-1 blockade in resectable lung cancer. N Engl J Med 2018; 378(21): 1976-86.
[http://dx.doi.org/10.1056/NEJMoa1716078] [PMID: 29658848]

[39] Tong M, Seeliger MA. Targeting conformational plasticity of protein kinases. ACS Chem Biol 2015; 10(1): 190-200.
[http://dx.doi.org/10.1021/cb500870a] [PMID: 25486330]

[40] Hancock JF. Ras proteins: different signals from different locations. Nat Rev Mol Cell Biol 2003; 4(5): 373-85.
[http://dx.doi.org/10.1038/nrm1105] [PMID: 12728271]

[41] Mazmanian SK, Liu G, Ton-That H, Schneewind O. Staphylococcus aureus sortase, an enzyme that anchors surface proteins to the cell wall. Science 1999; 285(5428): 760-3.
[http://dx.doi.org/10.1126/science.285.5428.760] [PMID: 10427003]

[42] Vigushin DM, Poon GK, Boddy A, *et al.* Phase I and pharmacokinetic study of d -limonene in patients with advanced cancer. Cancer Chemother Pharmacol 1998; 42(2): 111-7.
[http://dx.doi.org/10.1007/s002800050793] [PMID: 9654110]

[43] Muhsin M, Graham J, Kirkpatrick P. Gefitinib. Nat Rev Cancer 2003; 3(8): 556-7.
[http://dx.doi.org/10.1038/nrc1159]

[44] Grünwald V, Hidalgo M. Developing inhibitors of the epidermal growth factor receptor for cancer treatment. J Natl Cancer Inst 2003; 95(12): 851-67.
[http://dx.doi.org/10.1093/jnci/95.12.851] [PMID: 12813169]

[45] Wilhelm S, Carter C, Lynch M, *et al.* Discovery and development of sorafenib: a multikinase inhibitor for treating cancer. Nat Rev Drug Discov 2006; 5(10): 835-44.
[http://dx.doi.org/10.1038/nrd2130] [PMID: 17016424]

[46] Butrynski JE, D'Adamo DR, Hornick JL, *et al.* Crizotinib in ALK-rearranged inflammatory myofibroblastic tumor. N Engl J Med 2010; 363(18): 1727-33.
[http://dx.doi.org/10.1056/NEJMoa1007056] [PMID: 20979472]

[47] Harrison ML, Obermueller E, Maisey NR, *et al.* Tumor necrosis factor α as a new target for renal cell carcinoma: two sequential phase II trials of infliximab at standard and high dose. J Clin Oncol 2007; 25(29): 4542-9.
[http://dx.doi.org/10.1200/JCO.2007.11.2136] [PMID: 17925549]

[48] Reker D, Rodrigues T, Schneider P, Schneider G. Identifying the macromolecular targets of de novo-designed chemical entities through self-organizing map consensus. Proc Natl Acad Sci USA 2014; 111(11): 4067-72.
[http://dx.doi.org/10.1073/pnas.1320001111] [PMID: 24591595]

[49] Gómez-Bombarelli R, Wei JN, Duvenaud D, *et al.* Automatic chemical design using a data-driven continuous representation of molecules. ACS Cent Sci 2018; 4(2): 268-76.
[http://dx.doi.org/10.1021/acscentsci.7b00572] [PMID: 29532027]

[50] Jann B. The Blinder–Oaxaca decomposition for linear regression models. Stata J 2008; 8(4): 453-79.
[http://dx.doi.org/10.1177/1536867X0800800401]

[51] Manica M, Oskooei A, Born J, Subramanian V, Sáez-Rodríguez J, Rodríguez Martínez M. Toward explainable anticancer compound sensitivity prediction *via* multimodal attention-based convolutional encoders. Mol Pharm 2019; 16(12): 4797-806.
[http://dx.doi.org/10.1021/acs.molpharmaceut.9b00520] [PMID: 31618586]

[52] Cui L, Li L, Zhang A, Pan G, Bao D, Chang A. Biochar amendment greatly reduces rice Cd uptake in a contaminated paddy soil: a two-year field experiment. BioResources 2011; 6(3): 2605-18.

[53] Baratta MG, Schinzel AC, Zwang Y, *et al.* An in-tumor genetic screen reveals that the BET bromodomain protein, BRD4, is a potential therapeutic target in ovarian carcinoma. Proc Natl Acad

Sci USA 2015; 112(1): 232-7.
[http://dx.doi.org/10.1073/pnas.1422165112] [PMID: 25535366]

[54] Nappi AJ, Christensen BM. Melanogenesis and associated cytotoxic reactions: Applications to insect innate immunity. Insect Biochem Mol Biol 2005; 35(5): 443-59.
[http://dx.doi.org/10.1016/j.ibmb.2005.01.014] [PMID: 15804578]

[55] Liu Z, Robinson JT, Sun X, Dai H. PEGylated nanographene oxide for delivery of water-insoluble cancer drugs. J Am Chem Soc 2008; 130(33): 10876-7.
[http://dx.doi.org/10.1021/ja803688x] [PMID: 18661992]

[56] Meng XY, Zhang HX, Mezei M, Cui M. Molecular docking: a powerful approach for structure-based drug discovery. Curr Computeraided Drug Des 2011; 7(2): 146-57.
[http://dx.doi.org/10.2174/157340911795677602] [PMID: 21534921]

[57] Gainor JF, Dardaei L, Yoda S, *et al.* Molecular mechanisms of resistance to first-and second-generation ALK inhibitors in ALK-rearranged lung cancer. Cancer Discov 2016; 6(10): 1118-33.
[http://dx.doi.org/10.1158/2159-8290.CD-16-0596] [PMID: 27432227]

[58] Anderson KN, Schwab RB, Martinez ME. Reproductive risk factors and breast cancer subtypes: a review of the literature. Breast Cancer Res Treat 2014; 144(1): 1-10.
[http://dx.doi.org/10.1007/s10549-014-2852-7] [PMID: 24477977]

[59] Strickler JH, Starodub AN, Jia J, *et al.* Phase I study of bevacizumab, everolimus, and panobinostat (LBH-589) in advanced solid tumors. Cancer Chemother Pharmacol 2012; 70(2): 251-8.
[http://dx.doi.org/10.1007/s00280-012-1911-1] [PMID: 22744359]

[60] Blyszczuk P, Kania G, Dieterle T, *et al.* Myeloid differentiation factor-88/interleukin-1 signaling controls cardiac fibrosis and heart failure progression in inflammatory dilated cardiomyopathy. Circ Res 2009; 105(9): 912-20.
[http://dx.doi.org/10.1161/CIRCRESAHA.109.199802] [PMID: 19762681]

[61] Bakkouri WE, Kania RE, Guichard JP, Lot G, Herman P, Huy PTB. Conservative management of 386 cases of unilateral vestibular schwannoma: tumor growth and consequences for treatment. J Neurosurg 2009; 110(4): 662-9.
[http://dx.doi.org/10.3171/2007.5.16836] [PMID: 19099381]

[62] Vaughan CK, Mollapour M, Smith JR, *et al.* Hsp90-dependent activation of protein kinases is regulated by chaperone-targeted dephosphorylation of Cdc37. Mol Cell 2008; 31(6): 886-95.
[http://dx.doi.org/10.1016/j.molcel.2008.07.021] [PMID: 18922470]

[63] Chan ATC, Leung SF, Ngan RKC, *et al.* Overall survival after concurrent cisplatin-radiotherapy compared with radiotherapy alone in locoregionally advanced nasopharyngeal carcinoma. J Natl Cancer Inst 2005; 97(7): 536-9.
[http://dx.doi.org/10.1093/jnci/dji084] [PMID: 15812080]

[64] Sandilands A, O'Regan GM, Liao H, *et al.* Prevalent and rare mutations in the gene encoding filaggrin cause ichthyosis vulgaris and predispose individuals to atopic dermatitis. J Invest Dermatol 2006; 126(8): 1770-5.
[http://dx.doi.org/10.1038/sj.jid.5700459] [PMID: 16810297]

[65] Calabrese JM, Seila AC, Yeo GW, Sharp PA. RNA sequence analysis defines Dicer's role in mouse embryonic stem cells. Proc Natl Acad Sci USA 2007; 104(46): 18097-102.
[http://dx.doi.org/10.1073/pnas.0709193104] [PMID: 17989215]

[66] Gandhi L, Rodríguez-Abreu D, Gadgeel S, *et al.* Pembrolizumab plus chemotherapy in metastatic non–small-cell lung cancer. N Engl J Med 2018; 378(22): 2078-92.
[http://dx.doi.org/10.1056/NEJMoa1801005] [PMID: 29658856]

[67] Pastor MD, Nogal A, Molina-Pinelo S, *et al.* Identification of proteomic signatures associated with lung cancer and COPD. J Proteomics 2013; 89: 227-37.

[http://dx.doi.org/10.1016/j.jprot.2013.04.037] [PMID: 23665002]

[68] Yang R, Xu J, Xu L, *et al.* Cancer cell membrane-coated adjuvant nanoparticles with mannose modification for effective anticancer vaccination. ACS Nano 2018; 12(6): 5121-9. [http://dx.doi.org/10.1021/acsnano.7b09041] [PMID: 29771487]

[69] Zehir A, Benayed R, Shah RH, *et al.* Mutational landscape of metastatic cancer revealed from prospective clinical sequencing of 10,000 patients. Nat Med 2017; 23(6): 703-13. [http://dx.doi.org/10.1038/nm.4333] [PMID: 28481359]

[70] Mittica G, Ghisoni E, Giannone G, Aglietta M, Genta S, Valabrega G. Checkpoint inhibitors in endometrial cancer: preclinical rationale and clinical activity. Oncotarget 2017; 8(52): 90532-44. [http://dx.doi.org/10.18632/oncotarget.20042] [PMID: 29163851]

[71] Cohen EEW, Soulières D, Le Tourneau C, *et al.* Pembrolizumab versus methotrexate, docetaxel, or cetuximab for recurrent or metastatic head-and-neck squamous cell carcinoma (KEYNOTE-040): a randomised, open-label, phase 3 study. Lancet 2019; 393(10167): 156-67. [http://dx.doi.org/10.1016/S0140-6736(18)31999-8] [PMID: 30509740]

[72] Mughini-Gras L, Schaapveld M, Kramers J, *et al.* Increased colon cancer risk after severe Salmonella infection. PLoS One 2018; 13(1): e0189721. [http://dx.doi.org/10.1371/journal.pone.0189721] [PMID: 29342165]

[73] Cardenas-Goicoechea J, Wang Y, McGorray S, *et al.* Minimally invasive interval cytoreductive surgery in ovarian cancer: systematic review and meta-analysis. J Robot Surg 2019; 13(1): 23-33. [http://dx.doi.org/10.1007/s11701-018-0838-x] [PMID: 29992404]

[74] Seiler R, Ashab HAD, Erho N, *et al.* Impact of molecular subtypes in muscle-invasive bladder cancer on predicting response and survival after neoadjuvant chemotherapy. Eur Urol 2017; 72(4): 544-54. [http://dx.doi.org/10.1016/j.eururo.2017.03.030] [PMID: 28390739]

[75] Beaugerie L, Carrat F, Nahon S, *et al.* High risk of anal and rectal cancer in patients with anal and/or perianal Crohn's disease. Clin Gastroenterol Hepatol 2018; 16(6): 892-899.e2. [http://dx.doi.org/10.1016/j.cgh.2017.11.041] [PMID: 29199142]

[76] Toovey EW, Heller I, Webster DR. A method of transplanting gastric mucosa to the anterior abdominal wall of the rat for the local application of carcinogens. Cancer Res 1951; 11(12): 912-3. [PMID: 14886944]

[77] Ballo MT, Zagars GK, Pollack A, Pisters PWT, Pollock RA. Desmoid tumor: prognostic factors and outcome after surgery, radiation therapy, or combined surgery and radiation therapy. J Clin Oncol 1999; 17(1): 158-67. [http://dx.doi.org/10.1200/JCO.1999.17.1.158] [PMID: 10458229]

[78] Bulgaru AM, Mani S, Goel S, Perez-Soler R. Erlotinib (Tarceva®): a promising drug targeting epidermal growth factor receptor tyrosine kinase. Expert Rev Anticancer Ther 2003; 3(3): 269-79. [http://dx.doi.org/10.1586/14737140.3.3.269] [PMID: 12820772]

[79] Mendelsohn J, Baselga J. The EGF receptor family as targets for cancer therapy. Oncogene 2000; 19(56): 6550-65. [http://dx.doi.org/10.1038/sj.onc.1204082] [PMID: 11426640]

[80] Khokhar NZ, Lam AFY, Rusch VW, Sirotnak FM. Despite some expression of folate receptor α in human mesothelioma cells, internalization of methotrexate is predominantly carrier mediated. J Thorac Cardiovasc Surg 2002; 123(5): 862-8. [http://dx.doi.org/10.1067/mtc.2002.120352] [PMID: 12019370]

[81] Vigushin DM, Poon GK, Boddy A, *et al.* Phase I and pharmacokinetic study of d -limonene in patients with advanced cancer. Cancer Chemother Pharmacol 1998; 42(2): 111-7. [http://dx.doi.org/10.1007/s002800050793] [PMID: 9654110]

[82] Pinto-Bazurco Mendieta MAE, Negri M, Jagusch C, Müller-Vieira U, Lauterbach T, Hartmann RW. Synthesis, biological evaluation, and molecular modeling of abiraterone analogues: novel CYP17

inhibitors for the treatment of prostate cancer. J Med Chem 2008; 51(16): 5009-18. [http://dx.doi.org/10.1021/jm800355c] [PMID: 18672868]

[83] Hurwitz H, Fehrenbacher L, Novotny W, *et al.* Bevacizumab plus irinotecan, fluorouracil, and leucovorin for metastatic colorectal cancer. N Engl J Med 2004; 350(23): 2335-42. [http://dx.doi.org/10.1056/NEJMoa032691] [PMID: 15175435]

[84] Ahmad T, Eisen T. Kinase inhibition with BAY 43-9006 in renal cell carcinoma. Clin Cancer Res 2004; 10(18): 6388S-92S. [http://dx.doi.org/10.1158/1078-0432.CCR-040028] [PMID: 15448036]

[85] Theilmann RJ, Borders R, Trouard TP, *et al.* Changes in water mobility measured by diffusion MRI predict response of metastatic breast cancer to chemotherapy. Neoplasia 2004; 6(6): 831-7. [http://dx.doi.org/10.1593/neo.03343] [PMID: 15720810]

[86] Hughes KS, Schnaper LA, Berry D, *et al.* Lumpectomy plus tamoxifen with or without irradiation in women 70 years of age or older with early breast cancer. N Engl J Med 2004; 351(10): 971-7. [http://dx.doi.org/10.1056/NEJMoa040587] [PMID: 15342805]

[87] Hughes KS, Schnaper LA, Berry D, *et al.* Lumpectomy plus tamoxifen with or without irradiation in women 70 years of age or older with early breast cancer. N Engl J Med 2004; 351(10): 971-7. [http://dx.doi.org/10.1056/NEJMoa040587] [PMID: 15342805]

[88] Sasaki T, Rodig SJ, Chirieac LR, Jänne PA. The biology and treatment of EML4-ALK non-small cell lung cancer. Eur J Cancer 2010; 46(10): 1773-80. [http://dx.doi.org/10.1016/j.ejca.2010.04.002] [PMID: 20418096]

[89] Irfan SM, Bhurgri Y. Clinico-pathological features and outcomes in chronic phase chronic myeloid leukemia patients treated with hydroxyurea. Asian Pac J Cancer Prev 2009; 10(4): 591-4. [PMID: 19827875]

[90] Doll R. Cancers weakly related to smoking. Br Med Bull 1996; 52(1): 35-49. [http://dx.doi.org/10.1093/oxfordjournals.bmb.a011531] [PMID: 8746295]

[91] Speck-Planche A, Kleandrova VV, Luan F, Cordeiro MNDS. Chemoinformatics in anti-cancer chemotherapy: Multi-target QSAR model for the in silico discovery of anti-breast cancer agents. Eur J Pharm Sci 2012; 47(1): 273-9. [http://dx.doi.org/10.1016/j.ejps.2012.04.012] [PMID: 22538055]

CHAPTER 8

Human Topoisomerases and Caspases: Important Targets in Cancer Therapy

Sandeep Goyal[1,*], **Mukesh Gangar**[1,*], **Aditya Kulkarni**[1] and **Charu Kamal Yerneni**[2]

[1] *Aten Porus Lifesciences, Bangalore, India*

[2] *Flamma USA, Pennsylvania, USA*

Abstract: Cancer has always remained a major challenge to humanity with its rising morbidity and mortality rate making it uncontrollable. Current treatments for cancer offer limited efficacy and suffer from serious side effects. With a focus on making treatment safer and more effective, there is a need to identify novel targets and potent drugs for these targets. Recent years have witnessed significant progress in the discovery of targeted cancer therapy. On-going research in this field suggests that human topoisomerases and caspases are important molecular drug targets for anti-cancer drug development. Topoisomerases are DNA processing enzymes essentially required to maintain DNA topology during transcription, replication, recombination and chromosomal decatenation. Several new chemical classes of topoisomerase inhibitors including natural product derivatives are in clinical trials for the treatment of various human cancers. Several topoisomerase inhibitors such as topotecan, irinotecan, camptothecin, teniposide and doxorubicin are clinically approved for various cancers such as colon cancer, lung cancer, breast cancer, and many more. However, many of these inhibitors have also been associated with serious side effects during chemotherapy. Emerging data in recent years also suggests the role of topoisomerase inhibition in immunogenic cell death and activating anticancer immune responses making them potential combinatorial modalities for cancer immunotherapy. Caspases [1-12] belong to the family of cysteine-aspartic proteases responsible for the execution of cell death in apoptotic cells. Caspases play an important role in various non-lethal biological processes like cell proliferation, cell differentiation, intercellular communication, and cell migration. The dysregulation of apoptotic signalling pathways is considered one of the hallmarks of cancer. Hence the focus of cancer therapy is correcting this aberrant behaviour. Natural products such as alkaloids, flavonoids, diterpenoids, sesquiterpenes, and polyphenolics have been reported with various anticancer properties. In this chapter, we have discussed topoisomerases and the regulation of caspase functions through direct or indirect methods for anticancer drug discovery.

[*] **Corresponding authors Sandeep Goyal & Mukesh Gangar:** Aten Porus Lifesciences, Bangalore, India; E-mails: sandeep@atenporus.com & mukesh@atenporus.com

Motamarri Venkata Naga Lalitha Chaitanya, Galvina Pereira, & Heyam Saad Ali (Eds.)

Keywords: Apoptosis, Cancer, Caspases, Chromosomal decatenation, Cysteine-aspartic proteases, DNA topology, Topoisomerases.

INTRODUCTION

Cancer always remains one of the leading health problems globally for many decades, with a growing number of cases and fatalities every passing year. Cancer is the second leading cause of death globally. According to the WHO, an estimated 9.6 million people died in 2018 due to cancer. Available treatment options include chemotherapy, radiotherapy, surgery, immunotherapy, and targeted therapies [1]. Chemotherapy remains the primary approach for cancer treatments. However, the treatment efficiency is limited due to drug-associated toxicities on normal cells and adverse side effects. Therefore, the most effective and less toxic therapy for the treatment of cancer is required. Natural products and their analogues have been reported to demonstrate success in cancer therapy [2 - 5]. Natural products comprise a vast and rich source of bioactive compounds with diverse beneficial effects on our health and living. A lot of safe and useful drugs have been developed based on natural compounds [6, 7]. Scientists around the world are working to find the cure for cancer, wherein topoisomerases I & II and caspases play a very important role in this. In this chapter, we will briefly discuss the role of natural products and natural product-based human topoisomerases inhibitors and caspases modulators towards the therapeutics for cancer.

DNA TOPOISOMERASES

DNA topoisomerases are a group of cellular enzymes that control DNA topology and their proper functioning is essential for most processes taking place in the cell. These ubiquitous enzymes are involved in significant biological processes involving DNA in the cells *e.g.* DNA replication, transcription and recombination or chromosome condensation. To get the genetic information from the DNA it is necessary to separate the two DNA duplex strands and topoisomerases are essential for this and they also enable replicated chromosome release before partitioning and cell division. The utmost necessity of these topoisomerase enzymes is because of the continued need for the DNA duplex to be compacted and fit into a much smaller nucleus. During this process, there are chances for DNA entanglements and knots which can potentially pose serious concerns for the overall DNA functioning. DNA topoisomerases help to overcome these issues. These enzymes work by binding covalently to the DNA phosphorus group, splitting the DNA strand and finally reuniting them. Topoisomerase 1 and Topoisomerase 2 are well-established antitumor drug targets. DNA topoisomerase I was first discovered in 1971 by James Wang, as the omega (ω) protein from *Escherichia coli*. After that, several forms of DNA topoisomerases have been discovered to date and were characterised in all three domains of life (bacteria, eukarya and archaea). Both human topoisomerase I and human topoisomerase II are targets of anticancer drugs [8 - 12].

Classification and Terminology of Topoisomerases

Depending upon the structures and catalytic activity, there are two main types of topoisomerases: topoisomerases I (Top I) and topoisomerases II (Top II) are further divided into five categories: IA, IB, IC, IIA and IIB. Topoisomerase enzymes terminology is classified according to the number of strands they cut: type I enzymes cut one DNA strand and type II enzymes cut two DNA strands. Depending upon the catalytic activity and structural domain, these enzymes are further divided into three classes; A, B, and C (Fig. **1**). Type I-A enzymes have a tyrosine residue that remains linked to the 5′ end of the cut strand, I-B enzymes have a tyrosine residue that remains linked to the 3′ end and I-C enzymes also have the tyrosine residue that remains linked to the 3′ end. Human topoisomerase I belongs to the type-IB and human topoisomerase II belongs to type-2A topoisomerase [8].

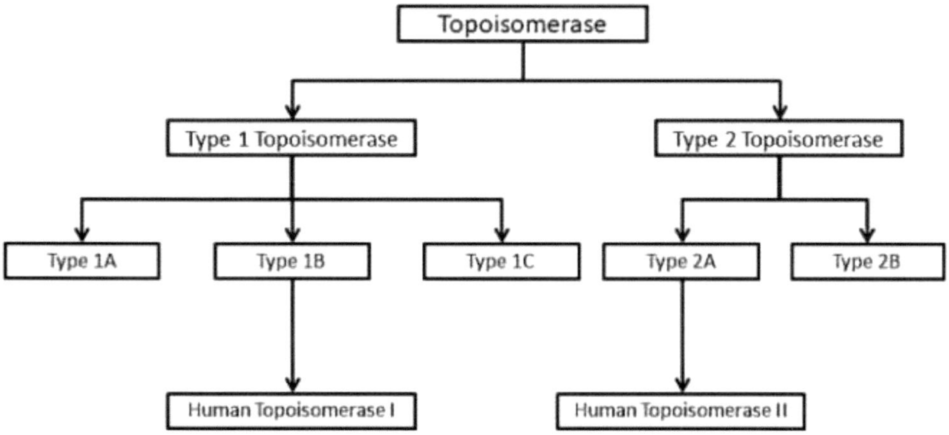

Fig. (1). Classification of Topoisomerases

Human topoisomerase I & II

Human topoisomerase I (hTop I) is a monomeric enzyme that belongs to Type-IB subfamily and has a molecular weight of 91 kDa. It consists of 765 amino acids which form four domains: an N-terminal domain, a linker domain, a core domain and a C-terminal domain as determined by X-ray crystallography [8].

Human topoisomerase I (hTop I) expression is higher in cancer cells as compared to healthy cells which make it a desired target for cancer, tumours or patients with the overexpression of Topoisomerase I. Human topoisomerase II (hTop II) has two homodimeric isoforms: a (MW 170 kDa) & b (MW 180 kDa) with 70% homogeneity in the amino acid sequence. It has four domains: two N-terminal domains, a core domain and a C-terminal domain. Human topoisomerase IIa expression increase is mainly observed in proliferating cells and it is crucial for cell survival [8].

Types of DNA Topoisomerase Inhibitors

Depending upon the mechanism of cell death through apoptosis, Topoisomerases inhibitors can be broadly classified into 2 categories:

Topoisomerase poisons: These compounds are based on the stabilisation of the topoisomerases enzyme–DNA covalent complex which prevents the relegation of the cut strand and ultimately results in DNA damage and cell death through apoptosis. Examples of topoisomerase poisons include doxorubicin (from the Anthracyclines class), it is approved for the treatment of various types of cancers including ovarian, lung, gastric and breast, thyroid cancer, multiple myeloma and others [8, 10].

Catalytic inhibitors: These inhibitors work by inhibiting the ability of the topoisomerase enzyme to attach to the DNA strand. This can be achieved in two ways: either the inhibitor is binding to the DNA duplex or the topoisomerase enzyme and ultimately these catalytic inhibitors will lead to cell death through apoptosis [8, 10].

Role of Natural Products as Topoisomerase Inhibitors

Natural products have been used as medicinal remedies since the very early times of mankind. The improvements in the use of natural products as medicine are drastic with the whole plant remedies used in ancient times for the isolation of active ingredients and further with the modification of the active ingredients to further improve the medicinal properties of the compounds. Medicinally active compounds derived from animals, plants and microbes have been used to treat human diseases since the dawn of medicine. It is estimated that about half of all the antitumor drugs available were actually natural products or their structural derivatives. Human Topoisomerases have been recognized and established as essential targets for cancer therapy. Many synthetic topoisomerase inhibitors have been identified with excellent anticancer activity and were subjected to clinical trials but owing to the undesired side effects of these synthetic drugs, they were restricted for universal use. The high cost of synthesis of these drugs adds to the burden of their use. To overcome the undesirable effects and high cost, natural products and their analogues are the best alternative and they can also be used for safe and long-term applications. Wide varieties of medicinal plants have shown anticancer activities both *in vitro* and/or *in vivo* through different pathways and mechanisms of action. There are several reports on different categories of Topoisomerase I and Topoisomerase II inhibitors including flavonoids, alkaloids, terpenes, coumarins, lignans and other secondary metabolites isolated from various sources, Table **1** summarizes some of the sources from which these compounds were isolated.

Table 1. Natural sources of various natural products with Inhibitor activity of human DNA Topoisomerases

Class of compounds	Natural source of Topoisomerases I inhibitors	Natural source of Topoisomerases II inhibitors
Flavanoids & Isoflavanoids	Roots of *Scutellaria amoena*, Roots of *Glycyrrhiza inflate*, *Ouratea semiserrata* [1, 13]	Resin of *Amburana cearensis*, Resin of *Garcinia hurburyi*, Leaves of *Annona dioca* [14],
Alkaloids	Roots of *Cryptolepis sanguinolenta*, *Lycoris radiate*, Fruits of *Evodia Rutaecarpa*, *Gelsemium sempervirens*, Roots of *Rubia cordifolia*, *Cynanchum Komarovii*, *Diospyros Morrisana*, Seeds of *Peganum harmala*, *Ocotea leucoxylon* [1, 15, 16]	*Ochrosia elliptica*, *Tabernaemontana divericata*, Roots of *Rubia cordifolia*, Barks of *Lunasia amara*, Roots of *Rauwolfia serpentine*, Bulb of *Eleutherine Americana* [1, 17]
Terpenoids	Roots of *Xylopia langsdorffiana*, Roots of *Peltodon longipes*, Twigs of *winchia Calophylla*, Roots of *orthosiphon Wulfenioides*, *Salvia miltiorrhiza*, Flower buds of *Daphne genkwa*, Fruit bodies of *Ganoderma amboinense*, *Fomitella fraxinea* [1, 18, 19]	Roots of *Xylopia langsdorffiana*, Branches and leaves of *Abies faxoniana*, Roots of *Stellera chamaejasme*, *Lobaria kurokawae Yoshim*, Roots of *Euphorbia kansui*, Bark of *Bischofia javanica*, Fruit bodies of *Ganoderma amboinense*, Sclerotium of *Poria cocos*, Barks of *Abies sachalinensis*, *Kokoona zeylanica*, *Salvia prionitis*, *Fomitella fraxinea* [1, 18, 20, 21]
Lignans	Leaves of *Koelreuteria henryi*, Roots of *Saururus chinensis*, Bark of *Machilus thunbergii* [1, 22]	Roots of *Stellera chamaejasme*, *Haplophyllum dauricum*, Roots and Rhizomes of *Podophyllum emodi*, Roots of *Saururus chinensis*, Bark of *Machilus thunbergii* [21, 23, 24]

Topoisomerase I inhibitors

Fig. (**2**) shows some of the potent natural products isolated from the different sources with Topoisomerase I inhibition activity.

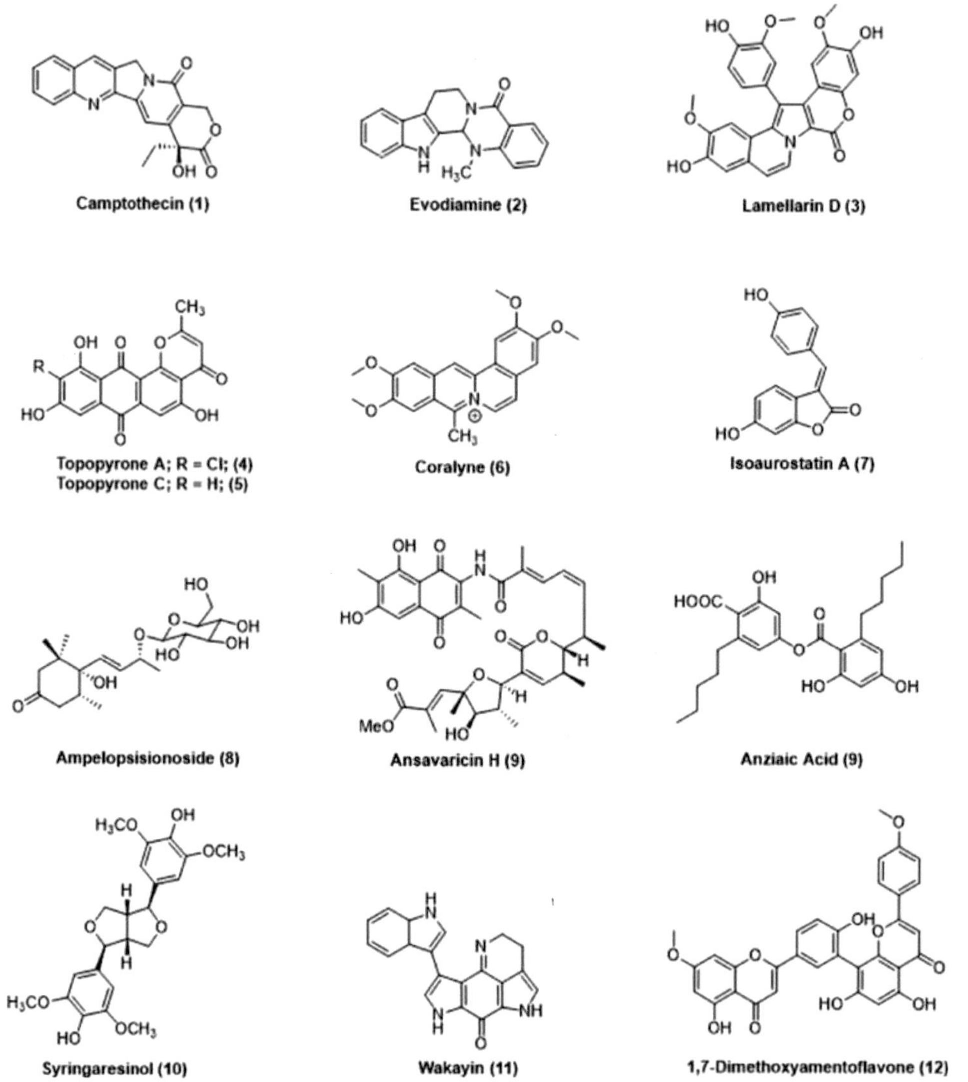

Fig. (2). Natural product based Topoisomerase I inhibitors.

Camptothecin (CPT), isolated from the Chinese tree *Camptotheca acuminata*, is a natural Topoisomerase I inhibitor. CPT acts by binding to a transient Topoisomerase I –DNA covalent complex, leading to an accumulation of DNA strand breaks on replication, and ultimately resulting in cell death [25, 26]. Evodiamine is a quinazolino carboline alkaloid isolated from the fruit of *Evodia rutaecarpa* Bentham and acts as Topoisomerase I inhibitor [27]. Lamellarins are a class of marine polycyclic alkaloids, lamellarin D (*LMD*) is a Topoisomerase I inhibitor with potent antitumor activity [27]. Topopyrones A–D is a family of anthraquinone polyphenols, isolated from the culture broth of the fungi *Phoma* sp, which were reported to be specific inhibitors of Topoisomerase I [27]. Coralyne, a protoberberine-type alkaloid, was reported to be a Topoisomerase I inhibitor [27]. Isoaurostatin A (IAS-A) is a weak Topoisomerase I inhibitor isolated from *Thermomonospora alba* [27]. Wakayin, a pyrroloiminoquinone alkaloid from the *ascidian Clavelina* species, was reported to be a Topoisomerase I inhibitor with potent cytotoxicity [27]. Several other drug candidates, such as rubitecan, lurtotecan, and exatecan, are currently under different stages of clinical evaluation [27].

Topoisomerase II inhibitors

Human DNA Topoisomerase II is one of the major targets in anticancer therapy and vast research is going on in this area. Many potent molecules have been identified in the past like synthetic compounds, semi-synthetic and natural product-based molecules. Herein we discuss Topoisomerase II inhibitors based on the natural products or compounds derived from natural products. A few examples of the Topoisomerase II inhibitors are discussed in Fig. (**3**). Etoposide (**14**) is a derivative of podophyllotoxin; its anticancer activity is based on Topoisomerase II poisoning. It is used for the treatment of SCLCs, lymphomas, acute myeloid leukaemia, and testicular and ovarian cancer [10]. Teniposide (**15**) is also a semisynthetic derivative of podophyllotoxin and its mechanism of action is similar to etoposide. It causes DNA double-stranded breakage *via* stabilisation of DNA-Topoisomerase II complexes. It was approved by the FDA in 1992. It is mainly used in the therapy of childhood acute lymphocytic leukaemia, glioma, CNS tumours and bladder cancer. Doxorubicin (**16**) and Epirubicinis (**17**) both are anthracycline derivatives and both work as Topoisomerase II poisons. Amrubicin (**19**) also is an anthracycline derivative with potent antitumor activity based on the Topoisomerase II inhibition. Mitoxantrone (**20**) is used as a chemotherapeutic drug in the treatment of acute leukaemia, lymphoma, prostate cancer and breast cancer. Amsacrine (**21**) and Vosaroxin (**22**) mechanism of action is also based on the Topoisomerase II poisoning. Dexrazoxane (**23**) is an ethylenediaminetetraacetic acid derivative and its mechanism of action is based on catalytic inhibition through the blocking of DNA dependent hydrolysis of ATP by Topoisomerase II which prevents the N-terminal clamp opening and consequently blocks the release of transported DNA segment. Merbarone (**24**) catalytic Topoisomerase II inhibitor, is a thiobarbiturate analogue [10].

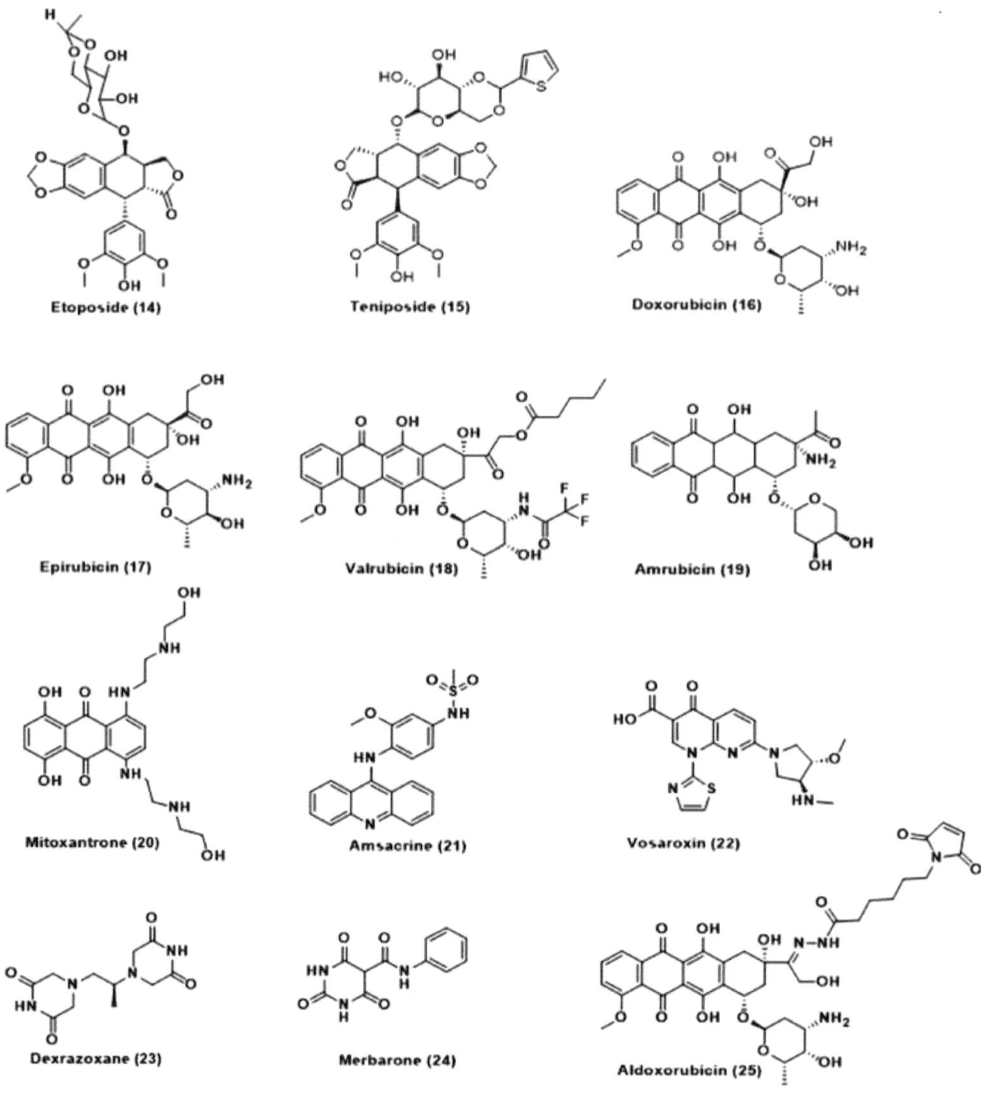

Fig. (3). Natural product based Topoisomerase II inhibitors.

CASPASES

Caspases (cysteine-aspartic proteases) are proteolytic enzymes important for maintaining homeostasis by regulating inflammation and cell death. Caspases play an important role in apoptosis, a major form of programmed cell death. Upon activation, they dismantle the cell from inside through the cleavage of structural and regulatory proteins. The suicidal mechanism is regulated by multiple interrelated pathways ensuring caspases are activated only in cells that require termination [28 - 32]. However, dysregulation of apoptosis contributes to the pathogenesis of several diseases including cancer [33 - 39]. Several studies demonstrate that natural products modulate apoptosis signalling pathways thereby improving cancer therapy [40 - 43].

Caspase Family

Caspases are a family of cysteine proteases that specifically hydrolyse peptide bonds containing aspartic acid residues. There are 12 known human caspases classified based on their roles in inflammation and apoptosis. Human caspase-1, caspase-4, caspase-5, caspase-11 and caspase-12 are involved in the coordination of inflammatory response whereas caspase-2, caspase-3, caspase-6, caspase-7, caspase-8, caspase-9 and caspase-10 are responsible for apoptosis (Fig. **4**)

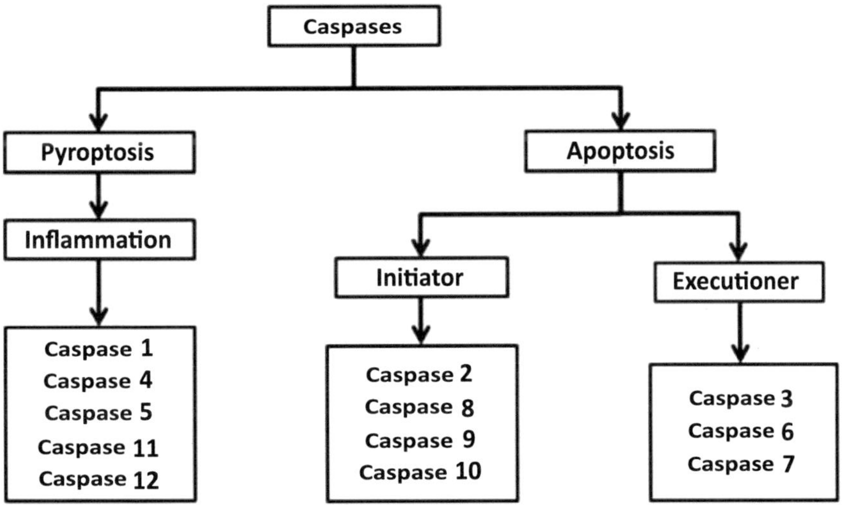

Fig. (4). Classification of human caspases.

The apoptotic caspases are further sub-classified into initiators and executioners caspases based on their mechanism of action and the presence or absence of specific protein domains: the prodomain, large (~20 kDa) catalytic domain, and small catalytic domain (~10 kDa). The identification of caspases and their role in apoptotic cell death was evident with the discovery of *ced-3* as an executioner of cell death during the development of the nematode *Caenorhabditis elegans*. The protein product of the *ced-3* gene was homologous to interleukin-1β converting enzyme (ICE), later known as cysteine protease caspase-1 [28 - 32, 44, 45].

Caspases Structure

Caspases are synthesized as inactive precursors or zymogens; consisting of a C-terminal catalytic domain and an N-terminal prodomain. The catalytic domains of caspases are comprised of small and large subunits, required for the active conformation of an enzyme. The catalytic cysteine residue resides within the large subunit while the small subunit contains specific residues that are essential for the structuring of the substrate-binding pockets and therefore are important for substrate recognition. The prodomains of caspases differ with respect to their structure and function.

Caspases Functions

Inflammatory Caspases

Caspase-1, -4, -5, and -12 comprise the inflammatory subset in humans, whereas caspase-1, -11, and -12 serve the same function in mice. Inflammatory caspases function as critical mediators of innate immune responses. Caspase 1, a prototypical member of the inflammatory caspase family has been identified as an important mediator of the innate immune response. Inflammatory caspases are synthesized as inactive zymogens (pro-caspases) in resting cells. Cellular stimulation *via* the engagement of pattern recognition receptors leads to its activation through the formation of inflammasomes.

Apoptotic Caspases

Apoptosis is a form of programmed cell death which involves controlled dismantling of intracellular components while avoiding inflammation and damage to neighbouring cells. Initiator caspases activate executioner caspases that subsequently coordinate their activities to demolish key structural proteins and activate other enzymes. The morphological hallmarks of apoptosis result include DNA fragmentation and membrane blabbing. The initiator caspases exist as inactive procaspase monomers that are activated by dimerization. The current model for activation of initiator caspase is proximity-induced dimerization. Homodimerzation is believed to be the initial event that triggers the activation of initiator caspases that mediate downstream signalling to effector molecules. The effector procaspases lacking long prodomains exist as inactive dimers in normal cells. Effector caspase activation induces conformational rearrangements in the active site which greatly increases their catalytic activity to produce a fully matured enzyme confirmation [28 - 32, 44, 45].

Role of Caspases in Cancer

Existing cancer therapies like chemotherapy or radiotherapy aim to activate apoptosis in cancer cells. However apoptotic caspases can play oncogenic roles through non-apoptotic functions. The loss of caspases promotes tumorigenesis through non-apoptotic pathways by affecting proliferation, invasion and migration. There is abundant experimental evidence which shows that a disturbance in the regulation of caspase activation and apoptosis underlies the pathogenesis of cancer. Evasion of apoptosis *via* caspases is considered one of the hallmarks of cancer. Therefore, many existing therapies for cancer aim to overcome apoptosis evasion by targeting different caspase pathways [33 - 39, 46 - 48].

NATURAL PRODUCTS IN CANCER THERAPY

Natural products are a valuable resource for drug discovery and development. Natural products from medicinal plants are one of the best reservoirs of novel chemical entities demonstrating structural diversity and new medicinal activities. According to reports, 50% of all drugs in clinical use are natural products or their derivatives which signify their importance.

More than 3000 plant species are reported for cancer therapy. Alkaloids, flavonoids, diterpenoids, sesquiterpenes, and polyphenolic represents a large and diverse group of natural products with anticancer properties [40 - 43]. The effects of selected promising natural products on regulating apoptosis and their therapeutic potential in cancer therapy are summarized Fig. (**5**) and Table **2**. These natural products have been reported to modulate the level of key proteins involved in apoptosis signalling pathways. Therefore, the identification of natural products has the ability to inhibit carcinogenesis without exerting cytotoxic effects in the normal cells. Camptothecin (**26**), a quinolone alkaloid isolated from the stem and bark of *Camptotheca acuminata* trees. Apart from Topoisomerase's inhibitory activity, it has also been shown to induce apoptosis in mice and human myeloid leukemia cells by upregulating pro-apoptotic proteins and down-regulating cell cycle proteins [49]. Evodiamine (**27**) is a quinazolinocarboline alkaloid found in a variety of herbs *Evodia rutaecarpa* and *Euonymus europaeus*. It exerts an anti-proliferative effect and increases the sensitivity of camptothecin to tumor cells [50]. Matrine (**28**), an alkaloid found in *Sophora flavescensait* possesses antitumor activity by inducing apoptosis in many cancers such as breast cancer, cervical cancer, gastric cancer, gallbladder cancer, hepatocellular carcinoma, lung cancer, prostate cancer, leukemia, melanoma and osteosarcoma [51]. Jaceosidin (**29**), is a trihydroxy flavone isolated from Japanese mugwort *Artemisia princeps* that also induces apoptotic cell death [52]. Triptolide (**30**), a diterpene isolated from *Tripterygium wilfordii* has shown anti-proliferative and pro-apoptotic activity in many cancer cells by downregulating NF-κB [53]. Oridonin (**31**), a kaurene-type diterpenoid from *Rabdosia rubescens* has been shown to possess antiproliferative effects *via* the modulation of apoptotic signalling pathways [54]. Costunolide (**32**), a sesquiterpene first isolated from *Saussurea costus* and Honokiol (**33**), a bioactive compound isolated from species of the genus *Mangolia* induce apoptosis and inhibit migration and invasion in cancer cells [55, 56]. Wedelolactone (**34**), a medicinal plant-derived natural compound from *Eclipta alba*, exhibits broad pharmacological effects by reduction of NF-κB-mediated transcription of genes [57].

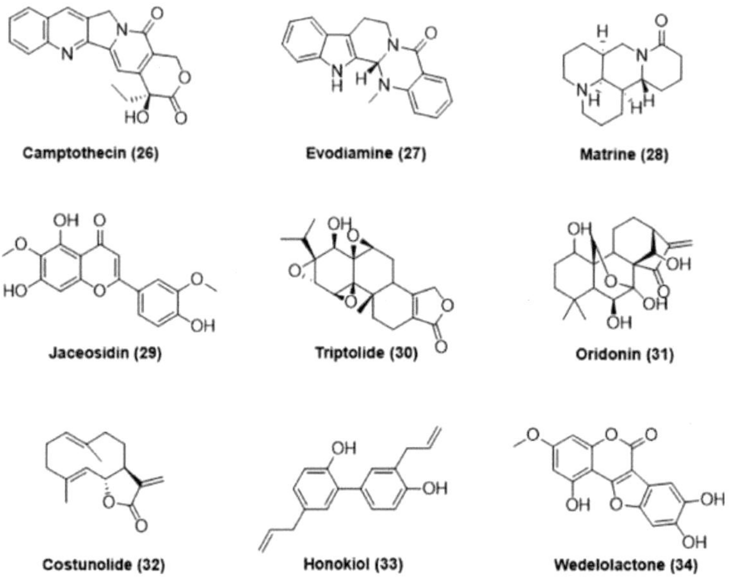

Fig. (5). Natural product inducing apoptosis in cancer cells.

Table 2. Natural products inducing apoptosis in tumor cells

Compound	Natural sources	Mode of action	Type of cancer
Camptothecin (Alkaloid)	*Camptotheca acuminate*	Upregulating pro-apoptotic proteins, *e.g.* JunB, c-Jun, Bak, Bax, Bfl1 and pRb2, and downregulating cell cycle proteins, *e.g.* CRAF-1, DP1, cyclinB1, cdk4, wee1	Hepatocellular carcinoma, human myeloid leukemia [42, 49]

(Table 2) cont.....

Compound	Natural sources	Mode of action	Type of cancer
Evodiamine (Alkaloid)	*Evodia rutaecarpa*	Cell-cycle arrest, antiinflammatory, antiproliferation, anticancer, antimetastatic	Leukemia, gastric, colorectal, breast, hepatocellular, melanoma, cervix, prostate, thyroid, and pancreatic cancer [41, 50]
Matrine (Alkaloid)	*Sophora flavescensait*	Cell-cycle arrest, anticancer, anti-inflammatory, anti-metastasis, antiviral	Leukemia, gastric, cervical, prostate, melanoma, breast, gall bladder, lung, hepatocellular, osteosarcoma, and esophageal cancer [42, 51]
Jaceosidin (Flavanoid)	*Artemisia princeps*	Cell-cycle arrest, anti-inflammation, antiproliferation	Cervical, human ovarian, epithelial, prostate, breast and glioblastoma [41, 52],
Triptolide (Diterpenoid)	*Tripterygium wilfordii*	Anti-proliferative, Anti-tumor, Pro-apoptotic, increase caspase activity, Immunosuppressive	Acute myeloid leukemia, prostate, Pancreatic, ovarian, lung, breast, gastric, osteosarcoma, colon, and neuroblastoma [42, 53]
Oridonin (Diterpenoid)	*Isodon rubescens*	Cell-cycle arrest, antiproliferation, antiinflammatory, autophagy, and immunomodulation	Breast, leukemia, prostate, melanoma, ovarian, pancreatic, cervical, gastric, colorectal, lung, and hepatocellular [41 - 54]
Costunolide (Sesquiterpenes)	*Inula helenium, Saussurea lappa, Magnolia grandiflora*	Cell-cycle arrest, antiproliferation, anti-inflammation, anticancer, antiviral, antifungal	Liver, ovarian, breast, bladder, melanoma, gastric, leukemia, prostate, and colorectal cancer [41, 55]
Honokiol (Lignan)	*Magnolia officinalis, Magnolia grandiflora, Magnolia spp.*	Cell-cycle arrest, anti-inflammatory, antiproliferation anticancer, antiangiogenesis, antiautophagy, immunomodulation	Glioblastoma, colon, melanoma, gastric, leukemia, prostate, pancreatic, ovarian, colorectal, breast, hepatocellular, lung head and neck squamous carcinoma [41, 56]
Wedelolactone (Polyphenolic)	*Eclipta alba, Wedelia, calandulaceae, Wedelia, chinensis, Eclipta prostrata*	Cell-cycle arrest, antiproliferation anti-inflammation, hepatoprotective, antioxidant	Myeloma, prostate, pancreatic, breast, neuroblastoma, carcinosarcoma, and leukemia [41, 57]

CONCLUSION

Natural products and their derivatives show high potency against Topoisomerase I, Topoisomerase II and caspases. Several natural products and their derivatives effectively manage the expression of key proteins involved in cancer therapy and hence hold great potential for the treatment of cancer with the benefits of having lower toxicity, and being safer and readily available without undergoing laborious multistep synthesis. The proper functioning of processes like DNA replication, transcription, recombination, repair mechanisms and apoptosis are vital for cell health and Topoisomerases/caspases enzymes play an important role in the proper functioning of all these processes. Owing to their significant cellular functions and mechanisms of action, these enzymes have been attracting medicinal chemists and scientists around the world toward the designing of new anticancer agents for nearly 3 decades. Despite having large data sets and Topoisomerase inhibitors/caspase modulators, challenges like drug resistance and undesired side effects demand the need for new and safer therapeutics. With the advancement of analytical and computational techniques, it becomes more convenient to the scientists to isolate new natural products, analyse their structures, test them for anti-cancer activity and design new analogues to improve their potency or other desired properties.

REFERENCES

[1] Fan M, Chen G, Sun B, *et al.* Screening for natural inhibitors of human topoisomerases from medicinal plants with bio-affinity ultrafiltration and LC–MS. Phytochem Rev 2020; 19(5): 1231-61. [http://dx.doi.org/10.1007/s11101-019-09635-x]

[2] Yuan S, Gopal JV, Ren S, Chen L, Liu L, Gao Z. Anticancer fungal natural products: Mechanisms of action and biosynthesis. Eur J Med Chem 2020; 202: 112502. [http://dx.doi.org/10.1016/j.ejmech.2020.112502] [PMID: 32652407]

[3] Talib WH, Alsalahat I, Daoud S, Abutayeh RF, Mahmod AI. Plant-Derived Natural Products in Cancer Research: Extraction, Mechanism of Action, and Drug Formulation. Molecules 2020; 25(22): 5319. [http://dx.doi.org/10.3390/molecules25225319] [PMID: 33202681]

[4] Greco G, Catanzaro E, Fimognari C. Natural Products as Inducers of Non-Canonical Cell Death: A Weapon against Cancer. Cancers (Basel) 2021; 13(2): 304. [http://dx.doi.org/10.3390/cancers13020304] [PMID: 33467668]

[5] Matulja D, Wittine K, Malatesti N, *et al.* Marine Natural Products with High Anticancer Activities. Curr Med Chem 2020; 27(8): 1243-307. [http://dx.doi.org/10.2174/0929867327666200113154115] [PMID: 31931690]

[6] Newman DJ, Cragg GM. Natural Products as Sources of New Drugs over the Nearly Four Decades from 01/1981 to 09/2019. J Nat Prod 2020; 83(3): 770-803. [http://dx.doi.org/10.1021/acs.jnatprod.9b01285] [PMID: 32162523]

[7] Harvey AL, Edrada-Ebel R, Quinn RJ. The re-emergence of natural products for drug discovery in the genomics era. Nat Rev Drug Discov 2015; 14(2): 111-29. [http://dx.doi.org/10.1038/nrd4510] [PMID: 25614221]

[8] Buzun K, Bielawska A, Bielawski K, Gornowicz A. DNA topoisomerases as molecular targets for anticancer drugs. J Enzyme Inhib Med Chem 2020; 35(1): 1781-99. [http://dx.doi.org/10.1080/14756366.2020.1821676] [PMID: 32975138]

[9] Capranico G, Marinello J, Chillemi G, Type I. Type I DNA Topoisomerases. J Med Chem 2017; 60(6): 2169-92. [http://dx.doi.org/10.1021/acs.jmedchem.6b00966] [PMID: 28072526]

[10] Delgado JL, Hsieh CM, Chan NL, Hiasa H. Topoisomerases as anticancer targets. Biochem J 2018; 475(2): 373-98.
[http://dx.doi.org/10.1042/BCJ20160583] [PMID: 29363591]

[11] Malpathak N, Baikar S. Secondary metabolites as DNA topoisomerase inhibitors: A new era towards designing of anticancer drugs. Pharmacogn Rev 2010; 4(7): 12-26.
[http://dx.doi.org/10.4103/0973-7847.65320] [PMID: 22228937]

[12] Pommier Y. Drugging topoisomerases: lessons and challenges. ACS Chem Biol 2013; 8(1): 82-95.
[http://dx.doi.org/10.1021/cb300648v] [PMID: 23259582]

[13] Han HJ, Tan NH, Zeng GZ, *et al.* Natural inhibitors of DNA topoisomerase I with cytotoxicities. Chem Biodivers 2008; 5(7): 1364-8.
[http://dx.doi.org/10.1002/cbdv.200890124] [PMID: 18649302]

[14] de Oliveira GP, da Silva TMG, Camara CA, Santana ALBD, Moreira MSA, Silva TMS. Isolation and structure elucidation of flavonoids from Amburana cearensis resin and identification of human DNA topoisomerase II-α inhibitors. Phytochem Lett 2017; 22: 61-70.
[http://dx.doi.org/10.1016/j.phytol.2017.09.006]

[15] Pal H, Katiyar S. Cryptolepine a plant alkaloid, inhibits the growth of nonmelanoma skin cancer cells through inhibition of topoisomerase and induction of DNA damage. Molecules 2016; 21(12): 1758.
[http://dx.doi.org/10.3390/molecules21121758] [PMID: 28009843]

[16] Chen GL, Tian YQ, Wu JL, Li N, Guo MQ. Antiproliferative activities of Amaryllidaceae alkaloids from Lycoris radiata targeting DNA topoisomerase I. Sci Rep 2016; 6(1): 38284.
[http://dx.doi.org/10.1038/srep38284] [PMID: 27922057]

[17] Stiborová M, Poljaková J, Martínková E, *et al.* Ellipticine oxidation and DNA adduct formation in human hepatocytes is catalyzed by human cytochromes P450 and enhanced by cytochrome b5. Toxicology 2012; 302(2-3): 233-41.
[http://dx.doi.org/10.1016/j.tox.2012.08.004] [PMID: 22917556]

[18] Scotti L, Bezerra Mendonca FJ, Ribeiro FF, *et al.* Natural product inhibitors of topoisomerases: review and docking study. Curr Protein Pept Sci 2018; 19(3): 275-91.
[PMID: 28079013]

[19] Fronza M, Lamy E, Günther S, Heinzmann B, Laufer S, Merfort I. Abietane diterpenes induce cytotoxic effects in human pancreatic cancer cell line MIA PaCa-2 through different modes of action. Phytochemistry 2012; 78: 107-19.
[http://dx.doi.org/10.1016/j.phytochem.2012.02.015] [PMID: 22436445]

[20] Wang GW, Lv C, Yuan X, *et al.* Lanostane-type triterpenoids from Abies faxoniana and their DNA topoisomerase inhibitory activities. Phytochemistry 2015; 116: 221-9.
[http://dx.doi.org/10.1016/j.phytochem.2015.04.012] [PMID: 25986863]

[21] Liu LP, Han K, Chen W, *et al.* Topoisomerase II inhibitors from the roots of Stellera chamaejasme L. Bioorg Med Chem 2014; 22(15): 4198-203.
[http://dx.doi.org/10.1016/j.bmc.2014.05.042] [PMID: 24931277]

[22] Wu CC, Huang KF, Yang TY, *et al.* The Topoisomerase 1 inhibitor Austrobailignan-1 isolated from Koelreuteria henryi induces a G2/M-phase arrest and cell death independently of p53 in non-small cell lung cancer cells. PLoS One 2015; 10(7): e0132052.
[http://dx.doi.org/10.1371/journal.pone.0132052] [PMID: 26147394]

[23] Kang K, Nho CW, Kim ND, *et al.* Daurinol, a catalytic inhibitor of topoisomerase IIα, suppresses SNU-840 ovarian cancer cell proliferation through cell cycle arrest in S phase. Int J Oncol 2014; 45(2): 558-66.
[http://dx.doi.org/10.3892/ijo.2014.2442] [PMID: 24841075]

[24] Nagarani B, Debnath S, Kumar S, Bhattacharjee C, Kumar G. Herbs used as anticancer agents. Int Res J Pharm 2011; 2: 20-4.

[25] Tang XJ, Han M, Yang B, *et al.* Nanocarrier improves the bioavailability, stability and antitumor activity of camptothecin. Int J Pharm 2014; 477(1-2): 536-45. [http://dx.doi.org/10.1016/j.ijpharm.2014.10.054] [PMID: 25445532]

[26] Liu YQ, Li WQ, Morris-Natschke SL, *et al.* Perspectives on biologically active camptothecin derivatives. Med Res Rev 2015; 35(4): 753-89. [http://dx.doi.org/10.1002/med.21342] [PMID: 25808858]

[27] Sheng C, Miao Z, Zhang W, Topoisomerase I. Topoisomerase I Inhibitors Derived from Natural Products: Structure–Activity Relationships and Antitumor Potency. Studies in Natural Products Chemistry 2016; 47: 1-28. [http://dx.doi.org/10.1016/B978-0-444-63603-4.00001-2]

[28] Pop C, Salvesen GS. Human caspases: activation, specificity, and regulation. J Biol Chem 2009; 284(33): 21777-81. [http://dx.doi.org/10.1074/jbc.R800084200] [PMID: 19473994]

[29] Van Opdenbosch N, Lamkanfi M. Caspases in cell death, inflammation and disease. Immunity 2019; 50(6): 1352-64. [http://dx.doi.org/10.1016/j.immuni.2019.05.020] [PMID: 31216460]

[30] McIlwain DR, Berger T, Mak TW. Caspase functions in cell death and disease. Cold Spring Harb Perspect Biol 2013; 5(4): a008656. [http://dx.doi.org/10.1101/cshperspect.a008656] [PMID: 23545416]

[31] Nicholson DW, Melino G. Caspases and cell death.Encyclopedia of Biological Chemistry. 2013; pp. 388-96. [http://dx.doi.org/10.1016/B978-0-12-378630-2.00498-9]

[32] Arandjelovic S, Ravichandran KS. Phagocytosis of apoptotic cells in homeostasis. Nat Immunol 2015; 16(9): 907-17. [http://dx.doi.org/10.1038/ni.3253] [PMID: 26287597]

[33] Fuchs Y, Steller H. Programmed cell death in animal development and disease. Cell 2011; 147(4): 742-58. [http://dx.doi.org/10.1016/j.cell.2011.10.033] [PMID: 22078876]

[34] Hensley P, Mishra M, Kyprianou N. Targeting caspases in cancer therapeutics. bchm 2013; 394(7): 831-43. [http://dx.doi.org/10.1515/hsz-2013-0128] [PMID: 23509217]

[35] Olsson M, Zhivotovsky B. Caspases and cancer. Cell Death Differ 2011; 18(9): 1441-9. [http://dx.doi.org/10.1038/cdd.2011.30] [PMID: 21455218]

[36] Ghavami S, Hashemi M, Ande SR, *et al.* Apoptosis and cancer: mutations within caspase genes. J Med Genet 2009; 46(8): 497-510. [http://dx.doi.org/10.1136/jmg.2009.066944] [PMID: 19505876]

[37] Strasser A, Cory S, Adams JM. Deciphering the rules of programmed cell death to improve therapy of cancer and other diseases. EMBO J 2011; 30(18): 3667-83. [http://dx.doi.org/10.1038/emboj.2011.307] [PMID: 21863020]

[38] Fulda S. Evasion of apoptosis as a cellular stress response in cancer. Int J Cell Biol 2010; 2010: 1-6. [http://dx.doi.org/10.1155/2010/370835] [PMID: 20182539]

[39] Carneiro BA, El-Deiry WS. Targeting apoptosis in cancer therapy. Nat Rev Clin Oncol 2020; 17(7): 395-417. [http://dx.doi.org/10.1038/s41571-020-0341-y] [PMID: 32203277]

[40] Amaral RG, dos Santos SA, Andrade LN, Severino P, Carvalho AA. Natural products as treatment against cancer: a historical and current vision. Clin Oncol (Las Vegas) 2019; 4: 1562.

[41] Millimouno FM, Dong J, Yang L, Li J, Li X. Targeting apoptosis pathways in cancer and perspectives with natural compounds from mother nature. Cancer Prev Res (Phila) 2014; 7(11): 1081-107. [http://dx.doi.org/10.1158/1940-6207.CAPR-14-0136] [PMID: 25161295]

[42] Wang Y, Zhong J, Bai J, *et al.* The Application of Natural Products in Cancer Therapy by Targeting Apoptosis Pathways. Curr Drug Metab 2018; 19(9): 739-49. [http://dx.doi.org/10.2174/1389200219666180511154722]

[43] Tewary P, Gunatilaka AAL, Sayers TJ. Using natural products to promote caspase-8-dependent cancer cell death. Cancer Immunol Immunother 2017; 66(2): 223-31. [http://dx.doi.org/10.1007/s00262-016-1855-0] [PMID: 27286684]

[44] Shalini S, Dorstyn L, Dawar S, Kumar S. Old, new and emerging functions of caspases. Cell Death Differ 2015; 22(4): 526-539, 526, 539. [http://dx.doi.org/10.1038/cdd.2014.216] [PMID: 25526085]

[45] Kesavardhana S, Malireddi RKS, Kanneganti TD. Caspases in cell death, inflammation and pyroptosis. Annu Rev Immunol 2020; 38(1): 567-95. [http://dx.doi.org/10.1146/annurev-immunol-073119-095439] [PMID: 32017655]

[46] Dabrowska C, Li M, Fan Y. Apoptotic Caspases in Promoting Cancer: Implications from Their Roles in Development and Tissue Homeostasis.Apoptosis in Cancer Pathogenesis and Anti-cancer Therapy Advances in Experimental Medicine and Biology. Cham: Springer 2016; Vol. 930. [http://dx.doi.org/10.1007/978-3-319-39406-0_4]

[47] Boice A, Bouchier-Hayes L. Targeting apoptotic caspases in cancer. Biochim Biophys Acta Mol Cell Res 2020; 1867(6): 118688. [http://dx.doi.org/10.1016/j.bbamcr.2020.118688] [PMID: 32087180]

[48] Yu Z, Li Q, An Y, Chen X, Liu Z. Role of apoptosis repressor with caspase recruitment domain (ARC) in cancer. Oncol Lett 2019; 18(6): 5691-8.

[49] Ullmannová V, Haskovec C. Gene expression during camptothecin-induced apoptosis in human myeloid leukemia cell line ML-2. Neoplasma 2004; 51(3): 175-80. [PMID: 15254669]

[50] Sun Q, Xie L, Song J, Li X. Evodiamine: A review of its pharmacology, toxicity, pharmacokinetics and preparation researches. J Ethnopharmacol 2020; 262: 113164. [http://dx.doi.org/10.1016/j.jep.2020.113164] [PMID: 32738391]

[51] Zhang H, Chen L, Sun X, Yang Q, Wan L, Guo C. Matrine: A promising natural product with various pharmacological activities. Front Pharmacol 2020; 11: 588. [http://dx.doi.org/10.3389/fphar.2020.00588] [PMID: 32477114]

[52] Nageen B, Rasul A, Hussain G, *et al.* S.; Sarfraz, I.; Riaz, A.; Selamoglu, Z. Jaceosidin: A natural flavone with versatile pharmacological and biological activities. Curr Pharm Des 2021; 27(4): 456-66. [http://dx.doi.org/10.2174/1381612826666200429095101] [PMID: 32348212]

[53] Noel P, Von Hoff DD, Saluja AK, Velagapudi M, Borazanci E, Han H. Triptolide and its derivatives as cancer therapies. Trends Pharmacol Sci 2019; 40(5): 327-41. [http://dx.doi.org/10.1016/j.tips.2019.03.002] [PMID: 30975442]

[54] Liu X, Xu J, Zhou J, Shen Q. Oridonin and its derivatives for cancer treatment and overcoming therapeutic resistance. Genes Dis 2021; 8(4): 448-62. [http://dx.doi.org/10.1016/j.gendis.2020.06.010] [PMID: 34179309]

[55] Li Q, Wang Z, Xie Y, Hu H. Antitumor activity and mechanism of costunolide and dehydrocostus lactone: Two natural sesquiterpene lactones from the Asteraceae family. Biomed Pharmacother 2020; 125: 109955. [http://dx.doi.org/10.1016/j.biopha.2020.109955] [PMID: 32014691]

[56] Ong CP, Lee WL, Tang YQ, Yap WH. Honokiol: A review of its anticancer potential and mechanisms. Cancers (Basel) 2019; 12(1): 48.
[http://dx.doi.org/10.3390/cancers12010048] [PMID: 31877856]

[57] Pan H, Lin Y, Dou J, *et al.* Wedelolactone facilitates Ser/Thr phosphorylation of NLRP3 dependent on PKA signalling to block inflammasome activation and pyroptosis. Cell Prolif 2020; 53(9): e12868.
[http://dx.doi.org/10.1111/cpr.12868] [PMID: 32656909]

CHAPTER 9

Cytotoxic Phytochemicals from Mushrooms as Potential Therapeutic Agents

Gana Manjusha Kondepudi[1,*], **Rashmi Saxena Pal**[2] and **Malakapogu Ravindra Babu**[2]

[1] *Vignan Institute of Pharmaceutical Technology, Visakhapatnam, Andhra Pradesh, India*

[2] *Department of Pharmacognosy, School of Pharmaceutical Sciences, Lovely Professional University, Phagwara, India*

Abstract: Cancer is a collective term for a group of deadly diseases that can affect and spread to various parts of the body. The main feature of cancer is the uncontrolled growth of cells due to a defect in the genes that control normal cell division and growth. As per the latest statistics, cancer is the second-leading cause of death globally, and almost 70% of these deaths are reported in low- and middle-income countries. Chemotherapy and irradiation are the most common cancer treatments; however, the development of resistance and severe side effects are the stumbling blocks of these methods. Hence, current research has focused more on developing novel drug leads from new sources like algae and fungi. Fungi, such as mushrooms, are an inexhaustible source of various anticancer biomolecules, and the 21st century saw a staggering interest in the anticancer potential of mushrooms among the western exploration clique. Their cellular and humoral immunity-boosting properties have made them better candidates for anticancer drug discovery. The mushrooms attributed with cytotoxic potential belong to various genera like *Vargenus Agrocybe, Amanita, Antrodia, Agaricus, Albatrellus Conocybe, Clitocybe, Cordyceps, Clavatia, Flammulina, Funlia, Fomes, Galerina, Gymnopilus, Ganoderma, Hypholoma, Inonotus, Inocybe, Lentinula, Lactarius, Panaeolus, Psilocybe, Plerurotus, Pholiotina, Pluteus, Russula, Suillus, Schizophyllum, Trametes, Xerocomus, and Weraroa.* Hence, the current chapter focuses on the botanical description, phytochemistry, mechanism of action, and clinical status of various vital mushrooms acting as essential libraries of anticancer drug leads.

Keywords: Anticancer, *Amanita*, *Antrodia*, *Agaricus*, *Albatrellus Conocybe*, Cancer, *Clitocybe*, *Cordyceps*, *Clavatia*, Cytotoxic Phytochemicals, Drug leads,*Vargenus Agrocybe*, *Flammulina*, *Funlia*, *Fomes*, *Galerina*, *Gymnopilus*, *Ganoderma*, *Hypholoma*, *Inonotus*, *Inocybe*, *Lentinula*, *Lactarius*, Mushrooms, *Panaeolus*, *Psilocybe*, *Plerurotus*, *Pholiotina*, *Pluteus*, *Russula*, *Suillus*, *Schizophyllum*, *Trametes*, *Xerocomus*, *Weraroa*.

* **Corresponding author Gana Manjusha Kondepudi:** Vignan Institute of Pharmaceutical Technology, Visakhapatnam, Andhra Pradesh, India; E-mail: manjusha.kondepudi.g@gmail.com

Motamarri Venkata Naga Lalitha Chaitanya, Galvina Pereira, & Heyam Saad Ali (Eds.)

INTRODUCTION

Cancer is one of the leading causes of death globally. Cancer is estimated to be responsible for approximately one in every six deaths worldwide. As per the National Cancer Registry Programme Report 2020, released by the Indian Council of Medical Research (ICMR), it was estimated that there would be 13.9 lakh cases of cancer in India in 2020, and that this number is probably going to ascend to 15.7 lakh by 2025. Continuous growth and uncontrolled proliferation of cells are the cardinal mechanisms behind the development of cancer. Despite the checkpoints that control a normal cell's behaviour, cancer cells continue to grow and divide in an unregulated manner, affecting and spreading to other organs. More than a hundred recognised types of cancer can differ considerably in their reaction to treatment. Though there are many kinds of cancer, only a few occur frequently, like breast, cervical, prostate, oral, and lung cancer (Fig. **1**).

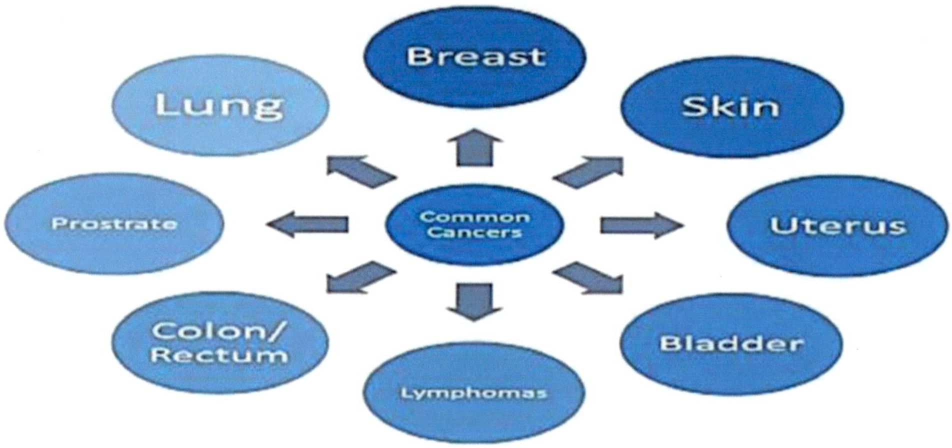

Fig. (1). The Most Common type of Cancers.

The battle against cancer has been reinforced with multidirectional approaches, including behavioural and dietary changes, chemotherapy, radiotherapy, medical procedures, and late immunotherapy. Miserably, these approaches have many ill effects, ranging from a suppressed immune system to decreased patient quality of life. This has encouraged researchers, prompting deliberate endeavours to discover better treatments that, aside from treating cancerous growth, help the immune system fight cancer and other opportunistic infections [1].

Complementary and alternative therapy is one of those therapies mentioned above that use plants, including algae and fungi. Among the enormous resources of fungi, higher basidiomycetes, distinctly mushrooms, constitute inexhaustible sources of therapeutically active agents [2]. Mushrooms are the spore-producing fruiting body of a fungus that grows above the soil or on a substrate. Several edible and non-edible mushrooms have been used for medicinal purposes since the dawn of civilization. Mushroom derived extracts are predominantly used alone or other herbal preparations to treat various ailments in traditional Chinese medicine (Fig. **2**).

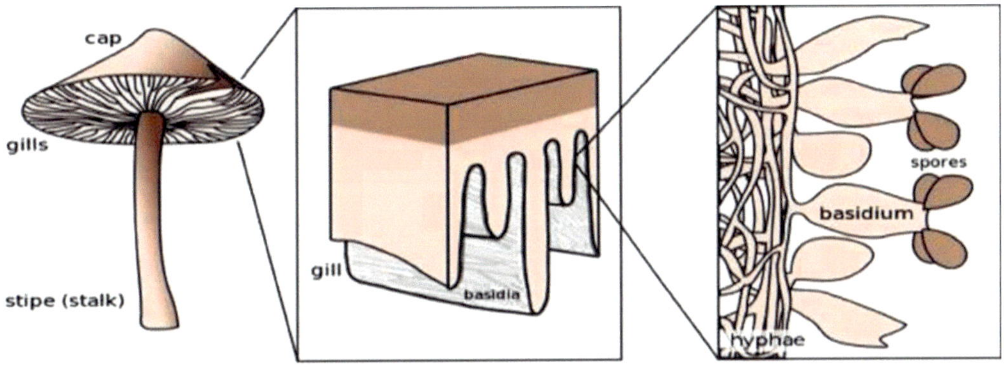

Fig. (2). Basidium Schematic Structure.

Among the enormous resources of fungi, higher basidiomycetes, distinctly mushrooms, constitute inexhaustible sources of therapeutically active agents [2]. Mushrooms are the spore-producing fruiting body of a fungus that grows above the soil or on a substrate. Since the beginning of time, people have used both edible and non-edible mushrooms as medicines. In traditional Chinese medicine, mushroom extracts are mostly used alone or with other herbal preparations to treat a wide range of illnesses. A plethora of biologically active substances, such as polysaccharides, minerals, vitamins, dietary fibers, and polyphenolic compounds, are found in mushrooms. Most ongoing studies have shown that mushrooms have around 130 therapeutic properties, such as antitumor, immunomodulating, antioxidant, cardiovascular, anti-hyperlipidemic, antimicrobial, detoxifying, anti-diabetic, and hepatoprotective [3].

The use of mushrooms in cancer treatment is well known in East Asian countries (Table **1**), the United States, and Canada. These biologically active compounds have been shown to influence the host's immune system and consequently could be used to treat a number of ailments and restore the cell immunity lost through radiotherapy and chemotherapy. But not enough research has been done on the interesting parts of medicinal mushrooms that help treat cancer and their benefits as a cancer support therapy [4].

Table 1. Medicinal properties of Mushrooms used in East Asia

Common Name	Biological Name	Family	Medicinal Activity
Caterpillar fungi	*Cordyceps sinensis*	Clavicipitaceae	Antitumour, antimetastatic, antioxidant, immunomodulatory, Anti-inflammatory, insecticidal, antimicrobial, hypolipidemic, hypoglycaemic, Anti-ageing, neuroprotective, renoprotective effects [5]
Tinder fungus	*Fomes fomentarius*	Polyporaceae	Hypoglycemic, anti-nociceptive, Anti-inflammatory, anti-infective and antitumor activities [6]
Wood conk, Agarikon	*Fomitopsis officinalis*	Polyporaceae	Antibacterial, Anti-viral, Anti-inflammatory, Anti-tumour activities [7]
Lacquered Bracket	*Ganoderma lucidum*	Ganodermataceae	Immunomodulation, anti-atherosclerotic, anti-inflammatory, analgesic, antitumor, chemo and radioprotective, sleep-promoting, antibacterial, antiviral (including anti-HIV), hypolipidemic, anti-fibrotic, hepatoprotective, antidiabetic, anti-androgenic, anti-angiogenic, anti-herpetic, antioxidative radical-scavenging, anti-ageing, hypoglycemic, estrogenic activity and anti-ulcer properties [8]
Hen of the woods, Dancing mushroom, Maitake	*Grifola frondose*	Meripilaceae	Antitumor, immunomodulatory, antidiabetic, anti-hyperlipidemia, antiviral activities [9]
Cinder conk, Clinker fungus	*Inonotus obliquus*	Hymenochaetaceae	Antioxidant, Anti-tumour, Antidiabetic, Anti-viral activities [10]
Snake butter	*Lentinula edodes*	Agaricaceae	Anti-inflammatory, Anti-tumour, Antihypertensive, Immunomodulant activities [11]
Birch polypore Razor strop	*Fomitopsis betulina (formerly Piptoporus betulinus)*	Polyporaceae	Antibacterial, anti-parasitic, antiviral, anti-inflammatory, anticancer, neuroprotective and immunomodulating properties [12].

Numerous medicinal mushrooms on the market guarantee anticancer benefits, yet these claims have not been checked in most cases. Consequently, the purpose of this chapter is to unite the accessible scientific data pertinent to the anticancer effects of medicinal mushrooms and their products so that the end-user can make a fair judgement concerning whether they may be effective or not. This chapter highlights the multitargeting novel anticancer bio-actives, their mechanism of action, and the clinical status of the anticancer leads present in mushrooms.

ANTICANCER METABOLITES IN MUSHROOMS.

Mushrooms are therapeutically active against cancerous cells because they contain several bioactive compounds. These bioactive compounds are categorised into two groups: 1) High molecular weight bioactive metabolites; 2) Bioactive metabolites with a low molecular weight (Fig. **3**).

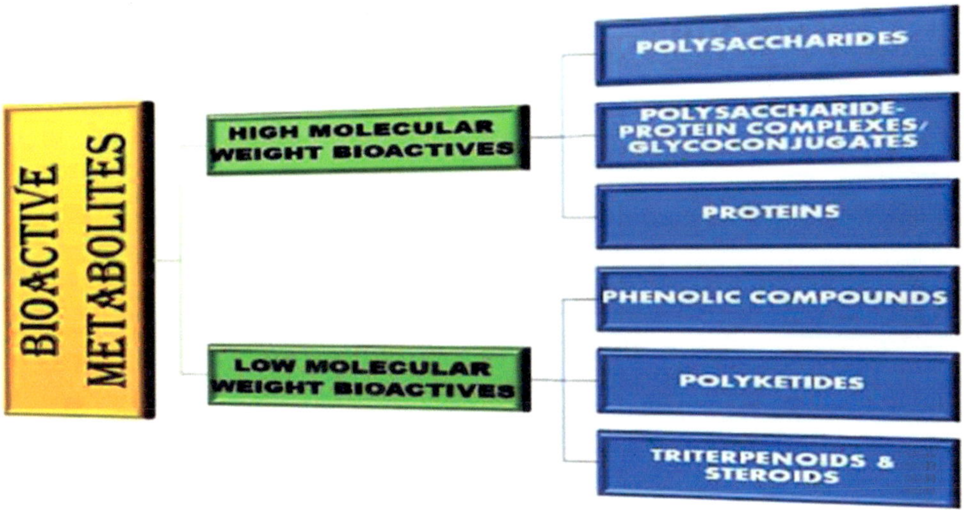

Fig. (3). Categories of bioactive compounds

Polysaccharides and Polysaccharide-Protein Complexes

Most of the plants, yeast, bacteria, and fungi are treasure troves of bioactive polysaccharides (carbohydrates). In mushrooms, these polysaccharides are found as glucans (-glucans and hetero-glucans) and glycans (heteroglycans). Polysaccharides made of D-glucose subunits are called glucans, and polysaccharides composed of monosaccharides as side chains are termed heteroglucans [4]. Simultaneously, polysaccharides containing sugars other than glucose in the structure are termed glycans (galactans, fucans, xylans, and mannans). Heteroglycans are composed of side chains of different sugars such as arabinose, mannose, fucose, galactose, and xylose as a single component or in combination [4]. In mushrooms, polysaccharides exist in the form of glucans. Some glucans are linear or branched, with a backbone of unlinked or linked glucose units, and some have side chains attached at various positions. The polysaccharide chain contains either (13) and (14) side chains or a mixture of (13) and (14) side chains [13].

These polysaccharides exhibit antimicrobial, antioxidant, anticancer, antidiabetic, anti-inflammatory, and immunomodulatory activities. Glucans, particularly - glucans, have antimicrobial and hypoglycemic properties, as well as the ability to boost immunity by activating macrophages [7]. Benefits of mushroom polysaccharides in the treatment of tumours and cancer were recognised after Chihara's publication on the fungal polysaccharides' antitumor activity in the 1960s [14].

It has been portrayed that the mushroom's immunomodulatory activity (Table **2**) was attributed to various polysaccharides of mushrooms and was probably going to influence the metastasis principally as per the alluded model of carcinogenesis [2].

More than 50 mushroom species have yielded potential polysaccharides with inhibitory effects on numerous tumour cells like sarcoma S-180, adenocarcinoma 755, and leukaemia L-1210. The most potent polysaccharides include lectins, polysaccharides, polysaccharide-peptides, and polysaccharide-protein complexes like lentinan from *Lentinus edodes, tremellan from Tremella fuciformis, schizophyllan from Schizophyllan commune, grifolan from Grifola frondosa, plueran from Pluerotus ostreatus, and ganodran* from *Ganoderma lucidus, etc.* (Table **2**). These polysaccharides are used in the treatment of various cancers [15].

Table 2. Common Polysaccharides and their Mechanism of Action

Mushroom Species	Bioactive Compounds	Mechanism of action	References
Lentinus edodes	Lentinan	Initiates immune response after the commencement of infection by increasing pro-inflammatory cytokines and exerts inflammation when an infection persists.	[18]
Ganoderma lucidus	Ganoderan	An antioxidant polysaccharide that was shown to prevent and control cerebral arteriosclerosis by regulating the NADPH oxidizing enzyme expression.	[19]
Pluerotus ostreatus	Plueran POPM-II	Effective in mild to severe atopic dermatitis. It is capable of improving hyperlipidemia in obese mice. Inhibits the proliferation of BGC 823 human. Gastric cancer cell line *in vitro/in vivo*.	[20, 21]

(Table 2) cont.....

Mushroom Species	Bioactive Compounds	Mechanism of action	References
Schizophyllan commune	Schizophyllan	Potential prebiotic with immunomodulating properties.	[22]
Grifola frondosa	Grifolan	Exerts antitumor effect, firstly by the activation of immunity against the origin of tumours and secondly, by inducing apoptosis of the tumour cells. Grifolan also can be used for the prevention of the oncogenesis by oral administration (cancer-preventing activity).	[23]
Trametes versicolor	Polysaccharopeptide and polysaccharopeptide Krestin	Inhibits adhesion, invasion, motility, and metastatic growth of tumour cells. Induces apoptosis. Adjuvant for immune-chemotherapy.	[24, 25]
Tremella fuciformis	Tremellan	Immunomodulant, antitumor, and antioxidant, anti-ageing, hypoglycemic, hypolipidemic drug	[26]

The polysaccharides' potent antitumor and anticancer activity is due to their complex structures. The structure and biological activity of a polysaccharide depend on the monosaccharide composition, configuration, and position of glycosidic linkages, the sequence of monosaccharides, and the nature, number, and location of adjoining non-carbohydrate groups [16]. The antitumor activity of polysaccharides bound to proteins or peptides is higher than that of the corresponding free glucans. Medicinal mushrooms show immunomodulatory activity because of the polysaccharides and varying combinations of polysaccharide-protein complexes, glycol-conjugated conjugate glycoproteins, glycopeptides, and proteoglycans.

The complexity of polysaccharides increases when they are bound covalently to other conjugate molecules, such as polypeptides and proteins. Glycoproteins are proteins that consist of glucans (oligosaccharide chains) attached covalently to polypeptide sidechains. They are made out of a protein centre encircled by various glucan chains bound to the protein moiety through O- or N-glycosidation. A core protein with one or more covalently attached, heavily glycosylated glycosaminoglycan chains is termed a proteoglycan [17].

Proteins

The second most sought-after functional component in mushrooms after polysaccharides is the proteins. Lectins, ribosome-inactivating proteins (R.I.P.s), fungal immunomodulatory proteins (F.I.P.s), and laccases are some of the mushroom proteins with notable biological activities (Table **3**) [27].

Table 3. Common Proteins and their Mechanism of Action

Mushroom Species	Bioactive Compounds	Mechanism of action	References
Agaricus bisporus, Pleurotus ostreatus, Tricholoma mongolicum, Agaricus subrufescens, Grifola frondosa, Russula lepida, Pholiota adiposa	Lectins	It binds to cell surface carbohydrates and causes cell agglutination. Antiproliferative and anti-tumour activities in cancer cell lines	[28, 29]
Hypsizigus marmoreus	Ribosome inactivating proteins (R.I.P.s)	Suppress the ribosomes by eliminating parts of adenosine residues from rRNA.	[30]
Ganoderma Species *Flammulina velutipes* *Volvariella volvacea* *Grifola frondosa* *Auricularia polytricha* *Pleurotus citrinopileatus* *Trametes versicolor*	Fungal Immunomodulatory Proteins (F.I.P.s)	Induce the significant activation and maturation of human dendritic cells, Antimetastatic effect Antitumor activity Potential immunomodulatory proteins	[31 - 33]

Alkaloids

Alkaloids are nitrogen-containing secondary metabolites that gained significance due to their anticancer properties. Indeed, even though ebb-and-flow research indicates that mushrooms are a magnificent bio-generator of alkaloids, the investigations were restricted. The most well-known mushroom alkaloids are the hallucinogenic indole derivatives found in magic mushrooms, which include bisnoryangonin, hispidin, baecystin, norbaecystin, psilocin, and psilocybin [34].

These alkaloids belong to the genera such as *Agarocybe, Amanita,* and *Conocybe.* GalHomer and Sperry [35] investigated the isolation of indole alkaloids derived from mushrooms as well as their biological activities.

The alkaloid compounds can be found in various amounts depending on mushroom species, their formative stages, climatic conditions, and the accessibility of soluble nitrogen and phosphorous in the soil [36]. A 50-year retroactive study of drug discovery from fungi gives a far-reaching record of fungal secondary metabolites and their contribution as drug leads with vast therapeutic potential [37]. However, little research has been conducted on the anticancer activity of mushroom alkaloids. Hence, there is a wide scope for research on isolating and evaluating multitargeting cytotoxic drugs (Table **4**), with leads from mushrooms [38].

Table 4. Common Indole alkaloids and their Mechanism of Action

Mushroom Species	Bioactive Compounds	Mechanism of Action	References
Hericium coralloides (Scop.) Pers	Corralocin B and C	Stimulate neurotrophin expression in human 1321N1 astrocytes. Corralocin B was reported to show antiproliferative activity against HUVEC (human umbilical vein endothelial cells) and MCF-7 and KB-3-1 human cancer cell lines.	[39]
Cortinarius infractus (Pers.) Fr	Infractopicrin and 10-hydroxyinfractopicrin	Acetylcholinesterase-inhibitory activity.	[40]
Boletus curtisii Berk	Sulfur-containing β-carboline derivatives, one of which is canthin-6-one	Possesses cytotoxic properties against leukemic cells.	[41]

Triterpenoids

Triterpenoids are oxidised lanostanes. In mushrooms, triterpenoids are widely reported as pharmacologically active components among Ganoderma species. The potential of Ganoderma triterpenoids against different cancer targets has been reported. Triterpenoids derived from Ganoderma lucidum suppress the invasive nature of the cancer cells directly. Based on the ligand bound to C-26, these triterpenoids are categorised into two groups. One group consists of the C-26 carboxyl group and is referred to as Gandoreic acids, and the other group consists of the C-26 hydroxyl group and is known as Ganoderma alcohols [42]. Several cytotoxic triterpenoid leads (Table **5**) have been reported to exert inhibitory action against human cancer cells [43].

Table 5. Common triterpenoids and their mechanism of action

Mushroom Species	Bioactive Compounds	Mechanism of action	References
Ganoderma lucidium	Ganoderic acid lucidimol ganoderiol ganodermanondiol ganodermanontriol	Induce apoptosis	[44]
Ganoderma tsugae	Tsugaric Acid tsugarioside tsugarioside	Effective against human hepatoma cells.	[45]
Ganoderma concinna	5α-lanosta-7,9(11),24-triene-3β-hydroxy-26-al, 5α-lanost--7,9(11),24-triene-15α-26-dihydroxy-3-one, and 8α,9α-epoxy-4,4,14α-trimethyl-3,7,11,15,20-pentaoxo-5α-pregnane	All three compounds were found to induce apoptosis.	[46]

(Table 5) cont.....

Mushroom Species	Bioactive Compounds	Mechanism of action	References
Ganoderma pfeifferi	Ganodermadiol Lucidadiol and Applanoxidic acid G	Antiviral activity against influenza virus type A and HSV type 1.	[47]
Ganoderma colossum	Colossolactone V Colossolactone VI Colossolactone VII Colossolactone VIII	Anti-HIV-1 protease activity.	[48]
Piptoporus betulinus	Piptolinic acids A-E	Potential cytotoxic agent against several human cancer cell lines.	[49]
Astraeus odoratus	Spiroastraodoric acid, astraodoric acids E and F	Cytotoxic agent	[50]

Polyphenolic Compounds

Medicinal mushrooms revealed diverse polyphenolic components known as the styrylpyrone class of phenols, gotten from polyketide pathways, which show significant pharmacological properties, including anticancer activity [51]. Styrylpyrone pigments are the most common constituents of the Phellinus and Inonotus species. Hispidin, a naturally occurring styrylpyrone, was first isolated from *Inonotus hispidus*. Ongoing investigations have shown that fruiting groups of Phellinus igniarius, *P. linteus*, and Inonotus obliquus contain exceptional styrylpyrone derivatives with numerous biological activities. However, only a few polyphenols are studied; hence, there is a need to explore mushroom phenolics' anticancer activities (Table **6**).

Table 6. Common phenolics and their mechanism of action

Mushroom Species	Bioactive Compounds	Mechanism of action	References
Phellinus igniarius	Inoscavin A Hispolon Phelligridins A-J Phelligridins (C-F)	Antioxidant, Cytotoxic activity.	[52, 53]

(Table 6) cont.....

Mushroom Species	Bioactive Compounds	Mechanism of action	References
Phellinus linteus	Hispolon	Induces apoptosis in human gastric cancer cells through a reactive oxygen species (R.O.S.)-mediated mitochondrial pathway. It can inhibit the metastasis of SK-Hep1 cells by reduced expression of MMP-2, MMP-9, and uPA through the suppression of various signalling pathways and of the activity of PI3K/Akt and Ras homologue gene family.	[52, 54]

CLINICAL STATUS OF SOME CYTOTOXIC NOVEL DRUGS LEADS DERIVED FROM MUSHROOMS

Medicinal mushrooms containing pharmacologically active substances have been used in a few human clinical trials and have shown promising results as adjuvant therapies when used in conjunction with conventional treatments [3]. Various industrially developed mushroom polysaccharides exist, for instance, Lentinan from *Lentinula edodes* and Schizophyllan (Sonifilan, Sizofiran, or S.P.G.). Polysaccharopeptide Krestin, peptidoglycans from Trametes versicolor, maitake D-portion from *Grifola frondosa*, and a Ganoderma polysaccharide from Ganoderma lucidum seem to intercede anti-tumor activity by the activation of the immune system and have continued through Phase I, II, and III clinical trials, fundamentally in Japan and China, while such trials are additionally happening in the U.S. and some European nations [55]. Several experimental and clinical trials have shown that various mushroom species, including Cordyceps sinensis, have promising cancer inhibitory and immunostimulatory activity [56]. *Flammulina velutipes* [57], *Inonotus obliquus*, and *Phellinus linteus* Among low-molecula--weight mushroom mixes, a couple of the various newfound mixes have advanced to clinical assessment. Irofulven is the most broadly contemplated compound in this gathering, yet it needs future clinical affirmation before being suggested for use as an enemy of disease drug [58].

CONCLUSION

Mushrooms are magnificently accepted remedies for diseases and the most favourite foods in several countries across the globe. On the other hand, cancer is a chronic disease that became resistant due to various unresolved genetic and epigenetic mechanisms, despite remarkable progress in the treatment methods. This is due to the serious side effects of those treatments, ranging from a suppressed immune system to a decreased patient's quality of life.

Hence, there is an urgent need to search for new drug leads that exert multiple actions. There is increasing evidence that medicinal mushrooms may contain various therapeutically significant compounds that have yet to be assessed by Western clinical researchers. Mycotherapy/biological immunotherapy treatments involving medicinal mushrooms meet many of the requirements of adjuvant cancer treatment and may act as a direct cure against cancer development. High-molecular-weight metabolites and low-molecular-weight metabolites are two broad categories of medicinal mushrooms.

High-molecular-weight metabolites such as polysaccharides and protein-polysaccharide complexes exhibit anticancer activity predominantly through the immune system's stimulation. Low-molecular-weight metabolites of mushrooms activate the immune system and control the cell signalling pathways responsible for cancer's pathogenesis. Additional investigations on the mechanisms of action and biological activities of the mushroom metabolites are required to develop them as potential anticancer drugs. New strategies and methods combined with biotechnology and other relevant disciplines are also required. *In vivo* experimentation with high-quality, long-term, double-blinded, clinical studies with large human volunteers will be needed to confirm these mushroom-derived cytotoxic leads' efficacy and safety. Future investigations must determine their structural suitability, mechanisms, and bioactive mushroom metabolism to promote them as potential drugs. There are additionally numerous issues with the correct identification, scientific classification, and nomenclature of medicinal mushrooms. There is a need to investigate tropical nations for mushrooms and examine their bioactive metabolites that can be used as potential solutions for anticancer treatments. Studies are justified to investigate this untapped resource for the isolation and production of novel anti-tumour compounds of therapeutic significance.

REFERENCES

[1] Ayeka PA. Potential of Mushroom Compounds as Immunomodulators in Cancer Immunotherapy: A Review. Hindawi Evidence-Based Complementary and Alternative Medicine 2018.

[2] Ferreira ICFR, Vaz JA, Vasconcelos MH, Martins A. Compounds from wild mushrooms with antitumor potential. Anticancer Agents Med Chem 2010; 10(5): 424-36. [http://dx.doi.org/10.2174/1871520611009050424] [PMID: 20545620]

[3] Wasser S. Medicinal mushroom science: Current perspectives, advances, evidences, and challenges. Biomed J 2014; 37(6): 345-56. [http://dx.doi.org/10.4103/2319-4170.138318] [PMID: 25179726]

[4] Phan C-W, Tan Y-Y, Sabaratnam V. Bioactive molecules in edible and medicinal mushrooms for human wellness.Bioactive molecules in foods, Reference Series in Phytochemistry, Springer international publishing. 2018. [http://dx.doi.org/10.1007/978-3-319-54528-8_83-1]

[5] Yue K, Ye M, Zhou Z, Sun W, Lin X. The genus *Cordyceps* : a chemical and pharmacological review. J Pharm Pharmacol 2013; 65(4): 474-93.

[http://dx.doi.org/10.1111/j.2042-7158.2012.01601.x] [PMID: 23488776]

[6] Kolundžić M, Grozdanić NĐ, Dodevska M, *et al.* Antibacterial and cytotoxic activities of wild mushroom Fomes fomentarius (L.) Fr., Polyporaceae. Ind Crops Prod 2016; 79: 110-5. [http://dx.doi.org/10.1016/j.indcrop.2015.10.030]

[7] Elkhateeb WA, Daba GM, Elnahas MO, Thomas P. Fomitopsis officinalis mushroom: ancient gold mine of functional components and biological activities for modern medicine. Egyptian Pharmaceutical Journal 2019; 18(4): 285-9. [http://dx.doi.org/10.4103/epj.epj_46_19]

[8] Sanodiya B, Thakur G, Baghel R, Prasad G, Bisen P. Ganoderma lucidum: a potent pharmacological macrofungus. Curr Pharm Biotechnol 2009; 10(8): 717-42. [http://dx.doi.org/10.2174/138920109789978757] [PMID: 19939212]

[9] He Y, Li X, Hao C, *et al.* Grifola frondosa polysaccharide: a review of antitumor and other biological activity studies in China. Discov Med 2018; 25(138): 159-76. [PMID: 29723488]

[10] Duru KC, Kovaleva EG, Danilova IG, Bijl P. The pharmacological potential and possible molecular mechanisms of action of *Inonotus obliquus* from preclinical studies. Phytother Res 2019; 33(8): 1966-80. [http://dx.doi.org/10.1002/ptr.6384] [PMID: 31209936]

[11] Choi EJ, Park ZY, Kim EK. Chemical Composition and Inhibitory Effect of Lentinula edodes Ethanolic Extract on Experimentally Induced Atopic Dermatitis *in Vitro* and *in Vivo*. Molecules 2016; 21(8): 993. [http://dx.doi.org/10.3390/molecules21080993] [PMID: 27483228]

[12] Pleszczyńska M, Lemieszek MK, Siwulski M, Wiater A, Rzeski W, Szczodrak J. Fomitopsis betulina (formerly Piptoporus betulinus): the Iceman's polypore fungus with modern biotechnological potential. World J Microbiol Biotechnol 2017; 33(5): 83. [http://dx.doi.org/10.1007/s11274-017-2247-0] [PMID: 28378220]

[13] De Silva DD, Rapior S, Fons F, Bahkali AH, Hyde KD. Medicinal mushrooms in supportive cancer therapies: an approach to anti-cancer effects and putative mechanisms of action. Fungal Divers 2012; 55(1): 1-35. [http://dx.doi.org/10.1007/s13225-012-0151-3]

[14] Chihara G, Maeda Y, Hamuro J, Sasaki T, Fukuoka F. Inhibition of mouse sarcoma 180 by polysaccharides from Lentinus edodes (Berk.) sing. Nature 1969; 222(5194): 687-8. [http://dx.doi.org/10.1038/222687a0] [PMID: 5768289]

[15] Ren L, Perera C, Hemar Y. Antitumor activity of mushroom polysaccharides: a review. Food Funct 2012; 3(11): 1118-30. [http://dx.doi.org/10.1039/c2fo10279j] [PMID: 22865023]

[16] Chen J, Seviour R. Medicinal importance of fungal β-(1#3), 1#6)-glucans. Mycol Res 2007; 111: 635-52. [http://dx.doi.org/10.1016/j.mycres.2007.02.011] [PMID: 17590323]

[17] Moradali MF, Mostafavi H, Ghods S, Hedjaroude GA. Immunomodulating and anticancer agents in the realm of macromycetes fungi (macrofungi). Int Immunopharmacol 2007; 7(6): 701-24. [http://dx.doi.org/10.1016/j.intimp.2007.01.008] [PMID: 17466905]

[18] Ahn H, Jeon E, Kim JC, *et al.* Lentinan from shiitake selectively attenuates AIM2 and non-canonical inflammasome activation while inducing pro-inflammatory cytokine production. Sci Rep 2017; 7(1): 1314. [http://dx.doi.org/10.1038/s41598-017-01462-4] [PMID: 28465544]

[19] Feng ZL, Fang TJ, Qian YX, Rong WH. The clinical research for Ganoderan's effect on preventing and treating cerebral arteriosclerosis through inhibiting NADPH oxidizing enzyme expression. Pak J

Pharm Sci 2014; 27(4) (Suppl.): 1107-11.
[PMID: 25016275]

[20] Jesenak M, Urbancek S, Majtan J, Banovcin P, Hercogova J. β -Glucan-based cream (containing pleuran isolated from *pleurotus ostreatus*) in supportive treatment of mild-to-moderate atopic dermatitis. J Dermatolog Treat 2016; 27(4): 351-4.
[http://dx.doi.org/10.3109/09546634.2015.1117565] [PMID: 26654776]

[21] Kanagasabapathy G, Malek SNA, Kuppusamy UR, Vikineswary S. Chemical composition and antioxidant properties of extracts of fresh fruiting bodies of Pleurotus sajor-caju (Fr.) Singer. J Agric Food Chem 2011; 59(6): 2618-26.
[http://dx.doi.org/10.1021/jf104133g] [PMID: 21348494]

[22] Singdevsachan SK, Auroshree P, Mishra J, Baliyarsingh B, Tayung K, Thatoi H. Mushroom polysaccharides as potential prebiotics with their antitumor and immunomodulating properties: A review. Bioactive Carbohydrates and Dietary Fibre 2016; 7(1): 1-14.
[http://dx.doi.org/10.1016/j.bcdf.2015.11.001]

[23] Jayachandran M, Xiao J, Xu B. A critical review on health promoting benefits of edible mushrooms through gut microbiota. Int J Mol Sci 2017; 18(9): 1934.
[http://dx.doi.org/10.3390/ijms18091934] [PMID: 28885559]

[24] Sun C, Rosendahl AH, Wang XD, Wu DQ, Andersson R. Polysaccharide-K (PSK) in cancer--old story, new possibilities? Curr Med Chem 2012; 19(5): 757-62.
[http://dx.doi.org/10.2174/092986712798992020] [PMID: 22204346]

[25] Jiménez-Medina E, Berruguilla E, Romero I, *et al.* The immunomodulator PSK induces *in vitro* cytotoxic activity in tumour cell lines *via* arrest of cell cycle and induction of apoptosis. BMC Cancer 2008; 8(1): 78.
[http://dx.doi.org/10.1186/1471-2407-8-78] [PMID: 18366723]

[26] Yang D, Liu Y, Zhang L. Tremella polysaccharide: The molecular mechanisms of its drug action. Prog Mol Biol Transl Sci 2019; 163: 383-421.
[http://dx.doi.org/10.1016/bs.pmbts.2019.03.002] [PMID: 31030755]

[27] Wong JH, Ng TB, Cheung RCF, *et al.* Proteins with antifungal properties and other medicinal applications from plants and mushrooms. Appl Microbiol Biotechnol 2010; 87(4): 1221-35. b
[http://dx.doi.org/10.1007/s00253-010-2690-4] [PMID: 20532758]

[28] Zhang GQ, Sun J, Wang HX, Ng TB. A novel lectin with antiproliferative activity from the medicinal mushroom Pholiota adiposa. Acta Biochim Pol 2009; 56(3): 415-21.
[http://dx.doi.org/10.18388/abp.2009_2475] [PMID: 19636442]

[29] Zhang G, Sun J, Wang H, Ng TB. First isolation and characterization of a novel lectin with potent antitumor activity from a Russula mushroom. Phytomedicine 2010; 17(10): 775-81.
[http://dx.doi.org/10.1016/j.phymed.2010.02.001] [PMID: 20378319]

[30] Wong JH, Wang HX, Ng TB. Marmorin, a new ribosome inactivating protein with antiproliferative and HIV-1 reverse transcriptase inhibitory activities from the mushroom Hypsizigus marmoreus. Appl Microbiol Biotechnol 2008; 81(4): 669-74.
[http://dx.doi.org/10.1007/s00253-008-1639-3] [PMID: 18751697]

[31] Lin YL, Liang YC, Tseng YS, *et al.* An immunomodulatory protein, Ling Zhi-8, induced activation and maturation of human monocyte-derived dendritic cells by the NF-κB and MAPK pathways. J Leukoc Biol 2009; 86(4): 877-89.
[http://dx.doi.org/10.1189/jlb.0708441] [PMID: 19498044]

[32] Lin CH, Sheu GT, Lin YW, *et al.* A new immunomodulatory protein from Ganoderma microsporum inhibits epidermal growth factor mediated migration and invasion in A549 lung cancer cells. Process Biochem 2010; 45(9): 1537-42.
[http://dx.doi.org/10.1016/j.procbio.2010.06.006]

[33] Kodama N, Mizuno S, Nanba H, Saito N. Potential antitumor activity of a low-molecular-weight protein fraction from Grifola frondosa through enhancement of cytokine production. J Med Food 2010; 13(1): 20-30.
[http://dx.doi.org/10.1089/jmf.2009.1029] [PMID: 20136432]

[34] Wieczorek PP, Witkowska D, Jasicka-Misiak I, Poliwoda A, Oterman M, Zielińska K. Bioactive alkaloids of hallucinogenic mushrooms. Studies in Natural Products Chemistry 2015; 46: 133-68.
[http://dx.doi.org/10.1016/B978-0-444-63462-7.00005-1]

[35] Homer JA, Sperry J. Mushroom-derived indole alkaloids. J Nat Prod 2017; 80(7): 2178-87.
[http://dx.doi.org/10.1021/acs.jnatprod.7b00390] [PMID: 28722414]

[36] Tsujikawa K, Kanamori T, Iwata Y, *et al.* Morphological and chemical analysis of magic mushrooms in Japan. Forensic Sci Int 2003; 138(1-3): 85-90.
[http://dx.doi.org/10.1016/j.forsciint.2003.08.009] [PMID: 14642723]

[37] Aly AH, Debbab A, Proksch P. Fifty years of drug discovery from fungi. Fungal Divers 2011; 50(1): 3-19.
[http://dx.doi.org/10.1007/s13225-011-0116-y]

[38] Chaitanya MVNL, Jose A, Ramalingam P, Mandal SC, Kumar PN. Multi-targeting cytotoxic drug leads from mushrooms. Asian Pac J Trop Med 2019; 12(12): 531-6.
[http://dx.doi.org/10.4103/1995-7645.272482]

[39] Wittstein K, Rascher M, Rupcic Z, *et al.* Corallocins A–C, nerve growth and brainderived neurotrophic factor inducing metabolites from the mushroom Hericium coralloides. J Nat Prod 2016; 79(9): 2264-9.
[http://dx.doi.org/10.1021/acs.jnatprod.6b00371] [PMID: 27588730]

[40] Geissler T, Brandt W, Porzel A, *et al.* Acetylcholinesterase inhibitors from the toadstool Cortinarius infractus. Bioorg Med Chem 2010; 18(6): 2173-7.
[http://dx.doi.org/10.1016/j.bmc.2010.01.074] [PMID: 20176490]

[41] Vieira Torquato HF, Ribeiro-Filho AC, Buri MV, *et al.* Canthin-6-one induces cell death, cell cycle arrest and differentiation in human myeloid leukemia cells. Biochim Biophys Acta, Gen Subj 2017; 1861(4): 958-67.
[http://dx.doi.org/10.1016/j.bbagen.2017.01.033] [PMID: 28161479]

[42] Liu J, Shimizu K, Kondo R. The effects of ganoderma alcohols isolated from Ganoderma lucidum on the androgen receptor binding and the growth of LNCaP cells. Fitoterapia 2010; 81(8): 1067-72.
[http://dx.doi.org/10.1016/j.fitote.2010.06.029] [PMID: 20603196]

[43] Cheng CR, Yue QX, Wu ZY, *et al.* Cytotoxic triterpenoids from Ganoderma lucidum. Phytochemistry 2010; 71(13): 1579-85.
[http://dx.doi.org/10.1016/j.phytochem.2010.06.005] [PMID: 20615519]

[44] Sliva D. Ganoderma lucidum (Reishi) in cancer treatment. Integr Cancer Ther 2003; 2(4): 358-64.
[http://dx.doi.org/10.1177/1534735403259066] [PMID: 14713328]

[45] Su HJ, Fann YF, Chung MI, Won SJ, Lin CN. New Lanostanoids of *Ganoderma t sugae*. J Nat Prod 2000; 63(4): 514-6.
[http://dx.doi.org/10.1021/np990367l] [PMID: 10785428]

[46] González AG, León F, Rivera A, *et al.* New lanostanoids from the fungus Ganoderma concinna. J Nat Prod 2002; 65(3): 417-21.
[http://dx.doi.org/10.1021/np010143e] [PMID: 11908995]

[47] Mothana RAA, Awadh Ali NA, Jansen R, Wegner U, Mentel R, Lindequist U. Antiviral lanostanoid triterpenes from the fungus Ganoderma pfeifferi. Fitoterapia 2003; 74(1-2): 177-80.
[http://dx.doi.org/10.1016/S0367-326X(02)00305-2] [PMID: 12628419]

[48] El Dine RS, El Halawany AM, Ma CM, Hattori M. Anti-HIV-1 protease activity of lanostane triterpenes from the vietnamese mushroom Ganoderma colossum. J Nat Prod 2008; 71(6): 1022-6. [http://dx.doi.org/10.1021/np8001139] [PMID: 18547117]

[49] Tohtahon Z, Xue J, Han J, Liu Y, Hua H, Yuan T. Cytotoxic lanostane triterpenoids from the fruiting bodies of Piptoporus betulinus. Phytochemistry 2017; 143: 98-103. [http://dx.doi.org/10.1016/j.phytochem.2017.07.013] [PMID: 28800422]

[50] Isaka M, Palasarn S, Srikitikulchai P, Vichai V, Komwijit S. Astraeusins A–L, lanostane triterpenoids from the edible mushroom Astraeus odoratus. Tetrahedron 2016; 72(23): 3288-95. [http://dx.doi.org/10.1016/j.tet.2016.04.057]

[51] Lee IK, Yun BS. Styrylpyrone-class compounds from medicinal fungi Phellinus and Inonotus spp., and their medicinal importance. J Antibiot (Tokyo) 2011; 64(5): 349-59. [http://dx.doi.org/10.1038/ja.2011.2] [PMID: 21304532]

[52] Huang GJ, Yang CM, Chang YS, *et al.* Hispolon suppresses SK-Hep1 human hepatoma cell metastasis by inhibiting matrix metalloproteinase-2/9 and urokinase-plasminogen activator through the PI3K/Akt and ERK signaling pathways. J Agric Food Chem 2010; 58(17): 9468-75. [http://dx.doi.org/10.1021/jf101508r] [PMID: 20698552]

[53] Wang Y, Shang XY, Wang SJ, *et al.* Structures, biogenesis, and biological activities of pyrano[4,3-c]isochromen-4-one derivatives from the Fungus Phellinus igniarius. J Nat Prod 2007; 70(2): 296-9. [http://dx.doi.org/10.1021/np060476h] [PMID: 17279797]

[54] Lu TL, Huang GJ, Lu TJ, *et al.* Hispolon from Phellinus linteus has antiproliferative effects *via* MDM2-recruited ERK1/2 activity in breast and bladder cancer cells. Food Chem Toxicol 2009; 47(8): 2013-21.
[http://dx.doi.org/10.1016/j.fct.2009.05.023] [PMID: 19477214]

[55] Jakopovich I. New dietary supplements from medicinal mushrooms: Dr Myko San--a registration report. Int J Med Mushrooms 2011; 13(3): 307-13. [http://dx.doi.org/10.1615/IntJMedMushr.v13.i3.110] [PMID: 22135883]

[56] Holliday JC, Cleaver MP. Medicinal value of the caterpillar fungi species of the genus Cordyceps (Fr.) Link (Ascomycetes). Int J Med Mushrooms 2008; 10(3): 219-34. [http://dx.doi.org/10.1615/IntJMedMushr.v10.i3.30]

[57] Maruyama H, Ikekawa T. Immunomodulation and antitumor activity of a mushroom product, proflamin, isolated from Flammulina velutipes (W.Curt.:Fr.) Singer (Agaricomycetideae). Int J Med Mushrooms 2007; 9(2): 109-22.
[http://dx.doi.org/10.1615/IntJMedMushr.v9.i2.20]

[58] Alexandre J, Kahatt C, Bertheault-Cvitkovic F, *et al.* A phase I and pharmacokinetic study of irofulven and capecitabine administered every 2 weeks in patients with advanced solid tumors. Invest New Drugs 2007; 25(5): 453-62.
[http://dx.doi.org/10.1007/s10637-007-9071-6] [PMID: 17628744]

CHAPTER 10

Spirulina: A Living Library of Anticancer Phytochemicals

Awotunde Oluwasegun Samson[1,*], Omogbadegun Olu Richard[1] and Mugambwa Joseph Yusuf [1]

[1] *Department of Biochemistry, Habib Medical School IUIU, Kampala, Uganda*

Abstract: Cancer is a group of diseases involving abnormal cell growth with the potential to invade or spread to other parts of the body. It is one of the major causes of human death, especially in developing countries. Alternative cancer treatments using medicinal plants are exploited because plants produce phytochemical compounds, which are secondary metabolites used for natural defence but could also be useful in inhibiting cancer growth. Medicinal plants also have limited side effects and toxicity as compared to conventional chemotherapy and irradiation treatments. Hence there is a need to develop novel drugs from other sources like plants, fungi, and algae. Spirulina is a blue-green alga with three species: *Spirulina platensis, Spirulina fusiformis, and Spirulina maxima. Spirulina platensis* and *Spirulina maxima* are consumable by humans in the form of dietary supplements, as they are enriched with important nutrients and a library of phytochemicals that can improve immunity and levels of blood lipids, lower blood sugar and blood pressure, and prevent oxidation. These activities of Spirulina phytochemicals make them a good candidate for anticancer therapy. Therefore, this chapter describes the botanical classification, phytochemical composition, and anticancer characteristics of Spirulina and with a specific focus on *Spirulina platensis*.

Keywords: Anticancer, Alternative, Blue-green algae, Cancer, Chemotherapy, Chemical library, Dietary supplement, Fungi, Fatty acids, Medicinal, Oxidation, Phytochemicals, Spirulina *platensis*, Spirulina *platensis*, Spirulina *fusiformis*, Spirulina *maxima*, Toxicity.

INTRODUCTION

Cancer is a worldwide major deadly disease that threatens humans' health. A notable treatment for cancer treatment is killing or inhibiting the development of cancerous cells (chemotherapy). However, it is noteworthy that these drugs are associated with toxicity that might be very unpleasant. Recently, increased interest in marine biological resources as sources of bioactive materials has been witnessed, especially in microalgae and seaweeds such as *Spirulina.*

* **Corresponding author Awotunde Oluwasegun Samson:** Department of Biochemistry, School of Health Sciences, Soroti University, Soroti. Uganda; E-mail: derockng@gmail.com

Motamarri Venkata Naga Lalitha Chaitanya, Galvina Pereira, & Heyam Saad Ali (Eds.)

Spirulina is a microscopic and filamentous cyanobacterium with a simple structure but a complex composition that derives its name from the spiral or helical nature of its filaments. It is a microalga that belongs to the class Cyanophyceae. *Spirulina* refers to the dried biomass of *Arthrospira platensis*, an oxygenic photosynthetic bacterium that can be found worldwide in fresh and marine waters.

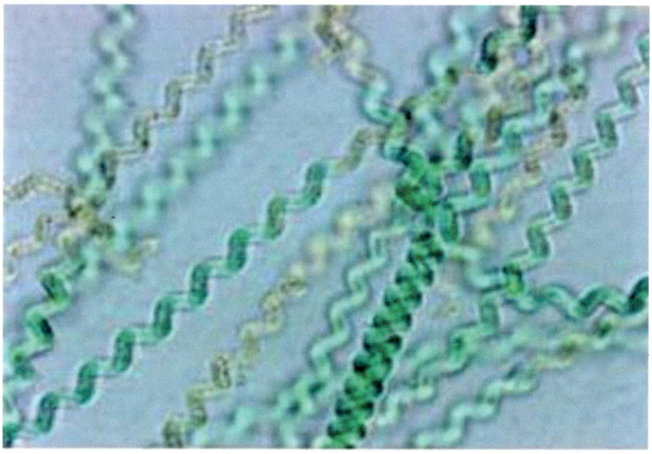

Fig. (1). Filamentous Structure of Cyanobacterium, *Spirulina platensis*

(Source: http://www.spirulinasource.com/library/health-library/)

It lacks cellulose, so it can be easily digested when used as food [1]. It has about 65% protein, 20% carbohydrates, 7% minerals, 5% lipids, 3% moisture, vitamins (B12), pro-vitamin A (-carotenes), and minerals, particularly iron1.Therefore, it is an important staple diet in humans that has been used as a source of protein and vitamin supplements without any significant side effects. Spirulina is rich in phenolic acids, tocopherols, and alpha-linolenic acid [1].

In recent times, the assessment of phytochemicals in macroalgae extracts has greatly contributed to the explanation of their important role in the prevention of human diseases. The identified phytochemicals in the alga are alkaloids, flavonoids, phenols, tannins, phlorotannin, terpenoids, pigments, glycosides, and steroids. These phytochemicals were thought to act as a defence mechanism, protecting them against reactive oxygen species (ROS) resulting from harsh environmental conditions [2, 3]. However, the phytochemicals are useful to humans; for example, Spirulina platensis extract revealed therapeutic cancer prevention activity [4]. As a result of its phytochemical composition, Spirulina thus possesses potent antibacterial, anticancer, antioxidant, antifungal, anti-inflammatory, antidiabetic, neuroprotective, hepatoprotective, and antiviral properties [5 - 7]. It was stated that most natural substances derived from marine algae have therapeutic and medicinal properties, such as anticancer, antibacterial, and antioxidant properties [8]. Among numerous species of Spirulina, three species, including *Spirulina platensis* (*Arthrospira platensis*), Spirulina maxima (*Arthrospira maxima*), and Spirulina fusiformis (*Arthrospira fusiformis*), are the most widely investigated because they are edible and have high nutritional and medicinal values [9].

Table 1. Nutritional and phytochemical Profile of *Cyanobacterium, Spirulina Powder*

Chemical composition %		**Physical properties**		**Pigments**
protein	60-65	Appearance	Fine powder	Chlorophyll α
Carbohydrates	15-20	Colour	Blue green	c-phycocyanin (C-PC)
Lipid	4-5	Odor and taste	mild like weed	Allophycocyanin (APC)
Minerals	6-7	Particle size	64 mesh through	Phycoerithrin (PE)
Moisture	2-3	Digestibility	83-84%	Cartonese. Betacarotene xanthophyll

(Source; http://www.spirulinasource.com/library/health-library/)

Developing a therapy for cancer treatment without harming the rest of the body is the greatest challenge in designing cancer drug therapy. Therefore, there are many difficulties in the treatment of cancer; these challenges include decreasing treatment-related adverse effects, managing triple-negative breast cancer despite poor outcomes, the lack of a therapeutic target, and balancing treatment toxicity with the quality of life in patients with metastatic cancer who have already received inclusive therapy [10]. To reduce this problem, the use of medicinal plants such as Spirulina platensis has been suggested. Many toxicological studies have proven Spirulina's safety and it has been listed by the US Food and Drug Administration under the category "Generally Recognized as Safe" (GRAS) [11, 12].

Over the past years, studies have discovered new classes of antibiotics or cytotoxic metabolic compounds of microalgae majorly cyanobacteria and green algae [13]. Many crude extracts and compounds obtained from different algae have been estimated for their antitumor activities [14].

The aqueous extract of Spirulina platensis shows pharmaceutical properties, such as the ability to fight cancers, reduce the level of blood cholesterol, decrease nephrotoxicity of drugs and toxic metals, and protect against the harmful radiation effects [15]. The methanolic extract of Spirulina platensis was evaluated against the human breast cancer cell line (MCF-7) and the human cancer cell line L20B, after safeguarding the safety of isolated Spirulina platensis through the detection of the microcystin-producing gene *via* the PCR technique. The inhibition of cancerogenesis induced by biologically active compounds derived from spirulina was tested both *in vitro* and *in vivo* [16].

The data obtained strongly linked S. platensis's anti-cancer effects to its antioxidant activity. The *in vitro* studies showed that the cytotoxic effect of Spirulina involved a decrease in the proliferative capacity of tumorigenic cell lines that could result from mitochondrial activity disturbance [17]. *In vivo*, spirulina was shown to have anti-pre-carcinogenic potential; it significantly reduced the number of aberrant crypts formed in the colon. This dependency was shown using rats [18], and mice [19] in an *in vivo* model.

Evidence has shown that the combination of antioxidant and immune modulation characteristics of Spirulina may have a possible mechanism of tumour destruction and hence play a role in cancer prevention. While there are many animal and *in vitro* studies, there has only been one trial with human subjects. A study specifically examined the effects of Spirulina on oral carcinogenesis, in particular leucoplakia [20].

It is not surprising that few human studies exist to date as cancer prevention trials with lower cancer incidence as an endpoint have logistic problems, rendering them essentially impossible to conduct for most malignancies. The research carried out by Mathew *et al.* [21] on a cohort of 77 patients originates from previous trials on hamsters that showed tumour regression after topical application or enteral intake of Spirulina extract [22, 23].

They reported that 45% of their study cohort showed complete regression of leukoplakia after taking Spirulina supplements for 1 year. The authors also reported that despite supplementation, there was no increase in serum concentrations of retinal -carotene, and concluded that other constituents of Spirulina may have been responsible for the anticancer effects. While their findings appear promising, because it was an unblinded, nonrandomized trial, they cannot be considered evidence of a positive effect [24].

Blue-green algae and Spirulina display antitumor activity against many cancers both in human and animal systems, and their pharmaceutical importance includes their roles as antiproliferative, antitumor, antifungal, antibacterial, antimalarial, antiviral, antimycotics, cytotoxic, multi-drug resistance reversers, and immunosuppressive agents [25, 26].

Anticancer Properties of *Spirulina Platensis*

Researchers are focusing on utilising natural products in conventional cancer treatment [27]. The latest development in research helps develop various novel anticancer agents. Several natural products and their synthetic derivatives from marine organisms are identified as anticancer drugs [28]. The antioxidant properties of various forms of algae and their anti-inflammatory, antinociceptive, and anti-cancer effects were reviewed by Jin-Ching Lee *et al.* [29]. Spirulina, has three species, which are: *Spirulina platensis* (*Arthrospira platensis*), Spirulina maxima (*Arthrospira maxima*), and Spirulina fusiformis (*Arthrospira fusiformis*). An inhibitory effect of Spirulina algae on oral carcinogenesis was evaluated showing the chemo preventive effect of *Spirulina fusiformis* in reversing oral leukoplakia in pan tobacco chewers in Kerala, India [30].

Mathew *et al.* [20] studied the effect of spirulina platensis supplementation on pan tobacco chewers with oral leukoplakia in Kerala and discovered that lesions regressed and that the constituents of these Spirulina species might be responsible for these activities. The intravenous injection of radachlorin resulted in significant to complete tumour regression. Radachlorin is a photosensitizer isolated from Spirulina platensis [31]. The enhanced antitumor activity of natural killer (NK) cells was observed in rats by the hot-water extract of Spirulina platensis [32]. In male golden Syrian hamsters, Spirulina platensis extract causes regression of squamous cell carcinoma progression induced by 0.5% 7, 12-dimethylbenz[a]anthracene (DMBA) [33]. It was also observed that the ultrasonic extraction of Spirulina maxima exhibited potential anticancer activity. The extract is effective against different types of human cancer cell lines, such as lung (A549), liver (Hep B), stomach (AGS), and breast (MCF-7) cell lines [34].

Studies by Karkos *et al.* [35] stated that the anticancer properties *of Spirulina platensis* may be due to two important activities which are antioxidant and immune-modulation activities. *Spirulina platensis* shows antitumor, anticancer, and antimicrobial (antibacterial, antifungal, and antiviral) activities *via* the production of valuable products, phycobiliproteins including c-phycocyanin (C-PC), phycocyanobilin, and allophycocyanin (APC) [36].

Table 2. Anticancer Properties of *Spirulina platensis*

S/N	Author	Name of the Cancer	Mechanism	Name of the Compound / Extract	Animal model
1	42	Liver	Anticancer	Phycocyanin	Mice
2	38	Oral –squamous cell carcinoma	Cytotoxic and cytostatic activity	*Spirulina* Phycocyanin	Human and Hamster

(Table 2) cont.....

S/N	Author	Name of the Cancer	Mechanism	Name of the Compound / Extract	Animal model
3	39	Squamous cell carcinoma (DMBA induced)	Total tumor regression	*Spirulina* Dunaliella Extract	Hamster
4	39	Oral buccal pouches tumor	Immune response	*Spirulina* Dunaliella Extract administration Orally	Hamster
5	41	Hepatoma	Inhibited proliferation of abscisic hepatoma cells	*Spirulina* Polysaccharide Extract	Mice
6	46	HeLa cells	Cytotoxic	Water extract	*In vitro*
7	47	Colon (Dimethyhydrazi ne: DMH)	The no. of aberrant crypts reduced significantly	Whole *Spirulina* feed	Rats
8	30, 20	Oral leukoplakia	Combined antioxidant and immune modulation	*Spirulina* supplementation	Human
9	44	Leukemia	Inhibited growth of K562 leukemia cells	*Spirulina* C-Phycocyanin	Mice
10	48	Caspase dependent apoptosis	HeLa cells	C-phycocyanin (C-PC)	*In vitro*
11	49	human melanoma A375 cells and human breast adenocarcinoma MCF-7 cells	Apoptosis and antiproliferative agent	selenium-containing phycocyanin (Se-PC)	*In vitro*
12	32	B16 melanoma	natural killer (NK) cells dependent tumoricidal activity	Hot water extract	Human, mice
13	34	Lung, liver, stomach and breast cell lines	Not known	*Spirulina Maxima* ultrasonic Extraction	*In vitro*
14	33	Squamous cell carcinoma induced by 0.5% of 7, 12-dimethylbenz[a] anthracene (DMBA)	Tumor regression	Spirulina platensis extract	Hamsters
15	35	B16 melanoma cells - Indirectly helps in oral cancers	production of macrophage - tumor necrosis factor-(TNF-)	Polysaccharides from *S. Platensis*	*In vitro*

β- Carotene and Polysaccharides

Green and yellow vegetables are important foods for good health. Beta carotene NCI, USA is a well-known important natural anti-cancer antioxidant. Spinach and kale with their dark green leaves, broccoli, carrots, cantaloupes, squash, papayas, and pumpkin all contain this important substance. Spirulina is very rich in beta-carotene [37]. Beta-carotene significantly inhibits the formation of squamous cell carcinoma [38]. Spirulina and Dunaliella algae prevent tumour development. Studies related to the use of beta-carotene in animals indicate a smaller but statistically significant reduction in tumour number and size [39, 40]. The water-soluble polysaccharides isolated from Spirulina enhanced both the repair activity of radiation-damaged DNA and unscheduled DNA synthesis and exhibited enhanced endonuclease activity significantly [41]. The polysaccharides isolated from Spirulina platensis extract inhibited the DNA synthesis of sarcoma 180 and ascetic hepatoma cells and inhibited the proliferation of ascitic hepatoma cells in mice (a murine model) [41].

Phycocyanin (Pc)

Spirulina platensis possesses phycobiliproteins like C-PC, APC, and PE, and they are biologically active in the phycobilisome. Oral administration of PC from Spirulina causes an increase in the survival rate of mice with live tumour cells [42]. The phycocyanin isolated from Spirulina platensis exhibited anticancer activity against squamous cell carcinoma [38]. The effect of Spirulina and Dunaliella extracts on oral cancers in hamsters A study found that tumours induced by DMBA (dimethylbenz(a)-athracine)-induced squamous cell carcinoma in hamsters regressed [43].The oral administration of Spirulina and Dunaliella extract prevented tumour development in hamsters due to the immune response. Algae extract prevents cancer development and destroys developing malignant cells, and algae extract is not toxic to normal cells. The inhibition of growth and cell viability of human leukaemia K562 cells by C-phycocyanin (C-PC) isolated from Spirulina platensi was due to the involvement of different types of mechanisms [44].

Spirulina platensis - Haematopoiesis

Drugs and their components display potential effects on the immune system and immune response which contributes to some extent to treatment of diseases and killing of cancerous cells. Therefore, the role of *Spirulina platensis* and its components in enhancing the efficiency of immune response is important along with anticancer properties of *Spirulina platensis* for the treatments and prevention of diseases including cancer. The purified polysaccharides and c-phycocyanin of *Spirulina platensis* influence the proliferation and differentiation of committed hematopoietic progenitor cells and can lower the anaemic degree of mice [45]. *Spirulina platensis* enhances the immune response by activating macrophage functions, IL - I production, phagocytosis, and particularly by the primary response [46]. *Spirulina platensis* extract showed that it enhances disease resistance, macrophage phagocytic function, and chicken macrophage functions (*in-vitro*).

CONCLUSION

As a result of this study, Spirulina biomass contained a significant amount of bioactive phytochemicals and thus could play an active role as an anticancer and antioxidant. It also exhibited anti-proliferative properties against the breast cancer adenocarcinoma cell line (MCF-7) and the mouse intestine carcinoma cell line (L20B). Thus, this suggests it to be a possible novel anticancer product from the blue-green algae.

REFERENCES

[1] Dillon JC, Phuc AP, Dubacq JP. Nutritional value of the alga Spirulina. World Rev Nutr Diet 1995; 77: 32-46.
[http://dx.doi.org/10.1159/000424464] [PMID: 7732699]

[2] Yuan YV, Walsh NA. Antioxidant and antiproliferative activities of extracts from a variety of edible seaweeds. Food Chem Toxicol 2006; 44(7): 1144-50.
[http://dx.doi.org/10.1016/j.fct.2006.02.002] [PMID: 16554116]

[3] Senguttuvan J, Paulsamy S, Karthika K. Phytochemical analysis and evaluation of leaf and root parts of the medicinal herb, Hypochaeris radicata L. for *in vitro* antioxidant activities. Asian Pac J Trop Biomed 2014; 4 (Suppl. 1): S359-67.
[http://dx.doi.org/10.12980/APJTB.4.2014C1030] [PMID: 25183112]

[4] Zaid AAA, Hammad DM, Sharaf EM. Antioxidant and anticancer activity of Spirulina platensis water extracts. Int J Pharmacol 2015; 11(7): 846-51.
[http://dx.doi.org/10.3923/ijp.2015.846.851]

[5] S A, v SB, Saritha , Shantaram MS. SEAWEED EXTRACTS EXHIBIT ANTICANCER ACTIVITY AGAINST HeLa CELL LINES. Int J Curr Pharm Res 2016; 9(1): 114.
[http://dx.doi.org/10.22159/ijcpr.2017v9i1.16632]

[6] Monteiro LS, Bastos KX, Barbosa-Filho JM, de Athayde-Filho PF, Diniz MFFM, Sobral MV. Medicinal plants and other living organisms with antitumor potential against lung cancer. Evid Based Complement Alternat Med 2014; 2014: 1-15.
[http://dx.doi.org/10.1155/2014/604152] [PMID: 25147575]

[7] Ramamoorthy A, Premakumari S. Effect of supplementation of Spirulina on hypercholesterolemic patients. J Food Sci Technol 1996; 33(2): 124-8.

[8] Tannoury MYA, Saab M, Josiane ME, Nafez N, Harb HY, Assaf MD. *In vitro* Cytotoxic Activity of Laurencia papillosa, marine red Algae from the Lebanese Coast. J Appl Pharm Sci 2017; 7(03): 175-9.

[9] Deng R, Chow TJ. Hypolipidemic, antioxidant, and antiinflammatory activities of microalgae Spirulina. Cardiovasc Ther 2010; 28(4): e33-45.
[http://dx.doi.org/10.1111/j.1755-5922.2010.00200.x] [PMID: 20633020]

[10] Yezhelyev MV, Gao X, Xing Y, Al-Hajj A, Nie S, O'Regan RM. Emerging use of nanoparticles in diagnosis and treatment of breast cancer. Lancet Oncol 2006; 7(8): 657-67.

[http://dx.doi.org/10.1016/S1470-2045(06)70793-8] [PMID: 16887483]

[11] Tarantino L M. Agency Response Letter GRAS Notice No. GRN000127, FDA Home page. 2003.

[12] Belay A. The potential application of Spirulina (Arthrospira) as a nutritional and therapeutic supplement in Health management. Journal of the American Nutraceutical Association 2002; 5: 27-48.

[13] Fayyad RJ, Dwaish AS. Examination the growth of blue-green alga, Chroococcus turigidus in different traditional media formulations. IES J 2016; 22(95): 51-60. a

[14] Mohamed S, Hashim SN, Rahman HA. Seaweeds: A sustainable functional food for complementary and alternative therapy. Trends Food Sci Technol 2012; 23(2): 83-96. [http://dx.doi.org/10.1016/j.tifs.2011.09.001]

[15] Kumar V, Bhatnagar AK, Srivastava JN. Antibacterial activity of crude extracts of Spirulina platensis and its structural elucidation of bioactive compound. J Med Plants Res 2011; 5: 7043-8.

[16] Ismail M, Hossain MF, Tanu AR, Shekhar HU. Effect of spirulina intervention on oxidative stress, antioxidant status, and lipid profile in chronic obstructive pulmonary disease patients. BioMed Res Int 2015; 2015: 1-7. [http://dx.doi.org/10.1155/2015/486120] [PMID: 25685791]

[17] Koníčková R, Vaňková K, Vaníková J, *et al.* Anti-cancer effects of blue-green alga Spirulina platensis, a natural source of bilirubin-like tetrapyrrolic compounds. Ann Hepatol 2014; 13(2): 273-83. [http://dx.doi.org/10.1016/S1665-2681(19)30891-9] [PMID: 24552870]

[18] Chen F, Zhang Q. [Inhibitive effects of spirulina on aberrant crypts in colon induced by dimethylhydrazine]. Chin J Prev Med 1995; 29(1): 13-7. [PMID: 7600882]

[19] Madrigal-Bujaidar E, Alvarez-Gonzalez I, Islas-Islas V, *et al.* Inhibitory effect of spirulina maxima on the azoxymethane-induced aberrant colon crypts and oxidative damage in mice. Pharmacogn Mag 2015; 11(44) (Suppl. 4): 619. [http://dx.doi.org/10.4103/0973-1296.172973] [PMID: 27013804]

[20] Mathew B, Sankaranarayanan R, Nair PP, *et al.* Evaluation of chemoprevention of oral cancer with *spirulina fusiformis*. Nutr Cancer 1995; 24(2): 197-202. [http://dx.doi.org/10.1080/01635589509514407] [PMID: 8584455]

[21] Mathew B, Sankaranarayanan R, Nair PP, *et al.* Evaluation of chemoprevention of oral cancer with *spirulina fusiformis*. Nutr Cancer 1995; 24(2): 197-202. [http://dx.doi.org/10.1080/01635589509514407] [PMID: 8584455]

[22] Schwartz J, Shklar G. Regression of experimental hamster cancer by beta carotene and algae extracts. J Oral Maxillofac Surg 1987; 45(6): 510-5. [http://dx.doi.org/10.1016/S0278-2391(87)80011-3] [PMID: 3108474]

[23] Schwartz J, Shklar G, Reid S, Trickier D. Prevention of experimental oral cancer by extracts of Spirulina–Dunaliella algae. Nutr Cancer 1988; 11(2): 127-34. [http://dx.doi.org/10.1080/01635588809513979] [PMID: 3129701]

[24] Pignolet O, Jubeau S, Vaca-Garcia C, Michaud P. Highly valuable microalgae: biochemical and topological aspects. J Ind Microbiol Biotechnol 2013; 40(8): 781-96. [http://dx.doi.org/10.1007/s10295-013-1281-7] [PMID: 23660999]

[25] Jalaja Kumari D, Babitha B, Jaffar SK, Guru Prasad M, Ibrahim MD, Siddque Ahmed Khan MD. Potential health benefits of Spirulina platensis. International Journal of Advances In Pharmaceutical Sciences 2011; 21(1): 90-117.

[26] Dixit RB, Suseela MR. Cyanobacteria: potential candidates for drug discovery. Antonie van Leeuwenhoek 2013; 103(5): 947-61. [http://dx.doi.org/10.1007/s10482-013-9898-0] [PMID: 23532410]

[27] Blaylock RL. A review of conventional cancer prevention and treatment and the adjunctive use of nutraceutical supplements and antioxidants: Is there danger or a significant benefit? JANA 2000; 3: 17-35.

[28] Simmons TL, Andrianasolo E, McPhail K, Flatt P, Gerwick WH. Marine natural products as anticancer drugs. Mol Cancer Ther 2005; 4(2): 333-42. [http://dx.doi.org/10.1158/1535-7163.333.4.2] [PMID: 15713904]

[29] Lee JC, Hou MF, Huang HW, *et al.* Marine algal natural products with anti-oxidative, anti-inflammatory, and anti-cancer properties. Cancer Cell Int 2013; 13(1): 55. [http://dx.doi.org/10.1186/1475-2867-13-55] [PMID: 23724847]

[30] Mathew B, Sankaranarayanan R, Nair PP, *et al.* Evaluation of chemoprevention of oral cancer with *spirulina fusiformis*. Nutr Cancer 1995; 24(2): 197-202. [http://dx.doi.org/10.1080/01635589509514407] [PMID: 8584455]

[31] Privalov VA, Lappa AV, Seliverstov OV, *et al.* Clinical trials of a new chlorin photosensitizer for photodynamic therapy of malignant tumors Proceedings of SPIE, Optical Methods for Tumor Treatment and Detection: Mechanisms and Techniques in Photodynamic Therapy. 178-89. [http://dx.doi.org/10.1117/12.469355]

[32] Akao Y, Ebihara T, Masuda H, *et al.* Enhancement of antitumor natural killer cell activation by orally administered Spirulina extract in mice. Cancer Sci 2009; 100(8): 1494-501. [http://dx.doi.org/10.1111/j.1349-7006.2009.01188.x] [PMID: 19432881]

[33] Grawish ME, Zaher AR, Gaafar AI, Nasif WA. Long-term effect of Spirulina platensis extract on DMBA-induced hamster buccal pouch carcinogenesis (immunohistochemical study). Med Oncol 2009.
[PMID: 19156551]

[34] Sung-Ho O. Juhee Ahn, Do-Hyung Kang & Hyeon-Yong Lee. The Effect of Ultrasonificated Extracts of Spirulina maxima on the Anticancer Activity. Mar Biotechnol (NY) 2010. [http://dx.doi.org/10.1007/s10126-010-9282-2]

[35] Karkos P D. Spirulina in Clinical Practice: Evidence-Based Human Applications. Hindawi publishing corporation 2011; 2011: pp. 1-4.

[36] Abdulmumin A. Spirulina (Arthrospira): An Important Source of Nutritional and Medicinal Compounds. Journal of Marine Biology 2013; 2013

[37] Harald W. Spirulina, Micro food macro blessings. 4th edition., 2004.

[38] Schwartz J. Algae-derived Phycocyanin is both cytostatic and cytotoxic to oral squamous cell carcinoma (human or hamster). J Dent Res 1987; 66: 160.

[39] Schwartz J, Shklar G, Reid S, Trickier D. Prevention of experimental oral cancer by extracts of Spirulina–Dunaliella algae. Nutr Cancer 1988; 11(2): 127-34. [http://dx.doi.org/10.1080/01635588809513979] [PMID: 3129701]

[40] Annapurna V, *et al.* Bioavailability of spirulina carotenes in preschool children. by V. National Institute of Nutrition, Hyderabad, India. J Clin Biochem Nutr 1991; 10: 145-51. [http://dx.doi.org/10.3164/jcbn.10.145]

[41] Lisheng L, Baojiang G, Jihong R, Guangquan Q, Wu B. Inhibitive effect and mechanism of polysaccharide of spirulina platensis on transplanted tumor in mice Pub.Marine Sciences 1991; 33-8.

[42] Dainippon Ink & Chemicals, Inc. (DIC). Anti-tumoral agents containing phycobillin Japanese Patent #58- 65216, 1983.

[43] Shklar G, Schwartz J. Tumor necrosis factor in experimental cancer regression with alphatocopherol, beta-carotene, canthaxanthin and algae extract. Eur J Cancer Clin Oncol 1988; 24(5): 839-50. [http://dx.doi.org/10.1016/0277-5379(88)90192-7] [PMID: 3139418]

[44] Liu Y, Xu L, Cheng N, Lin L, Zhang C. Inhibitory effect of phycocyanin from Spirulina platensis on the growth of human leukemia K562 cells. J Appl Phycol 2000; 12(2): 125-30. [http://dx.doi.org/10.1023/A:1008132210772]

[45] Zhang C-W. Effects of polysaccharide and phycocyanin from spirulina on peripheral blood and hematopoietic system of bone marrow in mice. Proc of Second Asia Pacific Conf on Algal Biotech. 58.China. China: Nanjing Univ. 1994; p.

[46] Hayashi. Enhancement of antibody production in mice by dietary spirulina Kagawa Nutrition Univ. Japan. Pub. Journal of Nutr Science and Vitaminology Japan 1994.

[47] Chen F, Zhang Q. [Inhibitive effects of spirulina on aberrant crypts in colon induced by dimethylhydrazine]. Chin J Prev Med 1995; 29(1): 13-7. [PMID: 7600882]

[48] Li B, Zhang X, Gao M, Chu X. Effects of CD59 on antitumoral activities of phycocyanin from Spirulina platensis. Biomed Pharmacother 2005; 59(10): 551-60. [http://dx.doi.org/10.1016/j.biopha.2005.06.012] [PMID: 16271846]

[49] Chen T, Wong YS. In vitro antioxidant and antiproliferative activities of selenium-containing phycocyanin from selenium-enriched Spirulina platensis. J Agric Food Chem 2008; 56(12): 4352-8. [http://dx.doi.org/10.1021/jf073399k] [PMID: 18522403]

CHAPTER 11

Terpenoids A Potential Scaffold for Cancer Therapy: A Mechanistic Approach

Surya Kant Tripathi[1], **Stuti Biswal**[1], **Munmun Panda**[1] and **Bijesh Kumar Biswal**[1,*]

[1] *Cancer Drug Resistance Laboratory, Department of Life Science, National Institute of Technology Rourkela, Odisha-769008, India*

Abstract: Cancer remains the most devastating disease that threatens public health with increasing incidence year by year worldwide. The anti-cancer property of naturally derived compounds appears to be a promising approach in cancer therapy. Terpenoids, generally known as terpenes, belong to the most abundant secondary metabolites class and extensively occur in various medicinal plants, fruits, and vegetables. Most of the terpenoids are non-toxic in nature and a ubiquitous part of the human diet. To date, approximately 50,000 terpenoids have been known in nature, and most of them have their use in traditional as well as modern medicinal systems. Based on the number of cyclic structures, terpenoids have been classified into eight main classes such as hemiterpenoids, monoterpenoids, sesquiterpenoids, diterpenoids, sesterterpenoids, triterpenoids, tetraterpenoids, and polyterpenoids. Terpenoids have shown several biological and pharmaceutical significances, including anticancer activity. The literature study revealed that terpenoids exhibit anticancer activity against various human cancers *via* inhibiting the initiation and progression of tumor growth *in vitro* and *in vivo*. In addition, many terpenoids inhibit cell proliferation, invasion, metastasis, and angiogenesis which promote apoptosis of various cancer cells *via* inhibiting various deregulated oncogenic intracellular signaling pathways. Moreover, the pre-clinical anticancer efficacy of terpenoids supports their clinical application as an anticancer therapeutic. This chapter attempts to provide a comprehensive overview of recent advancements and mechanistic progress on terpenoids as cancer therapeutic.

Keywords: Apoptosis, Cytotoxicity, Cancer, Diterpenoids, Hemiterpenoids, Monoterpenoids, Oncogenic signaling pathways, Phytochemicals, Polyterpenoids, Sesquiterpenoids, Sesterterpenoids, Terpenoids, Triterpenoids, Tetraterpenoids.

TERPENOIDS

Phytochemicals originated from various traditional medicinal plants, are biologically active compounds, which have a remarkable contribution in the field

* **Corresponding author Bijesh Kumar Biswal:** Cancer Drug Resistance Laboratory, Department of Life Science, National Institute of Technology Rourkela, Odisha-769008, India; E-mail: biswalb@nitrkl.ac.in

Motamarri Venkata Naga Lalitha Chaitanya, Galvina Pereira, & Heyam Saad Ali (Eds.)

of present-day drug discovery [1]. Many phytochemicals that occur in our diets have been effectively known for their promising disease-preventing properties, including cancer [2]. Terpenoids, very minutely occurring phytochemicals of our diet but highly ubiquitous in nature, are among the largest class of biological agents [2]. At present, over 50,000 terpenoids have been known so far in nature [3]. Interestingly, most of the terpenoids are plant-purified volatile oil-based compounds and mainly occur in medicinal plant groups, including Acanthaceae, Araliaceae, Aristolochiaceae, Celastraceae, Compositae, Labiatae, Lauraceae, Magnoliaceae, Oleaceae, Pinaceae, Ranunculaceae, Rutaceae, Taxaceae, and Umbelliferae [4]. They are highly potent and target selective biologically active compounds, which have been extensively used to combat many deadly diseases. In addition, terpenoids are also known for their several medicinal activities, such as anticancer, antibacterial, anti-inflammatory, antimalarial, and antiviral [4]. Terpenoids also have their uses as blood sugar lowering agents, antiaging agents, immunomodulatory and neuroprotective agents, and in the treatment of many cardiovascular diseases [4]. Studies have revealed that many plant-isolated terpenoids have shown promising anticancer activity *via* inhibiting the initiation and progression of various cancers at an early stage [5]. While they also exhibit significant tumor-reducing potential in the late stages of cancer [5]. Mechanistically, terpenoids inhibit tumor growth *via* targeting various apoptotic and intracellular signaling pathways, cell cycle arrest, anti-angiogenic effect, inhibiting invasion, and metastasis in many types of cancer [6]. Compiling and renewing the recent updates on terpenoids related to an anticancer prospect can provide a newer reference for discovering novel anticancer therapeutics. Thus, this chapter provides recent updates on anticancer activity and diverse mechanisms involved in cancer prevention of terpenoids (Fig. **1**).

DIFFERENT FORMS OF TERPENOIDS

Terpenoids are structurally diverse compounds, and they are synthesized from mevalonic acid (MVA) through the mevalonate or non-mevalonate biosynthetic pathways. MVA is basically derived from different combinations of five carbon structural units (C5) named isoprene. Considering biochemical structural-based studies, terpenoids are mainly categorized into monoterpenoids (C10), diterpenoids (C20), triterpenoids (C30), tetraterpenoids (C40), polyterpenoids (>C40), hemiterpenoids (C5), sesquiterpenoids (C15), and sesterterpenoids (C25). In addition, triterpenoids, sesquiterpenoids, and polyterpenoids are the product of mevalonate biosynthetic pathways, while monoterpenoids, diterpenoids, tetraterpenoids, and sesterterpenoids are derived in non-mevalonate biosynthetic pathways. However, isopentenyl pyrophosphate (IPP) is a common precursor in synthesizing all forms of terpenoids. It has been observed that continuous polymerization of IPPs by the enzyme prenyltransferases yields prenyl pyrophosphates (terpenoids skeleton). Finally, in the third phase, another enzymatic modification in prenyl pyrophosphates resulted in functional terpenoids.

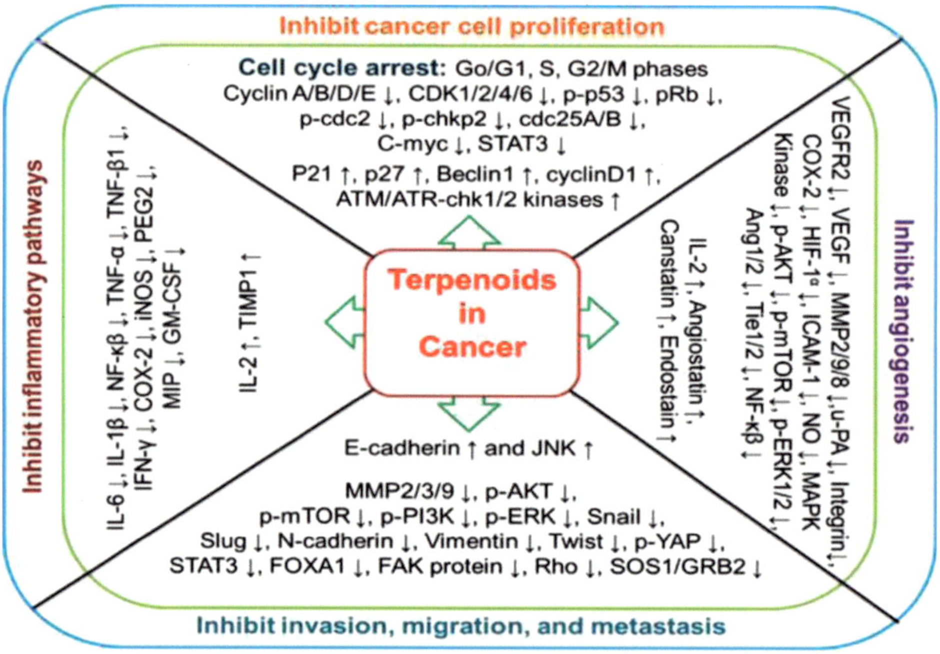

Fig. (1). Terpenoids regulated diverse mechanisms in cancer prevention.

Monoterpenoids

Monoterpenoid (C10) is the combined product of two isoprene residues with molecular a formula C10H16. They can be further classified into mono-, bi-, and a-cyclic groups. Monoterpenoids are mainly obtained from essential and fixed oils naturally occurring in plants. Monoterpenoids are well-known for their use in making perfumes due to their strong aroma and fragrance. In addition, they have shown vital biological activities, such as anticancer, anti-inflammatory, and antibacterial activity. For example, a monoterpenoid, Geraniol, shows a significant growth inhibitory effect against human hepatic carcinoma cell line HepG2 [7]. Mechanistically, the molecular target of Geraniol was 3-hydroxymethylglutaryl coenzyme A (HMG-CoA) reductase, a rate-limiting enzyme in the biosynthesis pathway of cholesterol. Geraniol showed a growth inhibitory effect by inhibiting the expression of HMG-CoA-reductase in the HepG2 cell line [7]. The chemical structure of some monoterpenoids is shown in Fig. (**2**).

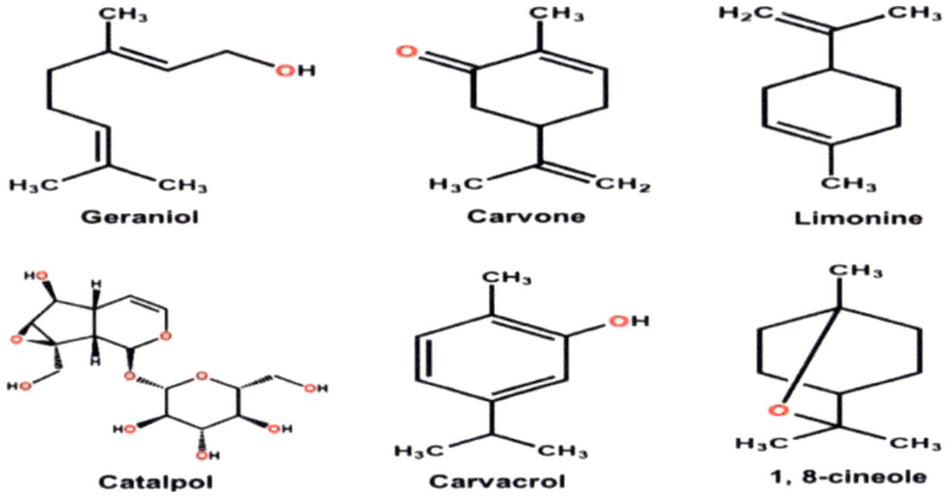

Fig. (2). Chemical structure of some monoterpenoids showing potent anticancer activity.

Diterpenoids

Diterpenoids (C20), a product of four isoprene residues with a molecular formula C20H32, are naturally plant-based versatile compounds. Other than plants, diterpenoids are also synthesized in some fungi and animals *via* HMG-CoA reductase pathway. Diterpenoids have been known for their effective biological activities, including anti-inflammatory and anticancer activities. Currently, many diterpenoids and their derivatives, such as andrographolide, cafeic acid, cafestol, kahweol, oridonin, paclitaxel (taxol), and triptolide have already been introduced as anticancer drugs to encounter various types of cancers. For example, a potent diterpenoid, Andrographolide (AG), obtained from *Andrographics paniculata* showed anti-inflammatory, cytotoxicity, and growth inhibitory effects against human HepG2 cell line by targeting cellular apoptotic, mitogen-activated protein kinase (MAPK), and c-Jun-N-terminal kinase (JNK) pathways [8]. Similarly, another highly potent diterpenoid paclitaxel has promising cytotoxicity against breast and ovarian cancers [9]. Sugiol, a diterpenoid, showed significant anticancer activity by inhibiting oncogenic protein signal transducer and the activator of transcription 3 (STAT3) activities and inducing ERK activity [10]. The chemical structure of some diterpenoids is shown in Fig. (**3**).

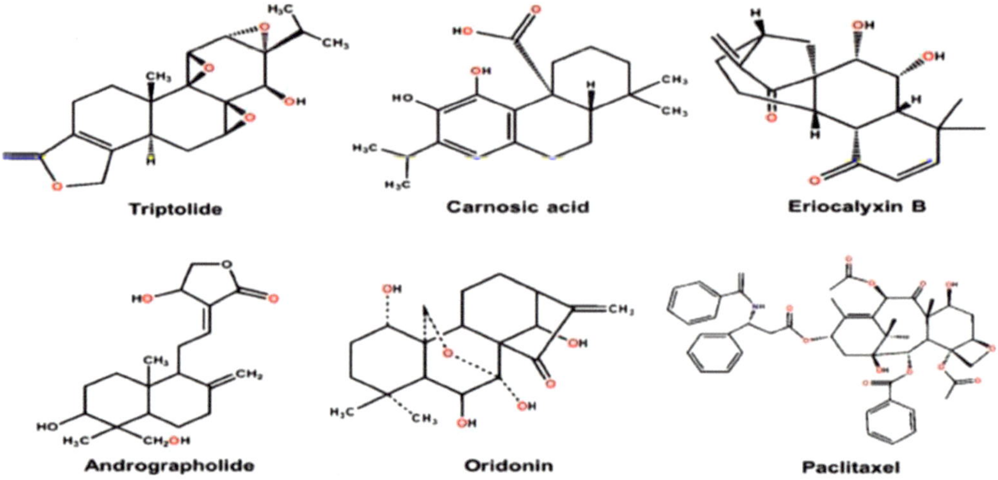

Fig. (3). Chemical structure of some diterpenoids showing potent anticancer activity.

Triterpenoids

Triterpenoids (C30), a product of six isoprene residues with a molecular formula C30H48, are naturally produced in plants, animals, and fungi *via* the squalene biosynthesis pathway. They are made up of multiple methyl groups, which further convert (oxidation reaction) into aldehydes, alcohols, and carboxylic acids. Triterpenoids are also found in another modified form named terpenoid glycosides (saponins), due to glycosylation of their multiple active sites. Oleanolic acid, Ursolic acid, Celastrol, Nimbolide, Asiatic acid, and Betulinic acid are potent triterpenoids, and they have promising anticancer activity against various cancers [11 - 13]. Mechanistically, terpenoids can regulate many signaling pathways, such as phosphatidylinositol 3-kinase/AKT pathway and hedgehog signaling pathway [14, 15]. The chemical structure of some monoterpenoids is shown in Fig. (**4**).

Tetraterpenoids

Tetraterpenoids (C40) are the combination product of eight isoprene residues with molecular a formula C40H64. Tetraterpenoids are mainly produced in plants, and carotenoids of eight isoprene subunits are their best example. They are basically derived from lycopene and lycopene has been documented for its multiple growth inhibitory effects against various cancers. Lycopene can regulate multiple anticancer mechanisms like intrinsic and extrinsic apoptotic pathways, growth factor signaling, cell cycle arrest, and modulation in antioxidant and phase II detoxifying enzymes [16 - 18]. β-carotene, a primary precursor of vitamin A is also documented for its cytotoxicity and anticancer activities in many *in vitro* and *in vivo* studies [19]. The chemical structure of some monoterpenoids is shown in Fig. (**5**).

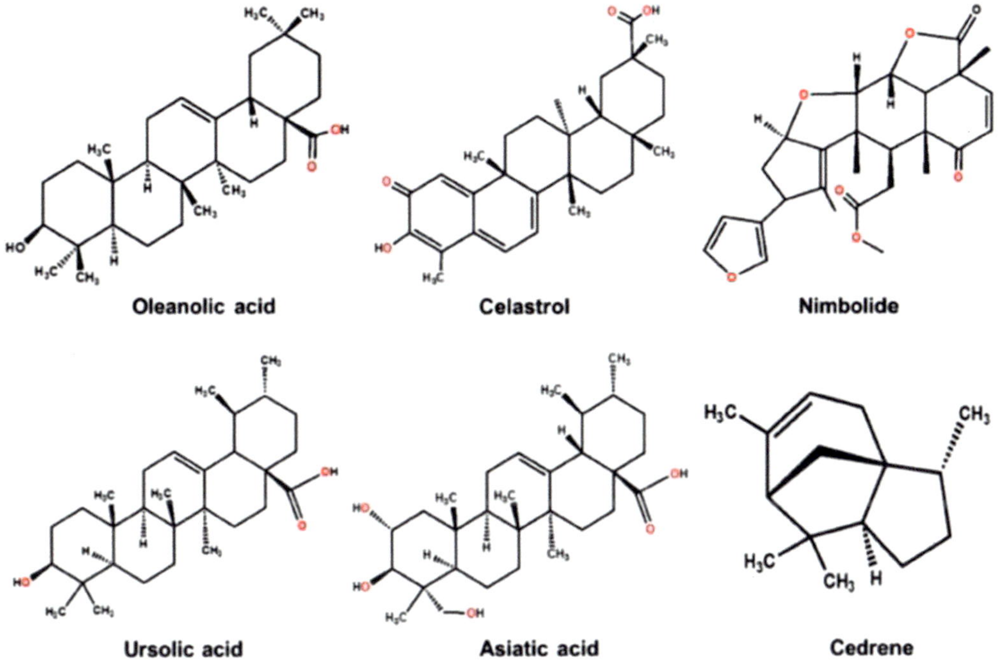

Fig. (4). Chemical structure of some triterpenoids showing potent anticancer activity.

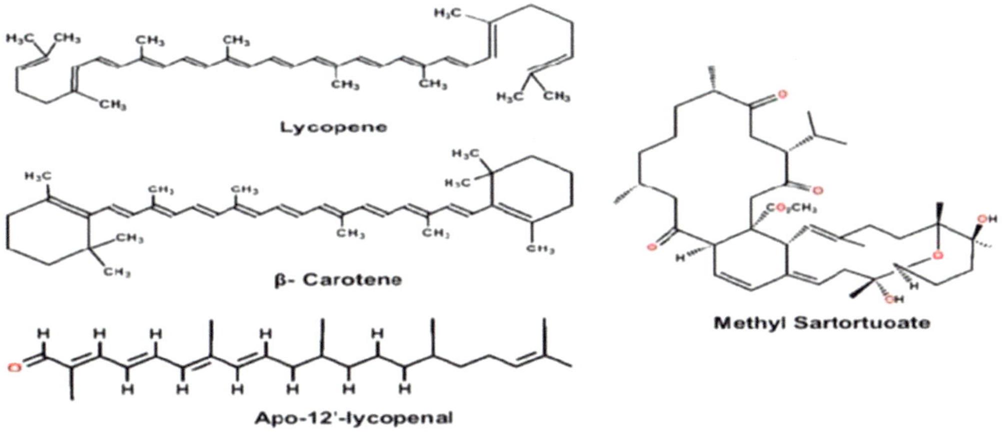

Fig. (5). Chemical structure of some tetraterpenoids showing potent anticancer activity.

Sesquiterpenoid

Sesquiterpenoids (C15), a product of three isoprene residues with a molecular formula C15H24, is mainly isolated from bryophytes, some gymnosperms, and many angiosperms. To date, almost 5000 sesquiterpenoids have been known so far, mostly related to the Asteraceae family. They can be classified into mono-, bi-, tri-, and a-cyclic groups. These compounds have been well-known for their significant medicinal properties, including anti-inflammatory and anticancer activity. For example, a sesquiterpenoid, α-Bisabolbol, shows potent cytotoxicity against human hepatic carcinoma cell line HepG2 [20]. It has been observed that α-Bisabolbol can induce apoptosis in HepG2 cell line by targeting both intrinsic and extrinsic mitochondrial apoptotic pathways. Treatment of α-Bisabolbol showed significant overexpression of pro-apoptotic markers, such as Bax, Bak, Caspase-3/8, and downregulation in anti-apoptotic markers like Bcl-2 [20]. The chemical structure of some monoterpenoids is shown in Fig. (**6**).

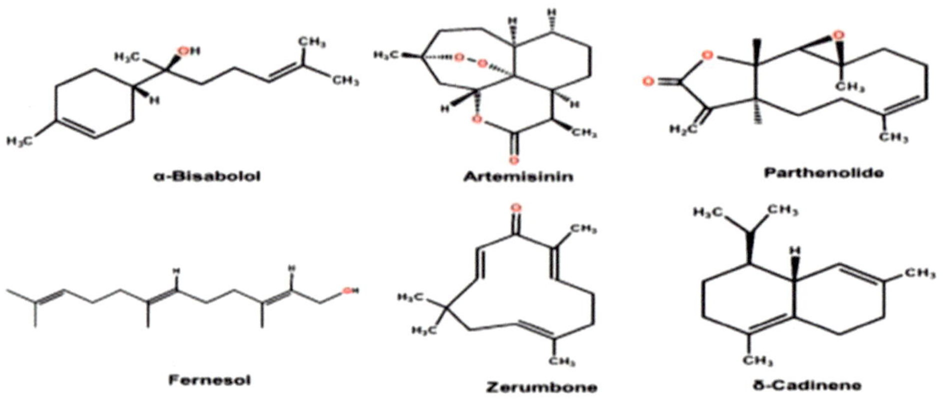

Fig. (6). Chemical structure of some sesquiterpenoids showing potent anticancer activity.

Sesterterpenoids

Sesterterpenoids (C25) are the derivative of five isoprene residues with the molecular formula C25H40. They can be further classified into mono-, bi-, tri-, and tetra-carbocyclic compounds. To date, more than 1,000 have been discovered mainly from plants, fungi, lichens, and insects. Sesterterpenoids have promising biological activities such as antibacterial, anti-fungal, anti-inflammatory, and anticancer potential. Almost all sesterterpenoid class exhibits anti-inflammatory, cytotoxicity, and growth inhibitory effects against various cancers *in vitro*. However, their anticancer mechanism is very limited and needs to be revealed to date. Leucosterlactone and leucosesterterpenone are two plant-based sesquiterpene; those have a potent anti-tumorigenic effect by inhibiting angiogenesis in endothelial cells *via* targeting fibroblast growth factor-2 (FGF-2) [21]. The chemical structure of some monoterpenoids is shown in Fig. (**7**).

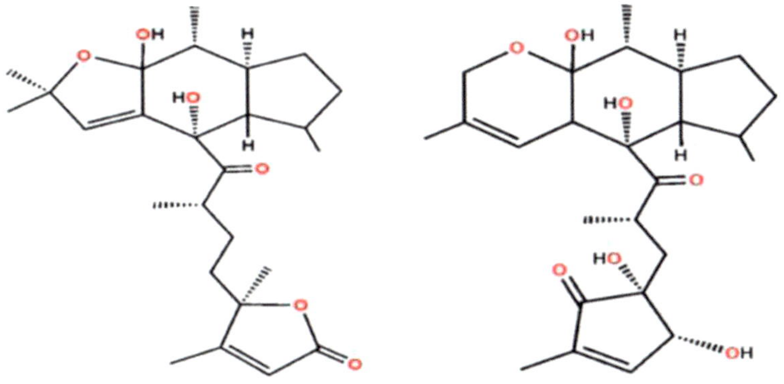

Leucosterlactone Leucosesterterpenone

Fig. (7). Chemical structure of some sesterterpenoids showing potent anticancer activity.

TERPENOIDS AND CANCER

Phytocompounds are plant-derived compounds playing a crucial role in various disease treatments, including cancer now-a-days. Terpenoids serve various pharmaceutical activities against different diseases, including anticancer activity. These different types of terpenoids show formidable activity in opposition to cancer. The anticancer activity of different types of terpenoids are shown by doing the mechanisms, such as inhibition of cell proliferation, arrest of the cell cycle, apoptosis induction, seize of angiogenesis, suppression of cell migration, invasion, and metastasis, repression of epithelial to mesenchymal transition, hampering several signaling pathways and inflammatory pathways. Here in this chapter, we elaborately explain how terpenoids targeted various mechanisms involved in cancer prevention (Table **1**).

TERPENOIDS REGULATE CANCER CELL DEATH PATHWAYS

Normal cells can maintain their intracellular reactive oxygen species (ROS) level, which protects cells from any harm or damage [39]. The normal level of ROS is crucial for many biological processes, and many antioxidant molecules in the cells steadily maintain ROS homeostasis through many detoxification processes [40]. While, during early stage of cancer, moderate increase in ROS may influence tumor microenvironment, leading to tumorigenesis, tumor cell survival, proliferation, invasion, migration, angiogenesis, and metastasis [40]. Despite moderate ROS level promotes tumorigenesis; its increase beyond a certain level promotes apoptosis, senescence, and death in cancer cells. Phytocompounds, including terpenoids, have been shown to regulate various cellular antioxidant molecules, which result in tumor growth inhibition and cancer cell death. A terpenoid named Taraxastane has been shown to induce ROS-mediated inhibition of DoTc2 cancer cells proliferation, invasion, migration, and metastasis [41]. Taraxastane induced DoTc2 cancer cell death was also associated with G2/M phase arrest and inhibition of the JNK/MAPK signaling pathway [41]. Thymol, another terpenoid, was found to induce intrinsic mitochondrial apoptotic pathway mediated cell death in bladder cancer cells [42]. Thymol induced bladder cancer cell death was associated with higher ROS level, activation of JNK/p38 pathway, G2/M phase cell cycle arrest, and inhibition of Akt pathway [42].

Table 1. Terpenoids targeted various mechanisms involved in cancer prevention.

	Name of terpenoid	Anticancer effect	Mechanism	Ref
Monoterpenoid	Catalpol	reduces cell proliferation, invasion, angiogenesis, and inflammation	VEGF↓, VEGFR2↓, bFGF↓, HIF-1α↓, IL-1β↓, IL-6↓, IL-8↓, COX-2↓, iNOS↓	[22]
	Carvacrol	induces cell cycle arrest and apoptosis	Cyclin D1↓, CDK4↓, p21↑, Notch-1↓, Jagged-1↓	[23]
	Carvone	induces apoptosis, arrests cell cycle, and inhibits cell invasion	p-p38 MAPK↓	[24]
	Abisilin	arrests cell cycle and inhibits cell proliferation and angiogenesis	ICAM-1↓, VEGF↓, Cyclin D1↓, Cyclin E1↓, Cyclin A2↓, pAMPK↑	[25]
Sesquiterpenoid	Furanodiene	inhibits adhesion, migration, and invasion	Integrin↓, vimentin↓, β-catenin↓, p-FAK↓, p-Akt↓, p-PI3K↓	[26]
	Artimisinin	inhibits cell proliferation and angiogenesis and induces apoptosis	P53↑, Mdm2↓, ERα↓, VEGF↓, VEGF↓, HIF-1α↓, Notch-1↓, Dll4↓, Jagged1↓, telomerase activity↓	[27, 28]
	Oridonin	arrests cell cycle and induces apoptosis	P21↑, P53↑, cdk2↓, cyclin B↓, Bax↑, Bcl2↓, PI3K/Akt/mTOR↓, and Ras/Raf↓	[29]
Diterpenoid	Andrographolide	Inhibits proliferation and angiogenesis and induces apoptosis	VEGF↓, COX-2↓, p300 HAT↓, Cytochrome C↑, Caspase 3↑, Caspase 9↑, Bax↑	[30]
	Triptolide	Inhibits cell proliferation, and EMT, induces cell cycle arrest and apoptosis	E-cadherin↑, N-cadherin↓, twist↓, snail↓, MAPK/ERK↓, Cyclin D1↓, CDK4/6 ↓	[31]
	Oleanolic acid	Inhibits cell proliferation, induces cell cycle arrest, and apoptosis	Cdk4↓, cyclin D↓, Bax↑, Caspase 8↑, Caspase 9↑, Caspase 3↑, Bcl2↓, Bcl-xl↓, PI3K/Akt↓	[32]

(Table 1) cont.....

	Name of terpenoid	Anticancer effect	Mechanism	Ref
Triterpenoid	Cedrelone	Inhibits cell proliferation and angiogenesis, induces cell cycle arrest and apoptosis	ERK/MAPK1↓, Bax↑, Caspase 3↑, Caspase 9↑, Bcl2↓,	[33]
	Celastrol	Inhibits proliferation and angiogenesis	MMP9↓, IL-1β↓, PDGF↓, TIMP4↓, Serpin E1↓, iNOS↓, eNOS↓, TYMP↓, CDH5↓, THBS2↓, LEP↓, MMP9↓,TNF↓	[34]
	Nimbolide	Inhibits cell proliferation and EMT and induces apoptosis	E-Cadherin↑, N-cadherin↓, Zeb↓, notch2↓, vimentin↓, snail↓, slug↓, Bax↑, Caspase 3↑, PI3K/AKT↓	[35]
	Methyl sartortuoate	induces cell cycle arrest and apoptosis	Bax↑, P53↑, Caspase 3↑, Caspase 8↑, Caspase 9↑, Bcl2↓, cdc2↓, p21↑, p53↑, p-JNK↑, p-p38↑	[36]
Tetraterpenoid	Lycopene	Inhibits angiogenesis, cell migration, invasion, and tube formation	VEGF↓, MMP2↓,u-PA↓, PI3K-Akt↓, ERK/p38↓	[37]
	Manoalide	Arrests cell cycle and induces apoptosis	Caspase 3↑, Caspase 8↑, Caspase 9↑	[38]

In addition, overproduction of ROS has been mostly associated with DNA damage, resulting in activation of the programmed cell death pathway (apoptosis) in cancer cells [43 - 45]. A normal cell has a much-maintained complex balance on apoptosis by regulating proteins of the Bcl-2 family (pro-apoptotic and anti-apoptotic) [46]. Loss of this balance on apoptosis due to the imbalance of Bcl-2 family proteins contributes to inhibition of apoptosis, thereby continuous proliferation of cancer cells [46]. Terpenoids are known to have a critical role in ROS overproduction, DNA damage, and induction of cell death pathways in various cancers. For example, two monoterpenoids named geraniol and geranyl acetate showed promising anticancer activity against colon cancer cell line colo-205 through induction of apoptotic pathways, G2/M phase cell cycle arrest, and DNA damage [47]. Another terpenoid named Oridonin induced intrinsic apoptotic pathway in hepatocellular carcinoma cell line HepG2 *via* enhancing ROS production, activation of apoptotic pathway proteins, such as caspase3/9 and cytochrome c, and tumor suppressor gene p53 [48].

Autophagy shows a novel intracellular degradative process, which is characterized for recycling of cellular wastes leads to cell death [49]. Initially, autophagy was discovered for their role in cell survival, while later on researches identified cytotoxic autophagy which has a significant role in cancer cell death [50]. Studies revealed that cancer cells have dysregulated autophagy, and phytocompounds, including terpenoids, have the ability to regulate autophagy [51, 52]. Ursolic acid

(UA), a pentacyclic triterpenoid, showed both apoptosis and autophagy at 20 μM treatment concentration [53]. Mechanistically, UA induced apoptosis and autophagy mediates inhibition of the AKT pathway, which causes energy stress leading to modulation in the glycolytic pathway and AMPK activation [53]. Another terpenoid named geraniol has been shown to induce both mitophagy (mitochondria eating) and autophagy *via* an increase of ATG proteins and AMPK expressions and a decrease in LC3I, LC3II, mTOR, and ER stress markers [54]. Kim and co-authors study revealed that geraniol showed autophagy-mediated antitumor activity by inhibiting the AKT pathway and activating AMPK signaling in prostate cancer cells [55].

TERPENOIDS REGULATE CELL CYCLE IN CANCER

Cell cycle arrest of cancer cells at different phases is one of the significant aspects in the development of a novel drug. Various terpenoids have been studies for cell cycle regulation in various types of cancer. Some examples are discussed here. A natural acyclic monoterpene, Geraniol induced G1 phase cell cycle arrest *via* reducing the activity of cyclins, such as cyclin A/B/D/E, CDK1, and CDK4 and enhancing the expression of p21 and p27 in PC-3 cell line of prostate cancer [55]. An important monoterpenoid, Carvone, has a promising effect on cell cycle regression in myeloma cells *via* G2/M phase cell cycle arrest [24]. Limonene checked cell cycle progression in human bladder cancer cell line T24 *via* arrest in the G2/M phase [56]. In addition, Thymol promoted the G2/M phase pause in the cell cycle *via* reduced production of cyclin A, cyclin B, and CDK2 and enhanced p21 expression in the T24 bladder cancer cell line [42]. While 1, 8-Cineole or eucalyptol is a monoterpene cyclic-ether. It arrested the HepG2 cells in the G0/G1 phase of the cell cycle *via* inhibiting cyclin-dependent kinase-2/4/6, cyclin A, and promoting p27 [57]. It was found that a polyhalogenated monoterpene, Mertensene, could induce G2/M phase arrest in the HT29 human colon adenocarcinoma cell line, inhibiting the phosphorylation of p53, p-retinoblastoma protein (Rb), p-cdc2, and p-chkp2 and expression of CDK2/4 proteins [58]. Abisilin1 is a complex of monoterpenoids that inhibited Hepa1-6 cell line growth *via* a significant reduction in relative mRNA expression of cyclin D1, E1, and A2 [25]. Treatment of linear monoterpenoid, Linalool, in HepG2 resulted in G0/G1 phase cell cycle arrest *via* low expression of Cdk4 and cyclin A/E levels. Additionally, the vigorous surge was observed in expression levels p21 and p27 [59]. Sesquiterpene lactones, Artemisinin (ART), and its derivatives dihydroartemisinin (DHA) and Artesunate, obtained from *Artemisia annua* L. showed anticancer activity *via* inhibiting the expression of CDK4 gene. While, DHA induced cell cycle arrest *via* reducing transcriptional activity of many cyclins and CDKs. Artesunate showed anticancer activity through G2/M phase cell cycle arrest of *via* autophagy initiation and upregulation of the Beclin1. The compound induced G2/M phase cell cycle arrest was also rcgulated by targeting Bub3, Mad3, and Mad2 regulator genes of the mitotic spindle checkpoint [60]. However, in human breast cancer cell line MCF-7, ART checked cell cycle by suppressing Retinoblastoma1 (Rb1), Cdk2/4, cyclin E1 (CCNE1), and cyclin D1 (CCND1) [61]. Guang and Xie's study documented that a sesquiterpene lactone, Parthenolide, promoted the G1 phase of cell cycle arrest by regulating cyclin D1 and p-cdk2 in human bladder cancer cell line 5637 [62]. The monocyclic sesquiterpene, Zerumbone, isolated from rhizomes of *Zingiber zerumbet* caused increased DNA content in cell cycle phase of S and G2/M in Hep-2 human laryngeal carcinoma cell line [63]. A sesquiterpenoid dimer Leariifolianoid-E could affect cell progression in the MCF-7 cell line by apprehending the G2/M phase of the cell cycle [64]. Geranyl farnesol, a linear sesterterpene derived from shoots of *Salvia lachnocalyx* showed sub-G1 phase arrest in MOLT-4 cells [65]. δ-Cadinene is a type of Cadinene family of sesquiterpene-induced sub-G1 phase arrest in OVCAR-3 ovarian cancer cell line [66]. Psilostachyin C is a sesquiterpene lactone arrested murine lymphoma cells in S phase at very short treatment period. While long time exposure of compound induced G1/G0 arrest [67]. An important diterpenoid lactone AG promoted G2/M phase cell cycle arrest *via* enhancing p21 and p27 and inhibiting cyclin kinases (Cyclin D1 and E2) in chondrosarcoma [68]. Totarol, a phenolic diterpenoid, derived from sap of *Podocarpus totara* showed anticancer activity by inhibiting cell growth through promoting G2/M phase cell cycle arrest in SGC-7901 human gastric carcinoma cell line [69]. Another, diterpenoid Oridonin, could hinder cell cycle progression *via* promoting S phase arrest in SGC996 and NOZ gallbladder cancer cell lines [70]. Another study suggested that Oridonin also induced cytotoxicity and G2/M phase cell cycle arrest *via* inhibiting cdc2, cdc25C, and cyclin B1 in OSCC cells [71]. A diterpenoid, Kaurenoic acid, arrested cell division at G1 phase in gastric cancer cell line [72]. *Pseudolarix kaemferi* bark purified, diterpenoid named Pseudolaric acids A and B (PA-A and B) promoted cell cycle arrest by blocking cells in the G2/M phase in HL-60 human leukemia cell line [73]. Dolabrane-type diterpenetagalsins caused S-G2 phase arrest by downregulating Cdc25A and Cdc25B and activating ATM/ATR-Chk1/Chk2kinases rapidly [74]. An abietane diterpenoid, Abietic acid (AA), promoted G0/G1 phase arrest *via* negatively modulating the cyclin D1 and cdk4 expression in PC-9 and H1975 cell lines [75]. A highly oxygenated tetracyclic triterpene, limonoid derivative from the Brazilian native Meliaceae plant catuaba is Cedrelone, which inhibits U87 glioma cell proliferation by arresting cells in G2/M phase [33]. According to Chao Gao *et al.* a triterpenoid Oleanolic acid (OA) regresses cell cycle of HepG2 liver cancer cells by halting G2/M phase [76]. Mechanistically, OA persuaded G2/M phase arrest *via* suppressing cdc2/cyclin B1 complex (MPF) and activating p21 in hepatocellular carcinoma [77]. The Cucurbitaceae family plants contain tetracyclic triterpenes called Cucurbitacins. The impact of Cucurbitacins on cell cycle arrest varies from one cancer cell type to other type. In non-small cell lung cancer (NSCLC), OS cells, melanoma cells, neuroblastoma, breast cancer cells, squamous cell carcinoma of cutaneous cell, glioblastomamultiforme, squamous cell carcinoma of larynx and pancreatic cancer cell lines, cucurbitacin B showed G2/M phase arrest. Cucurbitacin I repressed CDK1, cyclin B1, cyclin A, and CDC25C protein expression in SW480 carcinoma cells of colon. While Cucurbitacin D in endometrial and ovarian carcinoma cells upregulated p21Waf and p27Kipl proteins and downregulated cyclin A and B. Cucurbitacin E promoted G2/M phase *via* increasing the quantity of p27, p21, and p53 and blocking STAT3, CDK1, and cyclin B in T24 human bladder cancer, pancreatic carcinoma cells, ovarian cancer cell, and breast cancer cells. Cucurbitacin E also inhibited the formation of CDC2/cyclin B1 complex and increased GADD45 expression in malignant gliomas of human brain and colorectal cancers [78]. In HeLa cervical cancer cell, a triterpenoid glycoside glycyrrhizin isolated from licorice caused cell cycle arrest at the phase of G0/G1 [79]. Some other pentacyclic triterpenoids named Betulinic acid (BA) and Betulin (BT) had great impact on cell cycle in CLBL-1, CL-1 and D-17 canine cancer cell lines. They regulated the cell cycle by doing G0/G1 phase arrest in CLBL-1 cells. While their effect on CL-1 and D-17 cells are S phase arrest [80]. Another pentacyclic triterpenoid, Pomolic acid (PA), obtained from *Euscaphis japonica* inhibited the cell growth in human malignant melanoma SK-MEL-2 cells by arresting them in sub-G1 phase [81]. While, tetraterpenoid methyl sartortuoate, caused G2/M cell cycle arrest *via* downregulating cdc2 and upregulating p21, cdc2 inhibitor, and p53 expression in colon cancer cells [36].

TERPENOIDS TARGETING CELL SIGNALING PATHWAYS

Terpenoid has been found to display anticancer properties by regulating various phases of cancer development and progression, for example, suppression of cancer proliferation by promoting cell cycle arrest, apoptosis, and inhibition of cancer progression by affecting invasion, migration, and angiogenesis *via* targeting various cellular signaling pathways, such as PI3K/AKT, Ras/MAPK, Wnt/β-catenin, JAK/STAT3, NF-κB, and Notch-1 (Fig. **8**).

EGFR signaling Pathway

EGFR signaling pathway regulates cell proliferation, cell survival, differentiation, migration, and adhesion by activating either PI3K/Akt/mTOR or Ras/Raf/Mek/Erk pathway [82].

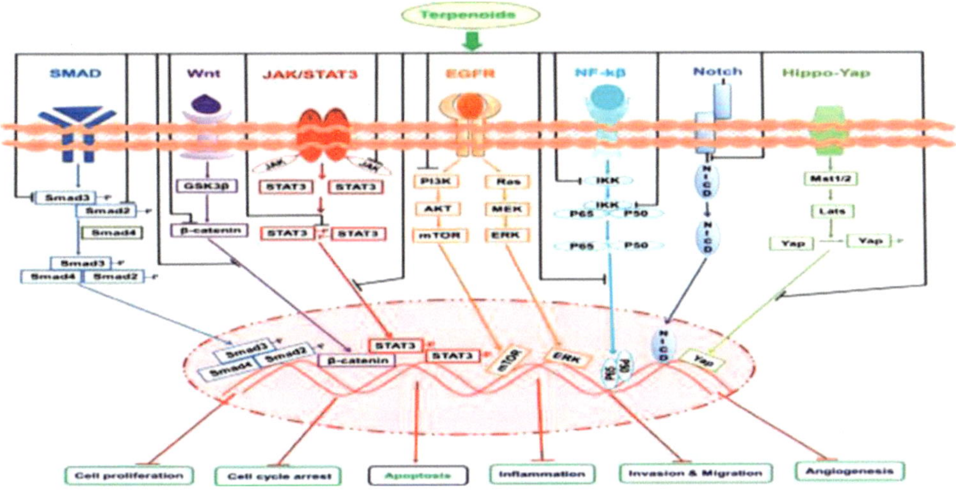

Fig. (8). Schematic representation of terpenoids targeted various cell signaling pathways in cancer prevention.

PI3K/AKT and RAS/RAF/MEK/ERK signaling Pathway

Numerous terpenoids exhibit anticancer effects against various kinds of human cancer by regulating PI3K/AKT signaling pathway. Triterpenoid UA showed anticancer potential against breast cancer by inducing apoptosis and autophagy through inhibition of PI3K/AKT pathway, leading to an upregulation of its downstream protein GSK-3β, which in turn downregulated cyclin D1 [83]. Another similar study had shown that treatment of breast cancer with UA resulted in energy stress, autophagy, and apoptosis by regulating AKT-induced glycolysis pathway that regulated phosphorylation levels of AMPK and ERK1/2 [53]. Interestingly, administration of UA in hepatocellular carcinoma inhibited p-AKT, p-MEK, and p-ERK1/2 levels, thereby enhancing cell cycle arrest and apoptotic cell death [84]. A terpenoid, Wentilactone B (WB), activated Ras signaling by binding of WB drug to Ras. It upregulated the phosphorylation levels of ERK and JNK, resulting in activation of Ras/Raf/ERK and Ras/Raf/JNK pathways [85]. Another study had shown that treatment with Oridonin remarkably suppressed PI3K and p-Akt levels and its downstream component, murine double minute 2 in prostate cancer [86]. A terpenoid, Alantolactone (ALT) displayed anticancer potential against gastric cancer cell line, BGC-823, by inducing apoptosis *via* suppression of AKT pathway in ROS-dependent manner [87]. An exciting study has investigated by Zhou *et al.* and they found that a new monoterpenoid compound, Tomentodione-M re-sensitized multidrug-resistant cancer cells by reducing P-glycoprotein levels through inactivation of the p38 MAPK pathway [88]. The anti-proliferative role of β-carotene was investigated by Zhu *et al.* in esophageal squamous cell carcinoma (ESCC) cells and found that β-carotene inhibited AKT/NF-κB pathway by reducing the phosphorylation levels of AKT and NF-κB [89]. Triterpenoids from *Liquidambaris* Fructus were associated with the PI3K/AKT pathway, inhibiting cell proliferation in hepatocellular carcinoma [90]. Treatment of ovarian cancer cells with Davanone inactivated the PI3K/AKT/MAPK pathway by downregulating the levels of p-PI3K, p-AKT, and upregulating p-MAPK level [91]. A defensive terpenoid, Cantharidin, reduced AKT and NF-κB levels. It downregulated other downstream molecules of the pathway, such as MMP-2 and MMP-9, and UPA resulted in inhibition of MAPK (p38, ERK, and JNK) signaling pathway in lung cancer [92]. ART had been found to inhibit cell growth in renal cell carcinoma *via* inhibiting the Akt pathway [93]. Some studies have shown that triptonide exhibits anticancer effects in pancreatic cancer by activating the MEKK4-MKK4-p38 MAPK pathway and prostate cancer by blocking the mTOR pathway [94, 95]. Interestingly, TPL overcomes cisplatin resistance in ovarian cancer cells through inhibition of Akt [96]. Jolkinolide B, a diterpenoid lactone, induced the detachment of breast cancer cells to fibronectin by modulating integrin/focal adhesion kinase (FAK) and ERK signaling pathways [97]. It also induced apoptosis by inhibiting PI3K/Akt/mTOR signaling pathway [98]. A triterpenoid compound, nimbolide activated the MAPK pathway to mediate its cytotoxic effect on HCC [99]. In addition, nimbolide also induced autophagy-mediated apoptotic cell death in breast cancer by upregulating caspases, Beclin 1 and LC3B, as well as downregulating Bcl-2, p62, and mTOR levels that occurred due to HDAC-2 inhibition [51]. Likewise, in SCC131 and SCC4 oral cancer cells, nimbolide exhibits a cytoprotective effect of autophagy by downregulating the levels of LC-3 II, Beclin-1, and autophagy-related 5 (ATG5) and upregulating Bax, cytosolic cytochrome c, and cleaved caspase-3. Treatment with nimbolide inhibited PI3K/Akt/GSK3 signaling increase the expression of miR-126 leading to activation of GSK-3β to contribute to inactivation of PI3K/Akt/GSK3 signaling by nimbolide [100]. Also, nimbolide reduced the colon cancer cell proliferation and invasion by inactivating the NF-κB pathway [101]. In HepG2 liver cancer cells, physalin A activated Nrf2 and its targeted genes by regulating ERK and p38 kinase [102]. Elemene showed a synergistic effect with an ERK 1/2 signaling pathway inhibitor PD98059 by inhibiting BGC-823 gastric cancer cell proliferation and inducing apoptosis through upregulation of p-ERK 1/2 and Bax levels, along with downregulation of Bcl-2 level [103].

Moreover, a tetraterpenoid, Gedunin, showed anticancer effect against ovarian cancer cells through arresting cell cycle at G2/M phase and ROS-induced apoptosis, mediated by MAPK and JAK/STAT3 pathways [104]. In addition, gedunin exhibited an anti-angiogenesis effect on hamster buccal pouch carcinomas by reducing the levels of miR-21, Vascular endothelial growth factor

(VEGF), and HIF-1α through inhibition of PI3K/Akt and NF-κB signaling pathways [105]. Kim *et al.* investigated the inhibitory effect of obacunone on MCF-7 cells of breast cancer by inhibiting the expression of NF-κB and cyclooxygenase-2 (COX-2) through activation of the MAPK pathway [106]. The inhibitory effect of bruceine D is exerted by inducing autophagy and apoptosis in lung cancer through activation of ROS-induced MAPK pathway [107], while the apoptotic effect of bruceine D in pancreatic cancer is mediated due to excess ROS generation and inhibition of PI3K/Akt pathway [108]. Meanwhile, Ailanthone exerts its cytotoxic activity on human leukemia cell line HL-60 by inhibiting cell proliferation, migration, and invasion through inhibition of Notch and PI3K/Akt signaling pathways and overexpression of miR-449a [109], while ailanthone exerts an inhibitory effect on liver cancer cells, Huh7 by inducing cell cycle arrest and regulating PI3K/Akt pathway [110]. Studies have also been found that limonin (LMN) reduced cell proliferation in HCC due to reduction of Akt activity resulted in suppression of phosphorylation levels of HK-2 [111]. At the same time, LMN attenuated the stemness of HCC cells by activating the PI3K/Akt pathway [112].

WNT/β-catenin Pathway

The anticancer effect of various terpenoids has been studied in several cancers by regulating the Wnt/β-catenin pathway. Zhu *et al.* have shown that parthenolide, a sesquiterpenoid downregulated the protein levels of TCF4/LEF1 by binding parthenolide to a ribosomal protein RPL10 [113]. Consequently, parthenolide also inhibited the Wnt/β-catenin pathway. Another *in vitro* study revealed that α-santalol could regulate Wnt//β-catenin signaling by blocking the localization of β-catenin from the cytosol to nucleus, thereby inhibiting migration rate of breast cancer cells [114]. Contrast to the previous study, another study suggested that treatment of cancer cells with terpenoid triptonide induced apoptosis by attenuating Wnt/β-catenin signaling *via* targeting the C-terminal transactivation domain of β-catenin and its nuclear co-factor involved with β-catenin [115]. β-elemene exhibited its anticancer potential in cervical cancer cells by attenuating the Wnt/β-catenin signaling pathway through downregulation of β-catenin levels and its downstream target proteins such as Cyclin D1, c-Myc, Bax, and MMP-2 [116]. A study investigated that limonin terpenoid inactivated the Wnt/β-catenin pathway by a unique mechanism. Mechanistically, limonin suppressed the methylation level of MIR216A that upregulated the expression of miR-216a-3p, which inhibited WNT3A by binding directly to it and inactivated the Wnt/β-catenin pathway [117].

STAT3 signaling Pathway

The inhibitory action of terpenoid on JAK/STAT signaling pathway has been confirmed in the study conducted by Li *et al.* Study suggested that parthenolide induced apoptosis and enhanced sensitivity in human gastric carcinoma cells toward DDP *via* suppression of STAT3 and its downstream molecules, including cyclin D1, p21, Bcl-2, and Bcl-XL [118]. Two other diterpenoids named Jolkinolide A (JA) and Jolkinolide B (JB) extracted from *Euphorbia fischeriana* roots exhibited antitumor activity by reducing VEGF expression *via* inhibition of Akt/STAT3/mTOR signaling pathway in lung cancer cells [119]. Another study has shown that treatment of cancer with 17-Hydroxy-jolkinolide B (HJB) purified from *Euphorbia fischeriana* inhibited the activation of STAT3 by inactivating JAK1, JAK2, and TYK2 [120]. Shan *et al.* have discovered 3-deoxy-2β, 16-dihydroxynagilactone E (B6) from *Podocarpus nagi* as a natural potent STAT3 inhibitor. Mechanistically, they have found that B6 reduced STAT3 phosphorylation by directly interacting with the regulatory domain of JAK2 and inhibited breast cancer cell proliferation, and induced apoptosis [121]. Emodin enhanced apoptosis by showing a synergistic effect with EGFR inhibitor (afatinib) on pancreatic cancer by inhibiting the phosphorylation of STAT3 [122]. Cucurbitacin B (CuB) potentiates the antiproliferative effect of gemcitabine in pancreatic cancer by inhibiting JAK2/STAT3 [123]. Besides, CuB inhibited neuroblastoma cell proliferation by regulating the expression of Cyclin B1, CDK1, Bcl-2, Bcl2-XL, p53, and p21 and induced apoptosis by downregulating p-JAK2, p-STAT3, p-ERK and activating JNK and p38 MAPK [124]. The cytotoxic effect of brusatol exerted by blocking the STAT3 pathway through inhibition of JAK1, JAK2, and Src, and also downregulated the nuclear STAT3 levels in head and neck squamous cell carcinoma [125]. Brusatol induced apoptotic cell death in pancreatic cancer by JNK/p38MAPK/NF-κB/Stat3/Bcl-2 signaling pathway [126]. Another terpenoid compound, Jolkinolide B inhibited leukemia cell growth *via* inhibition of the JAK2/STAT3 pathway [127]. Wang *et al.* investigated the anticancer effect of bruceine D in osteosarcoma stem cells by inhibiting STAT3 [128].

NF-κB signaling Pathway

Numerous terpenoids have been found as natural NF-κB inhibitors by inhibiting the NF-κB pathway. For instance, UA inhibited breast cancer cell proliferation and its progression by regulating PI3K/AKT and NF-κB signaling pathways [83]. A well-known sesquiterpene ART also caused inhibition of NF-κB [96]. Zhang's Research group mechanistically investigated the antiproliferative effect of AG on colon cancer was mediated through suppression of the TLR4/NF-κB/MMP-9 signaling pathway [129]. Nimbolide regulates NF-κB and MAPK signaling in prostate cancer cells [130]. Furthermore, treatment of lung adenocarcinoma with TPL re-sensitized to taxol by inhibiting NF-κB signaling and its downstream gene products such as Bcl-2, Bcl-xL, COX-2, FLICE-like inhibitory protein, and X-linked inhibitor of apoptosis protein [131]. Also, TPL enhanced sensitivity to gemcitabine in pancreatic cancer by attenuating the components of the TLR4/NF-κB pathway [132]. Dawood *et al.* mechanistically demonstrated that parthenolide showed hypersensitivity in breast cancer by directly binding to IkB kinase (IKK) results in inhibition of I-kappa-B-alpha (IκBα) degradation and also downregulated the hypoxia inducing factor 1-alpha (HIF-1α) [133]. Mechanistically, BA promoted the apoptotic cell death in prostate cancer by inhibiting IKK and IkBα phosphorylation that inhibited the nuclear translocation of NF-kB/p65 resulted in cytoplasmic accumulation [134].

NOTCH Signaling

To study the anticancer effect of related to, Xiang *et al.* study revealed the regulatory effect of terpenoid triptonide on Notch signaling in gastric cancer. They found that triptonide remarkably inhibited Notch1 protein level mediated by the ubiquitin-proteasome pathway. Consequently, downstream pathways proteins of Notch signaling RBPJ, IKKα, IKKβ, and phosphorylation of NF-κB were reduced [135]. Besides, another *in vitro* study has shown that treatment of breast cancer with BA-based terpenoid, 3-O-(E)-p-Coumaroylbetulinic acid (CB) inhibited the gamma-secretase, resulting in inhibition of cleavage of notch intracellular domain (NICD). Inhibition of NICD cleavage suppresses the expression of notch target genes, such as Hey1, Hes1, pro-caspase-3, CyclinD1, and E-cadherin. This resulted in inhibition of migration, cell cycle progression, and induction of apoptosis in the breast cancer cell and also suppression of stemness in breast cancer cell-derived mammosphere [136].

SMAD Signaling Pathway

The inhibitory action of terpenoid Oridonin on the Smad signaling pathway has been confirmed in a study conducted by Bu *et al.* In brief, it was observed that oridonin suppressed the expression of Smad2, Smad3, Smad4, PAI-1, and phosphorylation of smad2, smad3 in colon cancer. Also, oridonin downregulated the expression of Smad2, Smad3, Smad4, PAI-1, and p-Smad2, p-Smad3 in tumor-bearing nude mice model, thereby reduced tumor growth [137].

YAP Signaling

Li *et al.* reported that ART administration in hepatocellular carcinoma inhibited tumor growth, cell proliferation, invasion, and migration by downregulating Hippo-YAP signaling [138]. Another study has found that Limonin terpenoid inhibited stemness in cervical cancer cells, and invasion and migration in oral squamous cell carcinoma by mediating YAP trans-localization from nucleus to cytoplasm resulted in less transcriptional regulatory activity of YAP [139, 140].

TERPENOIDS: ANTI-ANGIOGENIC EFFECTS

Angiogenesis is an important process in the biotic system. In this process, new vascular system is formed from the existing vascular system *via* splitting and sprouting. Angiogenesis not only regulates different physiological activities like embryonic development, female reproductive cycle, wound healing but also in the formation of malignant tumor from benign state. After reaching the size of 2-3 mm tumor needs nutrient and oxygen supply from new formed blood vessels. Growth factors, such as VEGF, FGF, NRP1, and proteins, such as MMP, angiopoietins, integrins, prostaglandins are involved in angiogenesis process. VEGF stimulates the permeability of the vessel by interacting with VEGFR *via* promoting various signaling cascades. FGF helps in the differentiation and proliferation of endothelial cells. Survival signals are integrated by NRP1. For the genesis of matured blood vessels, angiopoietins are needed. MMP helps in the degradation of extracellular matrix proteins [141]. As angiogenesis has greater importance in cancer progression so it can be targeted for therapeutic treatment. In the therapeutic treatment, used drugs are expensive and become resistant for cancer cell after repeated use and they have limited resources. So to overcome this problem some natural compounds, including terpenoids, can be used for therapeutic treatment. Different types of terpenoids are there, which affect cancer cells by various processes. Studies suggested that various types of terpenoids can aim angiogenesis during tumorigenesis. Here, we are going to discuss recent studies that are focused on the action of terpenoids against angiogenesis during tumorigenesis. A monoterpenoid, Catalpol, suppressed angiogenesis by lowering the expression of factors promoting angiogenesis, such as VEGFR2, bFGF, and VEGF and upregulating the anti-angiogenic factors, such as angiostatin, canstatin and endostatin expression. Catalpol treatment suppressed HIF-1α nuclear translocation, which leads to downregulation of downstream HIF-1α angiogenic proteins in CT26 colon cancer cell line [22]. ART inhibits cancer spreading in different cancer cells through various mechanisms, including angiogenesis by regulating MMP2/7/9, avb3, integrins, urokinase plasminogen activator (u-PA), and VEGF expressions [142]. However, DHA showed an anti-angiogenic effect by suppressing VEGFR2 *via* blocking p65 translocation to the nucleus and elevating IkB-α protein in endothelial cells [143]. ART also impedes angiogenesis by regulating MAPK, PI3K/Akt/mTOR, and NF-κB signaling pathways. While in endothelial cells, DHA hinders proliferation by lowering ERK1/2 activation and expression. In addition, both ART and DHA regulate JNK and MAPK activation. ART inhibits angiogenesis by downregulating pro-angiogenic cytokine production and VEGFR2 expression [144]. Costunolide (CE) and dehydrocostuslactone (DE) are sesquiterpene lactones obtained from *Saussurealappa* and *Laurusnobilis* plants. According to Hao *et al.* CE and DE could suppress VEGF expression at non-harmful dose in human lung cancer A549 cells. By plugging VEGFR, KDR/Flk-1 signaling pathways, CE reduces angiogenesis at both *in vitro* and *in vivo* levels. In humans, an umbilical vein endothelial cell DE apprehends the origination of capillary-like tube *in vitro*. DE also affects angiogenesis in nude mice-based matrigel-plug [145]. Whereas AG and its derivative AGS-30 have potent anti-angiogenic activity in different cancer cell lines. Anti-angiogenic activity of AG was exhibited by inactivating pro-angiogenic factors, like VEGF and nitric oxide and increasing the expression anti-angiogenesis factors, including IL-2 and metallopeptidase inhibitor-1 of TIMP. However AG derivative AGS-30 inhibited the VEGF induced phosphorylation of Akt, mTOR, MEK1/2, ERK1/2, p38, and MAPK in endothelial cells of colon cancer. VEGF level in colon cancer cell HT-29 was sufficiently reduced by AGS-30. It was found that in the tumor microenvironment, AGS-30 impedes the formation of blood vessel, VEGF, and p-VEGF-2 levels [141]. Despite a potent anti-angiogenic property in AG, it has limitations like poor solubility in an aqueous solution and poor oral bioavailability. Therefore, the use of well-organized derivatives of AG can overcome the solubility-related issue. A 14-phenoxy andrographolide acetal derivative AGP-40 showed potent anti-angiogenic action in both *in vitro* and *in vivo* studies. The compound induced anti-angiogenesis in human umbilical vein endothelial cells (HUVECs) cells by regulating Erk/MEK and Akt/PI3K signaling pathways and suppressing the phosphorylation of Akt, PI3K, MEK, and Erk1/2 [146]. Kaurane diterpenoids named CHKA (3α-cinnamoyloxy-9ß-hydroxy-ent-kaura-16-en-19-oic acid) purified from *Wedelia chinensis* plant exhibited sufficient anti-angiogenic effect in Zebra fish embryo. Mechanistically, the compound CHKA inhibited Ang1/2, VEGF165, Kdr, and Tie1/2 in Zebrafish embryos. In the *ex vivo* study, CHKA apprehended sprouts formation, while *in vivo* study, it suppressed blood vessel formation. CHKA impeded VEGFR-2 phosphorylation at Tyr1175 induced by VEGF. The compound also apprehended phosphorylation of mTOR, ERK, and AKT. In addition, CHKA also restricts the activation of VEGFR-2 pathways HUVECs cells [147]. A complicated polyoxygenated diterpene, Taxol, from the bark of *Taxus brevifolia* showed an anti-angiogenic effect in malignant tumors by reducing VEGF formation and HIF1α expression [148]. Many types of terpenoids are found in *Euphorbia neriifolia* and showed anti-angiogenesis property. Out of which, two diterpenoids, Eurifoloid Q and 23(E)-eupha-8, 23–diene-3β, 25-diol-7-one were shown anti-angiogenesis by downregulating VEGFR/Akt signaling pathways [149]. A diterpenoid, Triptolide (TPL) isolated from *Tripterygium wilfordii* exhibited anticancer activity against oral cancer. In PANC-1 cells, TPL induced downregulation of VEGF expression in both *in vivo* and *in vitro* [150]. TPL also showed anti-angiogenic action by inhibiting VEGFR2 and Tie2 oriented angiogenic pathways. The compound TPL also showed anti-angiogenic property by apprehending the expression of COX-2 and VEGF in pancreatic carcinoma. *in vitro* study results suggested that TPL could inhibit MMP9 gene by its hypermethylation in human fibrosarcoma cell line HT-1080. In addition, TPL reduced the transcription rate of tie2 and angpt2 in an angiogenic zebrafish model. NF-κB pathway regulates VEGF level endogenously, and exposure of TPL showed inhibition of NF-κB transcription by controlling its downstream genes in human cell lines ATC and HUVECs, which was further proved by reduced expression of Upa, VEGF, and cyclin D1 [151]. Cafestol, a diterpenoids product of coffee beans, could inhibit angiogenesis by modulating the phosphorylation of FAK, Akt, and formation of NO. According to Moeenfard *et al.* Cafestolpalmitate (CP) and Kahweolpalmitate (KP) showed anti-angiogenic property by lowering VEGFR-2 and Akt expression in HMVECs. Both *in vivo* and *in vitro* anti-angiogenic action of KP was observed by Cardenas and colleagues. According to their findings, chick embryo chorioallantoic membrane (CAM) assay showed angiogenesis inhibition in all KP treated eggs at 50 mM and in transgenic zebrafish larvae at 25 μM treatment of KP. *In vitro*, mouse arotic ring assay showed inhibition of sprouting of an endothelial cell at the treatment of 5 μM only. The overall study suggested that KP exerts more potent anti-angiogenic activity than CP [152]. A tetracyclic triterpenoid, Ginsenoside Rg3, showed the promising anti-angiogenesis property. MVD (micro-vessel density), a marker for vascularization, was reduced in Ginsenoside Rg3 treated colorectal cancer cells. Ginsenoside Rg3 treatment negatively regulated the transcriptional expression of 22 pro-angiogenic genes ANGPT1/2, CCL13, CSF3, COL18A, CXCL1, EGF, FGF-2, Interleukin1A,1B, and 8, KDR, MMP1, PIGF, PGF, PLAUR,THPO, TEK, and TIMP1/2 [153]. While Ginsenoside Rg3 and ginsenoside Rb2 (tetracyclic triterpenoid ginsenosides isolated from *Panax ginseng*) reduced neo-vessel formation in B16 murine melanomas [148]. Despite promising anticancer potential in UA, it's less solubility in water limited its use as an anticancer agent in some extent. Therefore, to extend its effectiveness it is encapsulated in chitosan nanoparticles CH-UA-NPs. Interestingly, *in vitro* treatment of CH-UA-NPs in HUVECs cells hampered bFGF induced tube formation. According to Cárdenas *et al.* CH-UA-NPs sufficiently apprehends angiogenesis in CAM model [154]. Ganoderic acid F, a lanostane triterpene, showed anti-angiogenic effect in HUVECs through reduction of proliferation of endothelial cell and blockage of capillary tube induction [155]. Celastrol, a pentacyclic triterpenoid isolated compound from *Tripterygium wilfordii* showed inhibition of transcription of growth factors and receptors gene associated with angiogenesis. Transcriptional activation of CDH5, THBS2, LEP, MMP-9 and TNF gene was also found to be decreased after treatment with celastrol in colorectal cancer cells. However, celastrol treatment also decreased the expression of IL-1β, Serpin E1, PDGF, and TIMP-4 proteins [34]. Triterpenoid PA hindered the expression of EGFR regulated mTOR and p38-MAPK signaling pathways. PA also suppressed the EGF-enhanced VEGF/HIF1α expression in human mammary cancer cells, resulting in angiogenesis inhibition [156].

TERPENOIDS INHIBIT CANCER CELL MIGRATION, INVASION, AND METASTASIS

Metastasis is an important process in cancers, which helps in the spread of cancer cells from their origin tissue to other tissues and organs. Metastasis includes various steps such as loosening of epithelial cells from the primary tumor, invasion of tumor cells into the circulatory system, migration of cells to the neighboring tissue and then in the neighboring tissue, these cells spread away and form a colony. The beginning of metastasis needs invasion, which is done by the epithelial to mesenchymal transition (EMT) process. In this process, several proteins and signaling pathways play key roles [157]. The proteins involved in EMT are E-cadherin, N-cadherin, MMPs, snail, slug, and vimentin, while signaling pathways involved in EMT are PI3K/AKT, Hedgehog, NF-κB, Ras/MAPK, Notch, and Wnt/β-catenin, and TGF-β signaling pathways. E-cadherin is a protein of adherence junction formed between two epithelial cells. N-cadherin is a transmembrane protein highly expressed in mesenchymal cells. MMPs are matrix metalloproteases, which could degrade extracellular matrix and stroma to make a path for cancer cell migration. Snail and slug are the marker protein of mesenchymal cells, which could repress E-cadherin transcription *via* binding with E-cadherin promoter. In mesenchymal cells, a type-III intermediate filament is also expressed, named vimentin, which helps in the maintenance of organelles position [158]. As metastasis, invasion, and migration play a key role in cancer cell progression, so these processes can be targeted for therapeutic treatments, including chemotherapy. After several time periods, this chemotherapy becomes resistant to cancer cells *via* performing various processes, and chemotherapy has high cost and limited source. So to short out this problem, several researches are performed. There are different types of terpenoids, which exerted their effects against cell invasion, migration, and metastasis by targeting various dysregulated mechanisms. A monoterpenoid, Limonene, showed anticancer activity *via* inhibiting cell invasion and migration in human bladder cancer cell line T24 [56]. Carvacrol, a phenolic-based monoterpenoid, showed anti-invasive and anti-migratory effects on prostate cancer cells (DU145 and PC-3) through inhibiting fibrous-actin dynamics and protein MMP-2 expression and stopping the TRPM7 [159]. While sesquiterpene lactone, Lactucopicrin, showed potent anti-invasive and anti-migratory effects against Saos-2 cells *via* reducing the expression of MMP-9, MMP-3, and MMP-2 [160]. Helenalin, a sesquiterpene lactone, suppressed the phosphorylation of pAKT, pmTOR, and pPI3K, thus deactivating the PI3K/ AKT/mTOR signaling pathway. By deactivating this pathway, Helenalin blocks migration and invasion of HL-60 cells [161]. While, Farnesol, an acyclic hydrophobic sesquiterpene, showed anti-migratory and anti-invasive effects on HBL-52 carcinoma cells. The compound inhibited invasion and migration of cell through apprehending the expression of MMP-9 and MMP-2 in optic nerve sheath meningioma cell line HBL-52 [162]. ART derivative DHA showed anticancer activity in ovarian epithelial cancer cells. DHA suppressed cell invasion and migration by blocking the hedgehog pathway by downregulating the expression of Smo and GLI1 [163]. ART/Qinghaous also inhibited invasion and migration of cells in hepatocellular carcinoma *via* upregulating E-cadherin and downregulating snail, MMP-9, and N-cadherin. In addition, ART also regulated the phosphorylation of YAP Ser127 and retention of cytoplasm [138]. However, no potent effect on MMP-2 was found. A labdane diterpenoid, Coronarin D (CD), a purified product of *Hedychium coronarium* rhizomes showed promising anticancer activity. CD persuaded the migration and invasion of U251 cells. Mechanistically, CD blocked the activation of JNK/STAT3 signaling pathway in U251 glioma cells [164]. Marrubenol, a diterpenoid, derived from Marrubium genus plants was found to be effective at its IC50 dose by significantly suppressing migration in Saos-2 cells [165]. Also, diterpenoid TPL could block invasion and migration in both SAS and macrophage-like U937 cells. It was found that SAS cells showed higher E-cadherin levels after TPL treatment, while vimentin and snail levels were lowered, which indicated that TPL could inhibit EMT. In fibrosarcoma cell line HT-1080, TPL showed anti-invasive property by suppressing MMP-9 activity and expression [150]. According to Jao *et al.*, TPL apprehended the expression of MMP-9, MMP-2, and FAK protein and phosphorylation of Akt and ERK. In B16F10 murine melanoma cells, TPL showed anti-migratory and anti-invasive activity *via* blockage of MMP-9 and MMP-2 expression. TPL also showed this activity by apprehending FAK, AKT, Rho, and SOS1/GRB2 in B16F10 cells [166]. TPL also repressed migration and invasion of squamous cancer cells of esophagus by blocking EMT. TPL reversed EMT *via* controlling MAPK/ERK signaling pathway, upregulation of E-cadherin and downregulation of N-cadherin, snail, and twist in esophageal squamous cell cancer [31]. According to Yuan *et al.* TPL inhibited MMPs, Cav1, and CD147 expression, which led to the suppression of invasion and migration in human prostate cancer cells [167]. Moreover, terpenoid AG also regulates EMT in many cancers. It upregulates the epithelial-related markers and suppresses mesenchymal markers, including snail in osteosarcoma U-2 cells [168]. Eriocalyxin B, an ent-kaurene diterpenoid, showed anticancer activity against colon cancer cells. In SW1116 colon cancer cells, Eriocalyxin B showed anti-migratory and anti-invasive properties by inhibiting MMP-2 and MM-9. The inhibition of MMP-2 and MMP-9 was done by suppressing STAT3 *via* inactivating JAK2 in SW1116 cells [169]. A polyphenolic diterpenoid extracted from *Rosmarinus officinalis* named Carnosic acid showed anti-migratory and anti-invasive activities by the inhibiting MMP-9 in NSCLC cell line A549 [170]. *Pseudolarix kaempferi* plant trunk and root bark produces a diterpenoid called Pseudolaric acid B (PAB). Reduced formation of N-cadherin, snail, slug, fibronectin and vimentin and increased expression of E-cadherin in PAB treated pancreatic cancer cell line SW1990 leads to blockage of cell invasion and migration. PAB also blocked cell migration and invasion *via* promoting Hippo-YAP pathway and suppressing the EMT activation [171]. Triterpenoid OA also has anti-invasive and anti-migratory potential. Studies suggested that OA sufficiently inhibited HepG2 cells invasion and migration by inhibiting the phosphorylation of p38 and JNK [76]. Forkhead transcription factor A (FOXA1) protein is highly expressed and regulates proliferation, survival, migration, and invasion of cancer cells. According to Duan *et al.* OA induced anticancer activity by downregulation of FOXA1 and induced phosphorylation of Akt in thyroid cancer cells. Moreover, reduction of FOXA1 expression promoted the upregulation of E-cadherin and downregulation of vimentin, resulting seized migration and invasion of thyroid cancer cells [172]. Glycyrrhizic acid (GA), a triterpene glycoside, natural compound isolated from licorice has anticancer activity. In Leukemia TF-1 cells, GA suppressed TF-1 cells invasion and migration *via* inhibiting the mTOR/STAT3/AKT signaling pathway [173]. From Ginseng, a tetracyclic triterpenoid has been isolated called Ginsenoside Rg3. Ginsenoside Rg3 showed anti-migratory and anti-invasive property in colon cancer cell line Caco-2 *via* suppressing vimentin and MMP-9. CCAT1 induced growth, invasion, and migration of Caco-2 cells. Interestingly, Ginsenoside Rg3 repressed the CCAT1 and overcome migration and invasion of Caco-2 cells [174]. According to Wang *et al.* Ginsenoside Rg3 showed anti-cancer activity against nasopharyngeal carcinoma cells not only by inhibiting the expression of MMP-9 and MMP-2 but also by blocking the EMT. The blockage of EMT was done through reduced expression of transcription factors of EMT [175]. Nimbolide, a triterpenoid, purified from flowers and leaves of *Azadirachta indica*, showed anti-migratory and anti-invasive activity *via* upregulating E-cadherin and downregulating Snail and MMP-3 in NSCLC [176]. Cucurbitacin I or Elatericin B is a triterpenoid, showed anti-migratory and anti-invasive activity *via* inhibiting the MMP-9 and formation of pSTAT3 in colon cancer cells [177].

TERPENOIDS REGULATING KEY INFLAMMATORY PATHWAYS

Inflammation is known to serve a vital role in cancer development. Several natural compounds have shown anti-inflammatory properties and promise in the control of inflammation in cancer progression. Terpenoids are naturally occurring organic chemicals that have been extensively reported to suppress cancer progression in several cancers by inhibiting inflammatory signaling pathways. There are various types of naturally occurring terpenoids exhibiting anticancer potential by inhibiting inflammatory response through the inhibition of NF-κB signaling pathway [178, 179]. UA inhibited breast cancer progression by suppressing the inflammatory response. It inhibits the NF-κB pathway by downregulating the expression of IKKα, Iκβα, and phosphorylated NF-κB. UA also downregulated the levels of pro-inflammatory cytokines, including IL-1β, IL-18, TNF-α, Il-6, IL-18, and interferon (IFN)-γ expression [83]. Also, Obacunone exerts its anti-inflammatory effect on MCF-7 cells of breast cancer by inhibiting the expression of NF-κB and COX-2 through the activation of the MAPK pathway [106]. In addition to other anticancer activities, AG also acts as a potent inhibitor of the inflammatory pathway by inhibiting the nuclear activation of NF-κB through covalent modification of reduced cysteine 62 of p50 [180, 181]. Furthermore, AG treatment with melanoma *in vitro* and *in vivo* showed a dramatic reduction in pro-inflammatory cytokine levels, such as IL-6, IL-1β, TNF-α, and GM-CSF, and a pro-angiogenic factor VEGF [182]. Another research group also found a dramatic decrease in serum pro-inflammatory cytokines, such as IL-1β, IL-6, TNF-α, GM-CSF and a pro-angiogenic factor VEGF after treatment with vernolide-A in angiogenesis-induced animals [183]. Another terpenoid, Avicin G, also showed inhibition of inflammatory responses in Jurkat cells *via* decreasing the accumulation of NF-κB in the nucleus that in turn downregulated the targeted products of NF-κB, such as inducible iNOS and COX-2 [184]. Several triterpenoids, such as asiatic acid, betulinic acid, boswellic acid, celastrol, and lupeol exerted anti-inflammatory effects, resulting in the inhibition of cancer cell proliferation by targeting many inflammatory enzymes, such as COX-2, 5-LOX, and MMPs [185].

CONCLUSION

In essence, terpenoids are plant-based compounds, which are playing a crucial role in prevention and cure of various diseases including cancer to date. Terpenoids serve as anticancer agents by mechanisms, such as inhibition of cell proliferation and angiogenesis, arrest of cell cycle, apoptosis induction, and suppression of cell migration, invasion and metastasis, and repression of EMT. Most of the terpenoids are pleiotropic in nature and can regulate several deregulated signaling pathways and inflammatory pathways in cancer. Therefore, we may see terpenoids as promising anticancer agents from natural resources. Although very few terpenoids have already been approved and introduced as anticancer drugs, many others are still need to be researched at preclinical and clinical level.

REFERENCES

[1] Egbuna C, Kumar S, Ifemeje JC, Ezzat SM, Kaliyaperumal S. Phytochemicals as Lead Compounds for New Drug Discovery. Elsevier 2019.

[2] Akihisa T, Yasukawa K, Tokuda H. Potentially cancer chemopreventive and anti-inflammatory terpenoids from natural sources. Studies in natural products chemistry 2003; 29: 73-126.

[3] Sun L, Li S, Wang F, Xin F. Research progresses in the synthetic biology of terpenoids. Biotechnol Bull 2017; 33: 64-75.

[4] Yang W, Chen X, Li Y, Guo S, Wang Z, Yu X. Advances in pharmacological activities of terpenoids. \ Natural Product Communications 2020; 15(3): 1934578X20903555.

[5] Kuttan G, Pratheeshkumar P, Manu KA, Kuttan R. Inhibition of tumor progression by naturally occurring terpenoids. Pharm Biol 2011; 49(10): 995-1007.
[http://dx.doi.org/10.3109/13880209.2011.559476] [PMID: 21936626]

[6] Shehzad A, Ul Islam S, Al-Suhaimi EA, Lee Y. Pleiotropic Effects of Bioactive Phytochemicals (Polyphenols and Terpenes). Functional Foods, Nutraceuticals and Natural Products. Lancaster, PA, USA: DEStech Publications, Inc. 2020.

[7] Polo MP, de Bravo MG. Effect of geraniol on fatty-acid and mevalonate metabolism in the human hepatoma cell line Hep G2. Biochem Cell Biol 2006; 84(1): 102-11.
[http://dx.doi.org/10.1139/o05-160] [PMID: 16462894]

[8] Ji L, Liu T, Liu J, Chen Y, Wang Z. Andrographolide inhibits human hepatoma-derived Hep3B cell growth through the activation of c-Jun N-terminal kinase. Planta Med 2007; 73(13): 1397-401.
[http://dx.doi.org/10.1055/s-2007-990230] [PMID: 17918040]

[9] Song Y, Xin X, Zhai X, Xia Z, Shen K. Sequential combination of flavopiridol with Taxol synergistically suppresses human ovarian carcinoma growth. Arch Gynecol Obstet 2015; 291(1): 143-50.
[http://dx.doi.org/10.1007/s00404-014-3408-0] [PMID: 25118834]

[10] Bajpai VK, Sonwal S, Hwang SK, *et al.* Sugiol, a diterpenoid: Therapeutic actions and molecular pathways involved. Pharmacol Res 2021; 163: 105313.
[http://dx.doi.org/10.1016/j.phrs.2020.105313] [PMID: 33246173]

[11] Lee YS, Jin DQ, Kwon EJ, *et al.* Asiatic acid, a triterpene, induces apoptosis through intracellular Ca2+ release and enhanced expression of p53 in HepG2 human hepatoma cells. Cancer Lett 2002; 186(1): 83-91.
[http://dx.doi.org/10.1016/S0304-3835(02)00260-4] [PMID: 12183079]

[12] Eichenmüller M, von Schweinitz D, Kappler R. Betulinic acid treatment promotes apoptosis in hepatoblastoma cells. Int J Oncol 2009; 35(4): 873-9.
[PMID: 19724925]

[13] Rabi T, Bishayee A. Terpenoids and breast cancer chemoprevention. Breast Cancer Res Treat 2009; 115(2): 223-39.
[http://dx.doi.org/10.1007/s10549-008-0118-y] [PMID: 18636327]

[14] Ruiz i Altaba A, Sánchez P, Dahmane N. Gli and hedgehog in cancer: tumours, embryos and stem cells. Nat Rev Cancer 2002; 2(5): 361-72.
[http://dx.doi.org/10.1038/nrc796] [PMID: 12044012]

[15] Evangelista M, Tian H, de Sauvage FJ. The hedgehog signaling pathway in cancer. Clin Cancer Res 2006; 12(20): 5924-8.
[http://dx.doi.org/10.1158/1078-0432.CCR-06-1736] [PMID: 17062662]

[16] Vaishampayan U, Hussain M, Banerjee M, *et al.* Lycopene and soy isoflavones in the treatment of prostate cancer. Nutr Cancer 2007; 59(1): 1-7.
[http://dx.doi.org/10.1080/01635580701413934] [PMID: 17927495]

[17] Kucuk O, Sarkar FH, Sakr W, *et al.* Phase II randomized clinical trial of lycopene supplementation before radical prostatectomy. Cancer Epidemiol Biomarkers Prev 2001; 10(8): 861-8. [PMID: 11489752]

[18] Kelkel M, Schumacher M, Dicato M, Diederich M. Antioxidant and anti-proliferative properties of lycopene. Free Radic Res 2011; 45(8): 925-40. [http://dx.doi.org/10.3109/10715762.2011.564168] [PMID: 21615277]

[19] Tripathi SK, Pandey K, Panda M, Spinella MJ, Rengasamy KRR, Biswal BK. The potential of retinoids for combination therapy of lung cancer: Updates and future directions. Pharmacol Res 2019; 147: 104331. [http://dx.doi.org/10.1016/j.phrs.2019.104331] [PMID: 31254665]

[20] Chen W, Hou J, Yin Y, *et al.* α-Bisabolol induces dose- and time-dependent apoptosis in HepG2 cells via a Fas- and mitochondrial-related pathway, involves p53 and NFκB. Biochem Pharmacol 2010; 80(2): 247-54. [http://dx.doi.org/10.1016/j.bcp.2010.03.021] [PMID: 20346922]

[21] Evidente A, Kornienko A, Lefranc F, *et al.* Sesterterpenoids with anticancer activity. Curr Med Chem 2015; 22(30): 3502-22. [http://dx.doi.org/10.2174/0929867322666150821101047] [PMID: 26295461]

[22] Zhu P, Wu Y, Yang A, Fu X, Mao M, Liu Z. Catalpol suppressed proliferation, growth and invasion of CT26 colon cancer by inhibiting inflammation and tumor angiogenesis. Biomed Pharmacother 2017; 95: 68-76. [http://dx.doi.org/10.1016/j.biopha.2017.08.049] [PMID: 28826099]

[23] Khan F, Singh VK, Saeed M, Kausar MA, Ansari IA. Carvacrol induced program cell death and cell cycle arrest in androgen-independent human prostate cancer cells *via* inhibition of notch signaling. Anti-Cancer Agents in Medicinal Chemistry 2019; 19(13): 1588-608.

[24] Ding X, Chen H. Anticancer effects of Carvone in myeloma cells is mediated through the inhibition of p38 MAPK signalling pathway, apoptosis induction and inhibition of cell invasion. J BUON 2018; 23(3): 747-51. [PMID: 30003746]

[25] Nevzorova YA, Grossmann J, Trautwein C. Anti-tumorigenic and anti-angiogenic effects of natural conifer Abies sibirica terpenoids *in vivo* and *in vitro.* Biomed Pharmacother 2017; 89: 386-95. [http://dx.doi.org/10.1016/j.biopha.2017.02.035] [PMID: 28254663]

[26] Ateba SB, Mvondo MA, Ngeu ST, *et al.* Natural terpenoids against female breast cancer: a 5-year recent research. Curr Med Chem 2018; 25(27): 3162-213. [http://dx.doi.org/10.2174/0929867325666180214110932] [PMID: 29446727]

[27] Mondal A, Chatterji U. Artemisinin represses telomerase subunits and induces apoptosis in hpv–39 infected human cervical cancer cells. J Cell Biochem 2015; 116(9): 1968-81. [http://dx.doi.org/10.1002/jcb.25152] [PMID: 25755006]

[28] Dong J, Chen Y, Yang W, Zhang X, Li L. Antitumor and anti-angiogenic effects of artemisinin on breast tumor xenografts in nude mice. Res Vet Sci 2020; 129: 66-9. [http://dx.doi.org/10.1016/j.rvsc.2020.01.005] [PMID: 31945670]

[29] Jiang JH, Pi J, Jin H, Cai JY. Oridonin–induced mitochondria–dependent apoptosis in esophageal cancer cells by inhibiting PI3K/AKT/mTOR and Ras/Raf pathways. J Cell Biochem 2019; 120(3): 3736-46. [http://dx.doi.org/10.1002/jcb.27654] [PMID: 30229997]

[30] Peng Y, Wang Y, Tang N, *et al.* Andrographolide inhibits breast cancer through suppressing COX-2 expression and angiogenesis *via* inactivation of p300 signaling and VEGF pathway. J Exp Clin Cancer Res 2018; 37(1): 248. [http://dx.doi.org/10.1186/s13046-018-0926-9] [PMID: 30314513]

[31] Yanchun M, Yi W, Lu W, *et al.* Triptolide prevents proliferation and migration of Esophageal Squamous Cell Cancer *via* MAPK/ERK signaling pathway. Eur J Pharmacol 2019; 851: 43-51. [http://dx.doi.org/10.1016/j.ejphar.2019.02.030] [PMID: 30779917]

[32] Li X, Song Y, Zhang P, *et al.* Oleanolic acid inhibits cell survival and proliferation of prostate cancer cells *in vitro* and *in vivo* through the PI3K/Akt pathway. Tumour Biol 2016; 37(6): 7599-613. [http://dx.doi.org/10.1007/s13277-015-4655-9] [PMID: 26687646]

[33] Cao Y, Zhang L, Wang Y. Antitumor activity of Cedrelone in temozolomide-resistant human glioma cells is accompanied by mitochondrial mediated apoptosis, inhibition of angiogenesis, cell cycle disruption and modulation of ERK/MAPK signalling pathway. J BUON 2019; 24(3): 1204-9. [PMID: 31424680]

[34] Gao Y, Zhou S, Pang L, *et al.* Celastrol suppresses nitric oxide synthases and the angiogenesis pathway in colorectal cancer. Free Radic Res 2019; 53(3): 324-34. [http://dx.doi.org/10.1080/10715762.2019.1575512] [PMID: 30773944]

[35] Subramani R, Gonzalez E, Arumugam A, *et al.* Nimbolide inhibits pancreatic cancer growth and metastasis through ROS-mediated apoptosis and inhibition of epithelial-to-mesenchymal transition. Sci Rep 2016; 6(1): 19819. [http://dx.doi.org/10.1038/srep19819] [PMID: 26804739]

[36] Lan Q, Li S, Lai W, *et al.* Methyl sartortuoate inhibits colon cancer cell growth by inducing apoptosis and G2/M-phase arrest. Int J Mol Sci 2015; 16(8): 19401-18. [http://dx.doi.org/10.3390/ijms160819401] [PMID: 26287184]

[37] Chen ML, Lin YH, Yang CM, Hu ML. Lycopene inhibits angiogenesis both *in vitro* and *in vivo* by inhibiting MMP-2/uPA system through VEGFR2-mediated PI3K-Akt and ERK/p38 signaling pathways. Mol Nutr Food Res 2012; 56(6): 889-99. [http://dx.doi.org/10.1002/mnfr.201100683] [PMID: 22707264]

[38] Wang HR, Tang JY, Wang YY, *et al.* Manoalide preferentially provides antiproliferation of oral cancer cells by oxidative stress-mediated apoptosis and DNA damage. Cancers (Basel) 2019; 11(9): 1303. [http://dx.doi.org/10.3390/cancers11091303] [PMID: 31487907]

[39] Liou GY, Storz P. Reactive oxygen species in cancer. Free Radic Res 2010; 44(5): 479-96. [http://dx.doi.org/10.3109/10715761003667554] [PMID: 20370557]

[40] Aggarwal V, Tuli H, Varol A, *et al.* Role of reactive oxygen species in cancer progression: molecular mechanisms and recent advancements. Biomolecules 2019; 9(11): 735. [http://dx.doi.org/10.3390/biom9110735] [PMID: 31766246]

[41] Hu J, Zhang Y, Guo P, Tang N, Lu Y, Jin Z. Taraxastane inhibits the proliferation, migration and invasion of human cervical cancer by inducing ROS-mediated necrosis like cell death, cell cycle arrest and modulation of JNK/MAPK signaling pathway. Official journal of the Balkan Union of Oncology 2020; 25(2): 716-22.

[42] Li Y, Wen J, Du C, *et al.* Thymol inhibits bladder cancer cell proliferation *via* inducing cell cycle arrest and apoptosis. Biochem Biophys Res Commun 2017; 491(2): 530-6. [http://dx.doi.org/10.1016/j.bbrc.2017.04.009] [PMID: 28389245]

[43] Kumari S, Badana AK, G MM, G S, Malla R. Reactive oxygen species: a key constituent in cancer survival. Biomark Insights 2018; 13 [http://dx.doi.org/10.1177/1177271918755391] [PMID: 29449774]

[44] Yang H, Villani RM, Wang H, *et al.* The role of cellular reactive oxygen species in cancer chemotherapy. J Exp Clin Cancer Res 2018; 37(1): 1-10. [http://dx.doi.org/10.1186/s13046-017-0664-4] [PMID: 29301578]

[45] Srinivas US, Tan BWQ, Vellayappan BA, Jeyasekharan AD. ROS and the DNA damage response in cancer. Redox Biol 2019; 25: 101084.

[http://dx.doi.org/10.1016/j.redox.2018.101084] [PMID: 30612957]

[46] Czabotar PE, Lessene G, Strasser A, Adams JM. Control of apoptosis by the BCL-2 protein family: implications for physiology and therapy. Nat Rev Mol Cell Biol 2014; 15(1): 49-63. [http://dx.doi.org/10.1038/nrm3722] [PMID: 24355989]

[47] Qi F, Yan Q, Zheng Z, Liu J, Chen Y, Zhang G. Geraniol and geranyl acetate induce potent anticancer effects in colon cancer Colo-205 cells by inducing apoptosis, DNA damage and cell cycle arrest. J BUON 2018; 23(2): 346-52. [PMID: 29745075]

[48] Huang J, Wu L, Tashiro S, Onodera S, Ikejima T. Reactive oxygen species mediate oridonin-induced HepG2 apoptosis through p53, MAPK, and mitochondrial signaling pathways. J Pharmacol Sci 2008; 107(4): 370-9. [http://dx.doi.org/10.1254/jphs.08044FP] [PMID: 18719315]

[49] Denton D, Kumar S. Autophagy-dependent cell death. Cell Death Differ 2019; 26(4): 605-16. [http://dx.doi.org/10.1038/s41418-018-0252-y] [PMID: 30568239]

[50] Gozuacik D, Kimchi A. Autophagy and cell death. Curr Top Dev Biol 2007; 78: 217-45. [http://dx.doi.org/10.1016/S0070-2153(06)78006-1] [PMID: 17338918]

[51] Pooladanda V, Bandi S, Mondi SR, Gottumukkala KM, Godugu C. Nimbolide epigenetically regulates autophagy and apoptosis in breast cancer. Toxicol In Vitro 2018; 51: 114-28. [http://dx.doi.org/10.1016/j.tiv.2018.05.010] [PMID: 29778718]

[52] Kim K, Shin E, Jung J, *et al.* Ursolic acid induces apoptosis in colorectal cancer cells partially *via* upregulation of MicroRNA-4500 and inhibition of JAK2/STAT3 phosphorylation. Int J Mol Sci 2018; 20(1): 114. [http://dx.doi.org/10.3390/ijms20010114] [PMID: 30597956]

[53] Lewinska A, Adamczyk-Grochala J, Kwasniewicz E, Deregowska A, Wnuk M. Ursolic acid-mediated changes in glycolytic pathway promote cytotoxic autophagy and apoptosis in phenotypically different breast cancer cells. Apoptosis 2017; 22(6): 800-15. [http://dx.doi.org/10.1007/s10495-017-1353-7] [PMID: 28213701]

[54] Ashrafizadeh M, Ahmadi Z, Mohammadinejad R, Kaviyani N, Tavakol S. Monoterpenes modulating autophagy: A review study. Basic Clin Pharmacol Toxicol 2020; 126(1): 9-20. [http://dx.doi.org/10.1111/bcpt.13282] [PMID: 31237736]

[55] Kim SH, Bae HC, Park EJ, *et al.* Geraniol inhibits prostate cancer growth by targeting cell cycle and apoptosis pathways. Biochem Biophys Res Commun 2011; 407(1): 129-34. [http://dx.doi.org/10.1016/j.bbrc.2011.02.124] [PMID: 21371438]

[56] Ye Z, Liang Z, Mi Q, Guo Y. Limonene terpenoid obstructs human bladder cancer cell (T24 cell line) growth by inducing cellular apoptosis, caspase activation, G2/M phase cell cycle arrest and stops cancer metastasis. J BUON Off J Balk Union Oncol 2020; 25(1): 280-5. [PMID: 32277643]

[57] Rodenak-Kladniew B, Castro A, Stärkel P, Galle M, Crespo R. 1,8-Cineole promotes G0/G1 cell cycle arrest and oxidative stress-induced senescence in HepG2 cells and sensitizes cells to anti-senescence drugs. Life Sci 2020; 243: 117271. [http://dx.doi.org/10.1016/j.lfs.2020.117271] [PMID: 31926243]

[58] Tarhouni-Jabberi S, Zakraoui O, Ioannou E, *et al.* Mertensene, a halogenated monoterpene, induces G2/M cell cycle arrest and caspase dependent apoptosis of human colon adenocarcinoma HT29 cell line through the modulation of ERK-1/-2, AKT and NF-κB signaling. Mar Drugs 2017; 15(7): 221. [http://dx.doi.org/10.3390/md15070221] [PMID: 28726723]

[59] Rodenak-Kladniew B, Castro A, Stärkel P, De Saeger C, García de Bravo M, Crespo R. Linalool induces cell cycle arrest and apoptosis in HepG2 cells through oxidative stress generation and modulation of Ras/MAPK and Akt/mTOR pathways. Life Sci 2018; 199: 48-59.

[http://dx.doi.org/10.1016/j.lfs.2018.03.006] [PMID: 29510199]

[60] Li Z, Li Q, Wu J, Wang M, Yu J. Artemisinin and its derivatives as a repurposing anticancer agent: what else do we need to do? Molecules 2016; 21(10): 1331.
[http://dx.doi.org/10.3390/molecules21101331] [PMID: 27739410]

[61] Firestone GL, Sundar SN. Anticancer activities of artemisinin and its bioactive derivatives. Expert Rev Mol Med 2009; 11: e32.
[http://dx.doi.org/10.1017/S1462399409001239] [PMID: 19883518]

[62] George VC, Kumar DRN, Kumar RA. Relative *in vitro* potentials of parthenolide to induce apoptosis and cell cycle arrest in skin cancer cells. Curr Drug Discov Technol 2016; 13(1): 34-40.
[http://dx.doi.org/10.2174/1570163813666160224124029] [PMID: 26906908]

[63] Jegannathan SD, Arul S, Dayalan H. Zerumbone, a sesquiterpene, controls proliferation and induces cell cycle arrest in human laryngeal carcinoma cell line Hep-2. Nutr Cancer 2016; 68(5): 865-72.
[http://dx.doi.org/10.1080/01635581.2016.1159701] [PMID: 27045964]

[64] Qin JJ, Jin HZ, Huang Y, *et al.* Selective cytotoxicity, inhibition of cell cycle progression, and induction of apoptosis in human breast cancer cells by sesquiterpenoids from Inula lineariifolia Turcz. Eur J Med Chem 2013; 68: 473-81.
[http://dx.doi.org/10.1016/j.ejmech.2013.07.018] [PMID: 24044895]

[65] Hadavand Mirzaei H, Jassbi AR, Pirhadi S, Firuzi O. Study of the mechanism of action, molecular docking, and dynamics of anticancer terpenoids from *Salvia lachnocalyx*. J Recept Signal Transduct Res 2020; 40(1): 24-33.
[http://dx.doi.org/10.1080/10799893.2019.1710847] [PMID: 31913736]

[66] Hui L-M, Zhao G-D, Zhao J-J. δ-Cadinene inhibits the growth of ovarian cancer cells *via* caspase-dependent apoptosis and cell cycle arrest. Int J Clin Exp Pathol 2015; 8(6): 6046-56.
[PMID: 26261482]

[67] Martino R, Beer MF, Elso O, Donadel O, Sülsen V, Anesini C. Sesquiterpene lactones from Ambrosia spp. are active against a murine lymphoma cell line by inducing apoptosis and cell cycle arrest. Toxicol In Vitro 2015; 29(7): 1529-36.
[http://dx.doi.org/10.1016/j.tiv.2015.06.011] [PMID: 26086122]

[68] Zhang HT, Yang J, Liang GH, *et al.* Andrographolide induces cell cycle arrest and apoptosis of chondrosarcoma by targeting TCF–1/SOX9 axis. J Cell Biochem 2017; 118(12): 4575-86.
[http://dx.doi.org/10.1002/jcb.26122] [PMID: 28485543]

[69] Xu T, Huang L, Liu Z, *et al.* A natural diterpenoid, induces selective antitumor activity in SGC-7901 human gastric carcinoma cells by triggering apoptosis, cell cycle disruption and suppression of cancer cell migration. Official Journal of the Balkan Union of Oncology 2019; 24(2): 686-92.

[70] Bao R, Shu Y, Wu X, *et al.* Oridonin induces apoptosis and cell cycle arrest of gallbladder cancer cells *via* the mitochondrial pathway. BMC Cancer 2014; 14(1): 217.
[http://dx.doi.org/10.1186/1471-2407-14-217] [PMID: 24655726]

[71] Wang H, Zhu L, Feng X, Zhang H, Luo Q, Chen F. Oridonin induces G2/M cell cycle arrest and apoptosis in human oral squamous cell carcinoma. Eur J Pharmacol 2017; 815: 282-9.
[http://dx.doi.org/10.1016/j.ejphar.2017.09.021] [PMID: 28935563]

[72] Cardoso PCS, Rocha CAM, Leal MF, *et al.* Effect of diterpenoid kaurenoic acid on genotoxicity and cell cycle progression in gastric cancer cell lines. Biomed Pharmacother 2017; 89: 772-80.
[http://dx.doi.org/10.1016/j.biopha.2017.02.085] [PMID: 28273639]

[73] Ma G, Chong L, Li XC, Khan IA, Walker LA, Khan SI. Selective inhibition of human leukemia cell growth and induction of cell cycle arrest and apoptosis by pseudolaric acid B. J Cancer Res Clin Oncol 2010; 136(9): 1333-40.
[http://dx.doi.org/10.1007/s00432-010-0784-0] [PMID: 20140742]

[74] Neumann J, Yang Y, Köhler R, *et al.* Mangrove dolabrane–type of diterpenes tagalsins suppresses tumor growth *via*ROS –mediated apoptosis and ATM/ATR–C hk1/Chk2–regulated cell cycle arrest. Int J Cancer 2015; 137(11): 2739-48.
[http://dx.doi.org/10.1002/ijc.29629] [PMID: 26061604]

[75] Liu X, Chen W, Liu Q, Dai J. Abietic acid suppresses non-small-cell lung cancer cell growth *via* blocking IKKβ/NF-κB signaling. OncoTargets Ther 2019; 12: 4825-37.
[http://dx.doi.org/10.2147/OTT.S199161] [PMID: 31354305]

[76] Gao C, Li X, Yu S, Liang L. Inhibition of cancer cell growth by oleanolic acid in multidrug resistant liver carcinoma is mediated *via* suppression of cancer cell migration and invasion, mitochondrial apoptosis, G2/M cell cycle arrest and deactivation of JNK/p38 signalling pathway. J BUON 2019; 24(5): 1964-9.
[PMID: 31786862]

[77] Wang X, Bai H, Zhang X, *et al.* Inhibitory effect of oleanolic acid on hepatocellular carcinoma *via* ERK–p53-mediated cell cycle arrest and mitochondrial-dependent apoptosis. Carcinogenesis 2013; 34(6): 1323-30.
[http://dx.doi.org/10.1093/carcin/bgt058] [PMID: 23404993]

[78] Cai Y, Fang X, He C, *et al.* Cucurbitacins: A systematic review of the phytochemistry and anticancer activity. Am J Chin Med 2015; 43(7): 1331-50.
[http://dx.doi.org/10.1142/S0192415X15500755] [PMID: 26503558]

[79] Farooqui A, Khan F, Khan I, Ansari IA. Glycyrrhizin induces reactive oxygen species-dependent apoptosis and cell cycle arrest at G_0/G_1 in HPV18$^+$ human cervical cancer HeLa cell line. Biomed Pharmacother 2018; 97: 752-64.
[http://dx.doi.org/10.1016/j.biopha.2017.10.147] [PMID: 29107932]

[80] Zhao J, Li R, Pawlak A, *et al.* Antitumor activity of betulinic acid and betulin in canine cancer cell lines. In Vivo 2018; 32(5): 1081-8.

[81] Li TH, Yan HX. Antitumor– and apoptosis–inducing effects of pomolic acid against SK–MEL–2 human malignant melanoma cells are mediated *via* inhibition of cell migration and sub–G1 cell cycle arrest. Mol Med Rep 2018; 17(1): 1035-40.
[PMID: 29115486]

[82] Nussinov R, Jang H, Tsai CJ. The structural basis for cancer treatment decisions. Oncotarget 2014; 5(17): 7285-302.
[http://dx.doi.org/10.18632/oncotarget.2439] [PMID: 25277176]

[83] Luo J, Hu YL, Wang H. Ursolic acid inhibits breast cancer growth by inhibiting proliferation, inducing autophagy and apoptosis, and suppressing inflammatory responses via the PI3K/AKT and NF-κB signaling pathways *in vitro*. Exp Ther Med 2017; 14(4): 3623-31.
[http://dx.doi.org/10.3892/etm.2017.4965] [PMID: 29042957]

[84] Kim GH, Kan SY, Kang H, *et al.* Ursolic acid suppresses cholesterol biosynthesis and exerts anti-cancer effects in hepatocellular carcinoma cells. Int J Mol Sci 2019; 20(19): 4767.
[http://dx.doi.org/10.3390/ijms20194767] [PMID: 31561416]

[85] Zhang Z, Miao L, Lv C, *et al.* Wentilactone B induces G2/M phase arrest and apoptosis *via* the Ras/Raf/MAPK signaling pathway in human hepatoma SMMC-7721 cells. Cell Death Dis 2013; 4(6): e657-7.
[http://dx.doi.org/10.1038/cddis.2013.182] [PMID: 23744357]

[86] Lu J, Chen X, Qu S, *et al.* Oridonin induces G_2/M cell cycle arrest and apoptosis via the PI3K/Akt signaling pathway in hormone-independent prostate cancer cells. Oncol Lett 2017; 13(4): 2838-46.
[http://dx.doi.org/10.3892/ol.2017.5751] [PMID: 28454475]

[87] Zhang X, Zhang HM. Alantolactone induces gastric cancer BGC–823 cell apoptosis by regulating reactive oxygen species generation and the AKT signaling pathway. Oncol Lett 2019; 17(6): 4795-

802.
[http://dx.doi.org/10.3892/ol.2019.10172] [PMID: 31186685]

[88] Zhou XW, Xia YZ, Zhang YL, *et al.* Tomentodione M sensitizes multidrug resistant cancer cells by decreasing P-glycoprotein *via* inhibition of p38 MAPK signaling. Oncotarget 2017; 8(60): 101965-83. [http://dx.doi.org/10.18632/oncotarget.21949] [PMID: 29254218]

[89] Zhu X, Zhang Y, Li Q, *et al.* β-Carotene Induces Apoptosis in Human Esophageal Squamous Cell Carcinoma Cell Lines *via* the Cav-1/AKT/NF-κB Signaling Pathway. J Biochem Mol Toxicol 2016; 30(3): 148-57.
[http://dx.doi.org/10.1002/jbt.21773] [PMID: 26733226]

[90] Zhang H, Kang Y, Li N, *et al.* Triterpenoids from Liquidambar Fructus induced cell apoptosis *via* a PI3K-AKT related signal pathway in SMMC7721 cancer cells. Phytochemistry 2020; 171: 112228. [http://dx.doi.org/10.1016/j.phytochem.2019.112228] [PMID: 31911265]

[91] Cai J, Zhong Y, Tian S. Naturally occurring davanone exhibits anticancer potential against ovarian cancer cells by inducing programmed cell death, suppression of cell migration and invasion and modulation of PI3K/AKT/MAPK signaling pathway.

[92] Hsia TC, Yu CC, Hsiao YT, *et al.* Cantharidin impairs cell migration and invasion of human lung cancer NCI-H460 cells *via* UPA and MAPK signaling pathways. Anticancer Res 2016; 36(11): 5989-98.
[http://dx.doi.org/10.21873/anticanres.11187] [PMID: 27793925]

[93] Yu C, Sun P, Zhou Y, *et al.* Inhibition of AKT enhances the anti-cancer effects of Artemisinin in clear cell renal cell carcinoma. Biomed Pharmacother 2019; 118: 109383.
[http://dx.doi.org/10.1016/j.biopha.2019.109383] [PMID: 31545251]

[94] Dong F, Yang P, Wang R, *et al.* Triptonide acts as a novel antiprostate cancer agent mainly through inhibition of mTOR signaling pathway. Prostate 2019; 79(11): 1284-93.
[http://dx.doi.org/10.1002/pros.23834] [PMID: 31212374]

[95] Tan B, Huang Y, Lan L, *et al.* Bruceine D induces apoptosis in human non-small cell lung cancer cells through regulating JNK pathway. Biomed Pharmacother 2019; 117: 109089.
[http://dx.doi.org/10.1016/j.biopha.2019.109089] [PMID: 31226632]

[96] Su T, Li F, Guan J, *et al.* Artemisinin and its derivatives prevent Helicobacter pylori-induced gastric carcinogenesis *via* inhibition of NF-κB signaling. Phytomedicine 2019; 63: 152968.
[http://dx.doi.org/10.1016/j.phymed.2019.152968] [PMID: 31280140]

[97] Sun C, Cui H, Yang H, *et al.* Anti-metastatic effect of jolkinolide B and the mechanism of activity in breast cancer MDA-MB-231 cells. Oncol Lett 2015; 10(2): 1117-22.
[http://dx.doi.org/10.3892/ol.2015.3310] [PMID: 26622636]

[98] Xu HY, Chen ZW, Hou JC, Du FX, Liu JC. Jolkinolide B induces apoptosis in MCF-7 cells through inhibition of the PI3K/Akt/mTOR signaling pathway. Oncol Rep 2013; 29(1): 212-8.
[http://dx.doi.org/10.3892/or.2012.2113] [PMID: 23129237]

[99] Hsueh KC, Lin CL, Tung JN, Yang SF, Hsieh YH. Nimbolide induced apoptosis by activating ERK-mediated inhibition of c-IAP1 expression in human hepatocellular carcinoma cells. Environ Toxicol 2018; 33(9): 913-22.
[http://dx.doi.org/10.1002/tox.22576] [PMID: 29962003]

[100] Sophia J, Kowshik J, Dwivedi A, *et al.* Nimbolide, a neem limonoid inhibits cytoprotective autophagy to activate apoptosis *via* modulation of the PI3K/Akt/GSK-3β signalling pathway in oral cancer. Cell Death Dis 2018; 9(11): 1087.
[http://dx.doi.org/10.1038/s41419-018-1126-4] [PMID: 30352996]

[101] Gupta SC, Prasad S, Sethumadhavan DR, Nair MS, Mo YY, Aggarwal BB. Nimbolide, a limonoid triterpene, inhibits growth of human colorectal cancer xenografts by suppressing the proinflammatory microenvironment. Clin Cancer Res 2013; 19(16): 4465-76.

[http://dx.doi.org/10.1158/1078-0432.CCR-13-0080] [PMID: 23766363]

[102] Shin JM, Lee KM, Lee HJ, Yun JH, Nho CW. Physalin A regulates the Nrf2 pathway through ERK and p38 for induction of detoxifying enzymes. BMC Complement Altern Med 2019; 19(1): 101. [http://dx.doi.org/10.1186/s12906-019-2511-y] [PMID: 31072358]

[103] Li P, Zhou X, Sun W, *et al.* Elemene induces apoptosis of human gastric cancer cell line BGC-823 *via* extracellular signal regulated kinase (ERK) 1/2 signaling pathway. Med Sci Monit 2017; 23: 809-17. [http://dx.doi.org/10.12659/MSM.903197] [PMID: 28196062]

[104] Sahai R, Bhattacharjee A, Shukla VN, *et al.* Gedunin isolated from the mangrove plant Xylocarpus granatum exerts its anti-proliferative activity in ovarian cancer cells through G2/M-phase arrest and oxidative stress-mediated intrinsic apoptosis. Apoptosis 2020; 25(7-8): 481-99. [http://dx.doi.org/10.1007/s10495-020-01605-5] [PMID: 32399945]

[105] Kishore T KK, Ganugula R, Gade DR, Reddy GB, Nagini S. Gedunin abrogates aldose reductase, PI3K/Akt/mToR, and NF-κB signaling pathways to inhibit angiogenesis in a hamster model of oral carcinogenesis. Tumour Biol 2016; 37(2): 2083-93. [http://dx.doi.org/10.1007/s13277-015-4003-0] [PMID: 26342697]

[106] Kim J, Jayaprakasha GK, Patil BS. Obacunone exhibits anti-proliferative and anti-aromatase activity *in vitro* by inhibiting the p38 MAPK signaling pathway in MCF-7 human breast adenocarcinoma cells. Biochimie 2014; 105: 36-44. [http://dx.doi.org/10.1016/j.biochi.2014.06.002] [PMID: 24927687]

[107] Fan J, Ren D, Wang J, *et al.* Bruceine D induces lung cancer cell apoptosis and autophagy *via* the ROS/MAPK signaling pathway *in vitro* and *in vivo*. Cell Death Dis 2020; 11(2): 126. [http://dx.doi.org/10.1038/s41419-020-2317-3] [PMID: 32071301]

[108] Lai ZQ, Ip SP, Liao HJ, *et al.* a naturally occurring tetracyclic triterpene quassinoid, induces apoptosis in pancreatic cancer through ROS-associated PI3K/Akt signaling pathway. Front Pharmacol 2017; 8: 936. [http://dx.doi.org/10.3389/fphar.2017.00936] [PMID: 29311937]

[109] Zhang Y, Zhang C, Min D. RETRACTED: Ailanthone up-regulates miR-449a to restrain acute myeloid leukemia cells growth, migration and invasion. Exp Mol Pathol 2019; 108: 114-20. [http://dx.doi.org/10.1016/j.yexmp.2019.04.011] [PMID: 31002772]

[110] Zhuo Z, Hu J, Yang X, *et al.* Ailanthone inhibits Huh7 cancer cell growth *via* cell cycle arrest and apoptosis *in vitro* and *in vivo*. Sci Rep 2015; 5(1): 16185. [http://dx.doi.org/10.1038/srep16185] [PMID: 26525771]

[111] Yao J, Liu J, Zhao W. By blocking hexokinase-2 phosphorylation, limonin suppresses tumor glycolysis and induces cell apoptosis in hepatocellular carcinoma. OncoTargets Ther 2018; 11: 3793-803. [http://dx.doi.org/10.2147/OTT.S165220] [PMID: 30013360]

[112] Tang Z, Tang Y, Li L, Liu T, Yang J. Limonin provokes hepatocellular carcinoma cells with stemness entry into cycle *via* activating PI3K/Akt signaling. Biomed Pharmacother 2019; 117: 109051. [http://dx.doi.org/10.1016/j.biopha.2019.109051] [PMID: 31177062]

[113] Zhu X, Yuan C, Tian C, *et al.* The plant sesquiterpene lactone parthenolide inhibits Wnt/β-catenin signaling by blocking synthesis of the transcriptional regulators TCF4/LEF1. J Biol Chem 2018; 293(14): 5335-44. [http://dx.doi.org/10.1074/jbc.M117.819300] [PMID: 29462785]

[114] Bommareddy A, Knapp K, Nemeth A, *et al.* Alpha-Santalol, a component of sandalwood oil inhibits migration of breast cancer cells by targeting the β-catenin pathway. Anticancer Res 2018; 38(8): 4475-80. [http://dx.doi.org/10.21873/anticanres.12750] [PMID: 30061212]

[115] Chinison J, Aguilar JS, Avalos A, *et al.* Triptonide effectively inhibits Wnt/β-catenin signaling *via* C-terminal transactivation domain of β-catenin. Sci Rep 2016; 6(1): 32779. [http://dx.doi.org/10.1038/srep32779] [PMID: 27596363]

[116] Wang L, Zhao Y, Wu Q, Guan Y, Wu X. Therapeutic effects of β-elemene *via* attenuation of the Wnt/β-catenin signaling pathway in cervical cancer cells. Mol Med Rep 2018; 17(3): 4299-306. [http://dx.doi.org/10.3892/mmr.2018.8455] [PMID: 29363722]

[117] Su Z, Wang C, Chang D, Zhu X, Sai C, Pei J. Limonin attenuates the stemness of breast cancer cells *via* suppressing MIR216A methylation. Biomed Pharmacother 2019; 112: 108699. [http://dx.doi.org/10.1016/j.biopha.2019.108699] [PMID: 30970511]

[118] Li H, Lu H, Lv M, Wang Q, Sun Y. Parthenolide facilitates apoptosis and reverses drug-resistance of human gastric carcinoma cells by inhibiting the STAT3 signaling pathway. Oncol Lett 2018; 15(3): 3572-9. [http://dx.doi.org/10.3892/ol.2018.7739] [PMID: 29467878]

[119] Shen L, Zhang SQ, Liu L, *et al.* Jolkinolide A and jolkinolide B inhibit proliferation of A549 cells and activity of human umbilical vein endothelial cells. Med Sci Monit 2017; 23: 223-37. [http://dx.doi.org/10.12659/MSM.902704] [PMID: 28087861]

[120] Wang Y, Ma X, Yan S, *et al.* 17-hydroxy-jolkinolide B inhibits signal transducers and activators of transcription 3 signaling by covalently cross-linking Janus kinases and induces apoptosis of human cancer cells. Cancer Res 2009; 69(18): 7302-10. [http://dx.doi.org/10.1158/0008-5472.CAN-09-0462] [PMID: 19706767]

[121] Shan H, Yao S, Ye Y, Yu Q. 3-Deoxy-2β,16-dihydroxynagilactone E, a natural compound from Podocarpus nagi, preferentially inhibits JAK2/STAT3 signaling by allosterically interacting with the regulatory domain of JAK2 and induces apoptosis of cancer cells. Acta Pharmacol Sin 2019; 40(12): 1578-86. [http://dx.doi.org/10.1038/s41401-019-0254-4] [PMID: 31201357]

[122] Wang Z, Chen H, Chen J, *et al.* Emodin sensitizes human pancreatic cancer cells to EGFR inhibitor through suppressing Stat3 signaling pathway. Cancer Manag Res 2019; 11: 8463-73. [http://dx.doi.org/10.2147/CMAR.S221877] [PMID: 31572001]

[123] Thoennissen NH, Iwanski GB, Doan NB, *et al.* Cucurbitacin B induces apoptosis by inhibition of the JAK/STAT pathway and potentiates antiproliferative effects of gemcitabine on pancreatic cancer cells. Cancer Res 2009; 69(14): 5876-84. [http://dx.doi.org/10.1158/0008-5472.CAN-09-0536] [PMID: 19605406]

[124] Zheng Q, Liu Y, Liu W, *et al.* Cucurbitacin B inhibits growth and induces apoptosis through the JAK2/STAT3 and MAPK pathways in SH-SY5Y human neuroblastoma cells. Mol Med Rep 2014; 10(1): 89-94. [http://dx.doi.org/10.3892/mmr.2014.2175] [PMID: 24789581]

[125] Lee JH, Rangappa S, Mohan CD, *et al.* Brusatol, a Nrf2 inhibitor targets STAT3 signaling cascade in head and neck squamous cell carcinoma. Biomolecules 2019; 9(10): 550. [http://dx.doi.org/10.3390/biom9100550] [PMID: 31575007]

[126] Xiang Y, Ye W, Huang C, *et al.* Brusatol inhibits growth and induces apoptosis in pancreatic cancer cells *via* JNK/p38 MAPK/NF-κb/Stat3/Bcl-2 signaling pathway. Biochem Biophys Res Commun 2017; 487(4): 820-6. [http://dx.doi.org/10.1016/j.bbrc.2017.04.133] [PMID: 28455228]

[127] Wang JH, Zhang K, Niu HY, *et al.* Jolkinolide B from Euphorbia fischeriana Steud induces in human leukemic cells apoptosis *via* JAK2/STAT3 pathways. Int J Clin Pharmacol Ther 2013; 51(3): 170-8. [http://dx.doi.org/10.5414/CP201807] [PMID: 23253949]

[128] Wang S, Hu H, Zhong B, *et al.* Bruceine D inhibits tumor growth and stem cell–like traits of osteosarcoma through inhibition of STAT3 signaling pathway. Cancer Med 2019; 8(17): 7345-58.

[http://dx.doi.org/10.1002/cam4.2612] [PMID: 31631559]

[129] Zhang R, Zhao J, Xu J, *et al.* Andrographolide suppresses proliferation of human colon cancer SW620 cells through the TLR4/NF-κB/MMP-9 signaling pathway. Oncol Lett 2017; 14(4): 4305-10. [http://dx.doi.org/10.3892/ol.2017.6669] [PMID: 28943944]

[130] Singh PR, Priya ES, Balakrishnan S, *et al.* Nimbolide inhibits androgen independent prostate cancer cells survival and proliferation by modulating multiple pro-survival signaling pathways. Biomed Pharmacother 2016; 84: 1623-34. [http://dx.doi.org/10.1016/j.biopha.2016.10.076] [PMID: 27889231]

[131] Jiang N, Dong XP, Zhang SL, You QY, Jiang XT, Zhao XG. Triptolide reverses the Taxol resistance of lung adenocarcinoma by inhibiting the NF-κB signaling pathway and the expression of NF-κ--regulated drug-resistant genes. Mol Med Rep 2016; 13(1): 153-9. [http://dx.doi.org/10.3892/mmr.2015.4493] [PMID: 26531258]

[132] Ma J-X, Sun Y-L, Yu Y, Zhang J, Wu H-Y, Yu X-F. Triptolide enhances the sensitivity of pancreatic cancer PANC-1 cells to gemcitabine by inhibiting TLR4/NF-κB signaling. Am J Transl Res 2019; 11(6): 3750-60. [PMID: 31312385]

[133] Dawood M, Ooko E, Efferth T. Collateral sensitivity of parthenolide *via* NF-κB and HIF-α inhibition and epigenetic changes in drug-resistant cancer cell lines. Front Pharmacol 2019; 10: 542. [http://dx.doi.org/10.3389/fphar.2019.00542] [PMID: 31164821]

[134] Shankar E, Zhang A, Franco D, Gupta S. Betulinic acid-mediated apoptosis in human prostate cancer cells involves p53 and nuclear factor-kappa B (NF-κB) pathways. Molecules 2017; 22(2): 264. [http://dx.doi.org/10.3390/molecules22020264] [PMID: 28208611]

[135] Xiang S, Zhao Z, Zhang T, *et al.* Triptonide effectively suppresses gastric tumor growth and metastasis through inhibition of the oncogenic Notch1 and NF-κB signaling pathways. Toxicol Appl Pharmacol 2020; 388: 114870. [http://dx.doi.org/10.1016/j.taap.2019.114870] [PMID: 31866380]

[136] Kushwaha PP, Singh AK, Shuaib M, *et al.* 3-O-(E)-p-Coumaroyl betulinic acid possess anticancer activity and inhibit Notch signaling pathway in breast cancer cells and mammosphere. Chem Biol Interact 2020; 328: 109200. [http://dx.doi.org/10.1016/j.cbi.2020.109200] [PMID: 32702347]

[137] Bu HQ, Shen F, Cui J. The inhibitory effect of oridonin on colon cancer was mediated by deactivation of TGF-β1/Smads-PAI-1 signaling pathway *in vitro* and vivo. OncoTargets Ther 2019; 12: 7467-76. [http://dx.doi.org/10.2147/OTT.S220401] [PMID: 31686852]

[138] Li Y, Lu J, Chen Q, *et al.* Artemisinin suppresses hepatocellular carcinoma cell growth, migration and invasion by targeting cellular bioenergetics and Hippo-YAP signaling. Arch Toxicol 2019; 93(11): 3367-83. [http://dx.doi.org/10.1007/s00204-019-02579-3] [PMID: 31563988]

[139] Zhao W, Wu M, Cui L, Du W. Limonin attenuates the stemness of cervical carcinoma cells by promoting YAP nuclear-cytoplasmic translocation. Food Chem Toxicol 2019; 125: 621-8. [http://dx.doi.org/10.1016/j.fct.2019.02.011] [PMID: 30738134]

[140] Yang G, Li Z, Chen L. Limonin suppresses the progression of oral tongue squamous cell carcinoma *via* inhibiting YAP transcriptional regulatory activity. Tissue Cell 2020; 65: 101346. [http://dx.doi.org/10.1016/j.tice.2020.101346] [PMID: 32746992]

[141] Li J, Li F, Tang F, *et al.* AGS-30, an andrographolide derivative, suppresses tumor angiogenesis and growth *in vitro* and *in vivo.* Biochem Pharmacol 2020; 171: 113694. [http://dx.doi.org/10.1016/j.bcp.2019.113694] [PMID: 31706845]

[142] Sheikh I, Sharma V, Tuli HS, *et al.* Cancer chemoprevention by flavonoids, dietary polyphenols and terpenoids. Biointerface Res Appl Chem 2020; 11(1): 8502-37.

[http://dx.doi.org/10.33263/BRIAC111.85028537]

[143] Dong F, Zhou X, Li C, *et al.* Dihydroartemisinin targets VEGFR2 *via* the NF-κB pathway in endothelial cells to inhibit angiogenesis. Cancer Biol Ther 2014; 15(11): 1479-88. [http://dx.doi.org/10.4161/15384047.2014.955728] [PMID: 25482945]

[144] Wei T, Liu J. Anti-angiogenic properties of artemisinin derivatives (Review). Int J Mol Med 2017; 40(4): 972-8. [http://dx.doi.org/10.3892/ijmm.2017.3085] [PMID: 28765885]

[145] Lin X, Peng Z, Su C. Potential anti-cancer activities and mechanisms of costunolide and dehydrocostuslactone. Int J Mol Sci 2015; 16(12): 10888-906. [http://dx.doi.org/10.3390/ijms160510888] [PMID: 25984608]

[146] Li J, Peng Y, Li S, *et al.* Anti-angiogenic activity of a new andrographolide derivative in zebrafish and HUVECs. Eur J Pharmacol 2016; 789: 344-53. [http://dx.doi.org/10.1016/j.ejphar.2016.07.043] [PMID: 27471159]

[147] Huang W, Liang Y, Wang J, *et al.* Anti-angiogenic activity and mechanism of kaurane diterpenoids from Wedelia chinensis. Phytomedicine 2016; 23(3): 283-92. [http://dx.doi.org/10.1016/j.phymed.2015.12.021] [PMID: 26969382]

[148] Lu K, Bhat M, Basu S. Plants and their active compounds: natural molecules to target angiogenesis. Angiogenesis 2016; 19(3): 287-95. [http://dx.doi.org/10.1007/s10456-016-9512-y] [PMID: 27154020]

[149] Qi WY, Gao XM, Ma ZY, Xia CL, Xu HM. Antiangiogenic activity of terpenoids from Euphorbia neriifolia Linn. Bioorg Chem 2020; 96: 103536. [http://dx.doi.org/10.1016/j.bioorg.2019.103536] [PMID: 31972463]

[150] Yang CY, Lin CK, Lin GJ, *et al.* Triptolide represses oral cancer cell proliferation, invasion, migration, and angiogenesis in co-inoculation with U937 cells. Clin Oral Investig 2017; 21(1): 419-27. [http://dx.doi.org/10.1007/s00784-016-1808-1] [PMID: 27073100]

[151] Naila A, Zhang YF. Triptolide: a critical review on antiangiogenesis in cancer and scope in therapeutics, Journal of Biomimetics. Journal of Biomimetics, Biomaterials and Biomedical Engineering 2015; 23: 37-46. [http://dx.doi.org/10.4028/www.scientific.net/JBBBE.23.37]

[152] Ren Y, Wang C, Xu J, Wang S. Cafestol and kahweol: A review on their bioactivities and pharmacological properties. Int J Mol Sci 2019; 20(17): 4238. [http://dx.doi.org/10.3390/ijms20174238] [PMID: 31480213]

[153] Tang Y-C, Zhang Y, Zhou J, *et al.* Ginsenoside Rg3 targets cancer stem cells and tumor angiogenesis to inhibit colorectal cancer progression *in vivo.* Int J Oncol 2018; 52(1): 127-38. [PMID: 29115601]

[154] Jin H, Pi J, Yang F, *et al.* Ursolic acid-loaded chitosan nanoparticles induce potent anti-angiogenesis in tumor. Appl Microbiol Biotechnol 2016; 100(15): 6643-52. [http://dx.doi.org/10.1007/s00253-016-7360-8] [PMID: 26883344]

[155] Nguyen VT, Tung NT, Cuong TD, *et al.* Cytotoxic and anti-angiogenic effects of lanostane triterpenoids from Ganoderma lucidum. Phytochem Lett 2015; 12: 69-74. [http://dx.doi.org/10.1016/j.phytol.2015.02.012]

[156] Park JH, Yoon J, Park B. Pomolic acid suppresses HIF1α/VEGF-mediated angiogenesis by targeting p38-MAPK and mTOR signaling cascades. Phytomedicine 2016; 23(14): 1716-26. [http://dx.doi.org/10.1016/j.phymed.2016.10.010] [PMID: 27912873]

[157] Seyfried TN, Huysentruyt LC. On the origin of cancer metastasis. Critical Reviews in Oncogenesis 2013; 18(1-2)

[158] Francou A, Anderson KV. The epithelial-to-mesenchymal transition in development and cancer. Annu Rev Cancer Biol 2020; 4(1): 197-220.
[http://dx.doi.org/10.1146/annurev-cancerbio-030518-055425] [PMID: 34113749]

[159] Luo Y, Wu JY, Lu MH, Shi Z, Na N, Di JM. Carvacrol alleviates prostate cancer cell proliferation, migration, and invasion through regulation of PI3K/Akt and MAPK signaling pathways. Oxid Med Cell Longev 2016; 2016: 1-11.
[http://dx.doi.org/10.1155/2016/1469693] [PMID: 27803760]

[160] Meng Q, Tang B, Qiu B. Growth inhibition of Saos-2 osteosarcoma cells by lactucopicrin is mediated *via* inhibition of cell migration and invasion, sub-G1 cell cycle disruption, apoptosis induction and Raf signalling pathway. J BUON 2019; 24(5): 2136-40.
[PMID: 31786886]

[161] Liu J, Zhao Y, Shi Z, Bai Y. Antitumor effects of helenalin in doxorubicin-resistant leukemia cells are mediated via mitochondrial mediated apoptosis, loss of mitochondrial membrane potential, inhibition of cell migration and invasion and downregulation of PI3-kinase/AKT/m-TOR signalling pathway. Official journal of the Balkan Union of Oncology 2019; 24(5): 2068-74.

[162] Zeng C, Guo B, Chen J, He W. Antitumor effects of Farnesol in optic nerve sheath menin-gioma cell line and its effects on cell cycle progression, au-tophagy, cell migration and invasion. 2019.

[163] Liu Y, Gao S, Zhu J, Zheng Y, Zhang H, Sun H. Dihydroartemisinin induces apoptosis and inhibits proliferation, migration, and invasion in epithelial ovarian cancer *via* inhibition of the hedgehog signaling pathway. Cancer Med 2018; 7(11): 5704-15.
[http://dx.doi.org/10.1002/cam4.1827] [PMID: 30338663]

[164] Zhou H, Liu J, Chen Z. Coronarin D suppresses proliferation, invasion and migration of glioma cells *via* activating JNK signaling pathway. Pathol Res Pract 2020; 216(2): 152789.
[http://dx.doi.org/10.1016/j.prp.2019.152789] [PMID: 31870592]

[165] Zhang Y, Ma R, Cheng S, Gu G. Marrubenol inhibits osteosarcoma cancer cell growth by inducing autophagic cell death and inhibiting cancer cell migration and invasion. J BUON 2018; 23(3): 729-34.
[PMID: 30003743]

[166] Jao HY, Yu FS, Yu CS, *et al.* Suppression of the migration and invasion is mediated by triptolide in B16F10 mouse melanoma cells through the NF-kappaB-dependent pathway. Environ Toxicol 2016; 31(12): 1974-84.
[http://dx.doi.org/10.1002/tox.22198] [PMID: 26420756]

[167] Yuan S, Wang L, Chen X, *et al.* Triptolide inhibits the migration and invasion of human prostate cancer cells *via* Caveolin-1/CD147/MMPs pathway. Biomed Pharmacother 2016; 84: 1776-82.
[http://dx.doi.org/10.1016/j.biopha.2016.10.104] [PMID: 27847199]

[168] Liu Y, Zhang Y, Zou J, *et al.* Andrographolide induces autophagic cell death and inhibits invasion and metastasis of human osteosarcoma cells in an autophagy-dependent manner. Cell Physiol Biochem 2017; 44(4): 1396-410.
[http://dx.doi.org/10.1159/000485536] [PMID: 29197865]

[169] Lu YM, Chen W, Zhu JS, Chen WX, Chen NW. Eriocalyxin B blocks human SW1116 colon cancer cell proliferation, migration, invasion, cell cycle progression and angiogenesis *via* the JAK2/STAT3 signaling pathway. Mol Med Rep 2016; 13(3): 2235-40.
[http://dx.doi.org/10.3892/mmr.2016.4800] [PMID: 26795301]

[170] Zhao L, Zhang J, Fan Y, Li Y. Antiproliferative activity of carnosic acid is mediated *via* inhibition of cell migration and invasion, and suppression of phosphatidylinositol 3-kinases (PI3K)/AKT/ mammalian target of rapamycin (mTOR) signaling pathway. Med Sci Monit 2019; 25: 7864-71.
[http://dx.doi.org/10.12659/MSM.917735] [PMID: 31631173]

[171] Li X, Zhao X, Song W, *et al.* Pseudolaric acid B inhibits proliferation, invasion and epithelial-t--mesenchymal transition in human pancreatic cancer cell. Yonsei Med J 2018; 59(1): 20-7. [http://dx.doi.org/10.3349/ymj.2018.59.1.20] [PMID: 29214772]

[172] Duan L, Yang Z, Jiang X, Zhang J, Guo X. Oleanolic acid inhibits cell proliferation migration and invasion and induces SW579 thyroid cancer cell line apoptosis by targeting forkhead transcription factor A. Anticancer Drugs 2019; 30(8): 812-20. [http://dx.doi.org/10.1097/CAD.0000000000000777] [PMID: 30882397]

[173] He S-Q, Gao M, Fu Y-F, Zhang Y-N. Glycyrrhizic acid inhibits leukemia cell growth and migration *via* blocking AKT/mTOR/STAT3 signaling. Int J Clin Exp Pathol 2015; 8(5): 5175-81. [PMID: 26191214]

[174] Li J, Qi Y. RETRACTED: Ginsenoside Rg3 inhibits cell growth, migration and invasion in Caco-2 cells by downregulation of lncRNA CCAT1. Exp Mol Pathol 2019; 106: 131-8. [http://dx.doi.org/10.1016/j.yexmp.2019.01.003] [PMID: 30633886]

[175] Wang D, Wu C, Liu D, *et al.* Ginsenoside Rg3 inhibits migration and invasion of nasopharyngeal carcinoma cells and suppresses epithelial mesenchymal transition. BioMed Res Int 2019; 2019: 1-11. [http://dx.doi.org/10.1155/2019/8407683] [PMID: 30915362]

[176] Lin H, Qiu S, Xie L, Liu C, Sun S. Nimbolide suppresses non-small cell lung cancer cell invasion and migration *via* manipulation of DUSP4 expression and ERK1/2 signaling. Biomed Pharmacother 2017; 92: 340-6. [http://dx.doi.org/10.1016/j.biopha.2017.05.072] [PMID: 28554129]

[177] Song J, Liu H, Li Z, Yang C, Wang C. Cucurbitacin I inhibits cell migration and invasion and enhances chemosensitivity in colon cancer. Oncol Rep 2015; 33(4): 1867-71. [http://dx.doi.org/10.3892/or.2015.3749] [PMID: 25625299]

[178] Salminen A, Lehtonen M, Suuronen T, Kaarniranta K, Huuskonen J. Terpenoids: natural inhibitors of NF-κB signaling with anti-inflammatory and anticancer potential. Cell Mol Life Sci 2008; 65(19): 2979-99. [http://dx.doi.org/10.1007/s00018-008-8103-5] [PMID: 18516495]

[179] Jain H, Dhingra N, Narsinghani T, Sharma R. Insights into the mechanism of natural terpenoids as NF-kB inhibitors: an overview on their anticancer potential. Exp Oncol 2016; 38(3): 158-68. [http://dx.doi.org/10.31768/2312-8852.2016.38(3):158-168] [PMID: 27685522]

[180] Xia YF, Ye BQ, Li YD, *et al.* Andrographolide attenuates inflammation by inhibition of NF-κ B activation through covalent modification of reduced cysteine 62 of p50. J Immunol 2004; 173(6): 4207-17. [http://dx.doi.org/10.4049/jimmunol.173.6.4207] [PMID: 15356172]

[181] Hidalgo MA, Romero A, Figueroa J, *et al.* Andrographolide interferes with binding of nuclear factor-κ B to DNA in HL-60-derived neutrophilic cells. Br J Pharmacol 2005; 144(5): 680-6. [http://dx.doi.org/10.1038/sj.bjp.0706105] [PMID: 15678086]

[182] Sheeja K, Guruvayoorappan C, Kuttan G. Antiangiogenic activity of Andrographis paniculata extract and andrographolide. Int Immunopharmacol 2007; 7(2): 211-21. [http://dx.doi.org/10.1016/j.intimp.2006.10.002] [PMID: 17178389]

[183] Pratheeshkumar P, Kuttan G. Vernolide-A inhibits tumour specific angiogenesis by regulating proinflammatory cytokines, VEGF, MMPs and TIMP. Eur J Pharmacol 2011; 656(1-3): 10-8. [http://dx.doi.org/10.1016/j.ejphar.2010.12.041] [PMID: 21256125]

[184] Haridas V, Arntzen CJ, Gutterman JU. Avicins, a family of triterpenoid saponins from *Acacia victoriae* (Bentham), inhibit activation of nuclear factor-κB by inhibiting both its nuclear localization and ability to bind DNA. Proc Natl Acad Sci USA 2001; 98(20): 11557-62. [http://dx.doi.org/10.1073/pnas.191363498] [PMID: 11572998]

[185] Shanmugam MK, Nguyen AH, Kumar AP, Tan BKH, Sethi G. Targeted inhibition of tumor proliferation, survival, and metastasis by pentacyclic triterpenoids: Potential role in prevention and therapy of cancer. Cancer Lett 2012; 320(2): 158-70. [http://dx.doi.org/10.1016/j.canlet.2012.02.037] [PMID: 22406826]

CHAPTER 12

Cytotoxic Phytochemical library of *Rosmarinus Officinalis*

Maida Engels S.E.[1,*], **Motamarri Venkata Naga Lalitha Chaitanya**[4], **Gnana Ruba Priya Muthaiah**[3], **Kuppuswamy Uma**[1] and **Rashmi Saxena Pal**[2]

[1] *PSG College of Pharmacy, Coimbatore, Tamil Nadu, India*

[2] *Department of Pharmacognosy, School of pharmacy, lovely professional university, Phagwara, Punjab- 144402, India*

[3] *College of Pharmaceutical Sciences, Department of Pharmaceutical Chemistry, Dayanandha Sagar University, Bangalore, Karnataka, India*

[4] *School of Pharmacy, Lovely Professional University Phagwara, 144402 Punjab, India*

Abstract: Globally, the prevalence of cancer has escalated at an alarming rate, and it has become a major health problem. The World Health Organization reported that one in six deaths is due to cancer. Despite the advantages of current chemotherapy available for cancer treatment, the development of resistance and severe side effects continuously insist cancer research focus on the discovery of new entities, especially from natural sources. In the last few decades, varieties of dietary herbs have been explored for their cytotoxic potential. Rosmarinus officinalis, a well-known culinary herb commonly known as rosemary, is not only used to enhance the flavour but also possesses medicinal values. The Rosmarinus officinalis plant extract and its essential oil are packed with different phenolic acids and terpenoids. Rosmarinus officinalis has anti-cancer, anti-proliferative, protective, anti-inflammatory, and anti-oxidant properties, according to several *in vitro* and *in vivo* studies. The antitumor activity of Rosmarinus officinalis is correlated with different molecular mechanisms such as reactive oxygen species scavenging, the on-co-suppressor gene expression, apoptosis, and immunomodulatory response regulation. So this chapter mainly focuses on the cytotoxic activities of Rosmarinus officinalis and the molecular mechanisms responsible for their anticancer activities. Also, possibilities of utilising the extracts, essential oils, and phytochemicals of Rosmarinus officinalis as potential therapeutic agents or complementary therapies with chemotherapeutic agents for cancer treatment have been discussed.

Keywords: Anticancer, Cancer, Cytotoxic Phytochemicals, Molecular mechanisms, Rosemary.

* **Corresponding author Maida Engels S.E.:** PSG College of Pharmacy, Coimbatore, Tamil Nadu, India; Email:maidase@gmail.com

Motamarri Venkata Naga Lalitha Chaitanya, Galvina Pereira, & Heyam Saad Ali (Eds.)

INTRODUCTION

Cancer is still continued to be a global burden that causes physical, emotional and financial strain on individuals, families, communities and health systems. In 2018, 9.6 million deaths and 1 in 6 deaths were reported due to cancer and it is the second leading cause of death worldwide. Leukemia, colorectal, prostate, lung, stomach and liver cancer are the most common types of cancer in men, while breast, lung, cervical, colorectal, and thyroid cancer are the most common among women. Blood cancer, and cancers related to the brain and lymph nodes are observed in children (Fig. **1**) [1].

Due to the prevailing resistance and side effects of anti-cancer agents, there is a need for the development of newer anti-cancer entities from natural sources like plants, algae and microbes. Many studies have been focused on developing newer anti-cancer drugs or leads from plant sources [2].

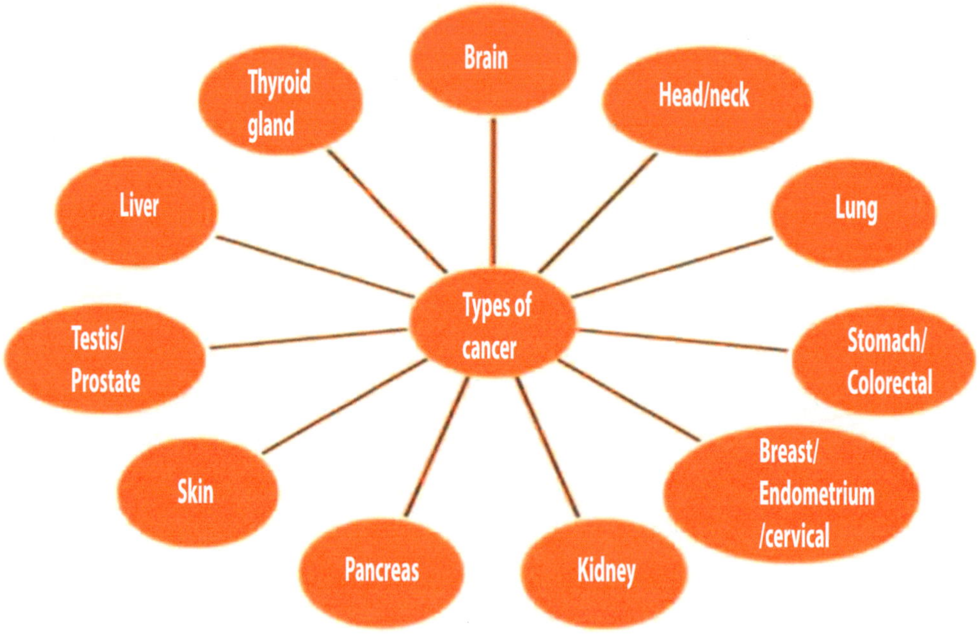

Fig. (1). Common types of cancer

Rosmarinus officinalis, commonly known as "Rusmari," belongs to the family Lamiaceae. This evergreen shrub is native to the Mediterranean and Portugal and grows all over the world. It grows 1-2 m high and has hard, narrow-linear, needle-shaped leaves that are packed with essential oil in their glandular scales. The tiny, two-lipped, bluish Labiatae flowers grow on the upper part of the branches. When rosemary leaves are crushed, they emit a camphoraceous and pungent aromatic odor.

The strong fragrance of this shrub is widely used in culinary flavoring, cosmetics, and toiletries. It was once used to expel negativity, improve memory, and season food. It is also believed that the benefits of rosemary are associated with the treatment of brain, liver, and eye problems, and that it has a wide range of therapeutic activities such as anticancer, cytotoxic, anti-inflammatory, anti-diabetic, anti-nociceptive, anti-microbial, diuretic, and hepatoprotective activities [3 - 9].

Taxonomy of *Rosmarinus officinalis*:

Domain: Eukaryota

Kingdom: Plantae

Phylum: Spermatophyta

Subphylum: Angiospermae

Class: Dicotyledonae

Order: Lamiales

Family: Lamiaceae

Genus: Rosmarinus

Species: Rosmarinus officinalis

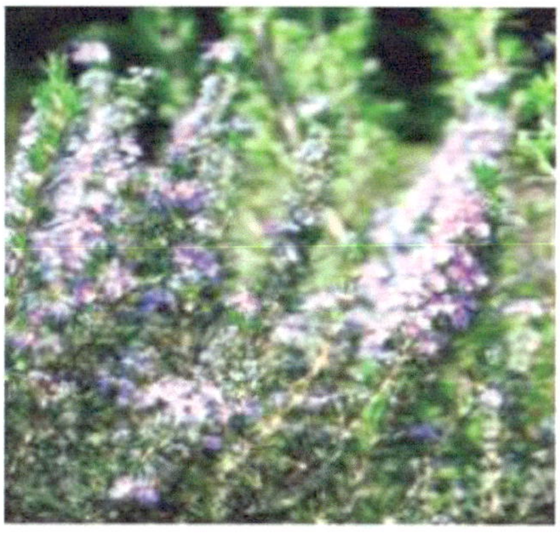

Fig. (2). *Rosmarinus officinalis*

Rosmarinus officinalis contains different classes of phytochemicals such as phenolic compounds, di and tri terpenoids. Table **1** and Fig. (**2**) describe the different phytoconstituents present in Rosmarinus *officinalis* and their pharmacological activities.

Table 1. Common pharmacological actions of *Rosmarinus officinalis*

Pharmacological activity	Extract/ essential oil/phytochemical responsible	References
Anti-inflammatory	Carnosol, Carnosic acid, Rosemary extract	[10]
Antibacterial	Caffeic acid, Extract, alpha pinene	[11 - 13]
Antifungal	Rosemary oil, Rosemary extract, Camphor	[14 - 16]
Skin cancer	Rosemary oil, Rosemary extract	[17, 18]
Wound healing	Rosemary oil, Rosemary cream	[19, 20]
Antioxidant	Chlorogenic acid, Caffeic acid, Oleanolic acid,	[21, 22]
Anti-Proliferation	Caffeic acid, Carnosic acid, Oleanolic acid, Rosemary extract, Carnosol	[23, 24]
Anti-cancer	Urosolic acid, Carnosic acid, Carnosol, Rosmnaol, Rosmarinic acid, Rosemary extracts.	[17, 25, 26]
Anti-viral	Oleanoilc acid, Rosmarinic acid, Eucalyptol	[27, 28]
Neuro protective	Rosmarinic acid, Urosolic acid.	[29]
Anti-anxiety	Rosmarinic acid	[30]
Anti-diabetic	Urosolic acid,	[31, 32]
Hypouricemic	Urosolic acid,	[33]
Anti-obesity and anti-atherosclerosis	Urosoilc acid,	[34]
Anti-microbial	Alpha pinene, luteolin.	[15]

Rosmarinus officinalis can be used in several forms such as fresh, dried, extract, and essential oil [35]. In ancient practice, the aerial parts of *Rosmarinus officinalis* are used to treat different ailments such as headaches, spasms, abdominal pain, arthritis, migraine, dizziness, and gout. Rosemary in the form of decoction, infusion and extract has been used to treat digestive, respiratory, inflammatory and cardiovascular disorders. It also has been used as a stomachic, wound healing, colorectic, diuretic, analgesic, anti-inflammatory and anti-depressant. Condensed water obtained from *Rosmarinus officinalis* is used to apply on the eyes. In ancient days, it was also used as memory enhancer.

CYTOTOXIC EFFECTS OF *ROSMARINUS OFFICINALIS*

In the last few decades, several reports have explored the anti-cancer activity of extracts, essential oils, and phytoconstituents of Rosmarinus officinalis [36]. Leaf extracts of rosemary were found to have high anti-proliferative and cytotoxic activity against HeLa, MCF-7, and Jurkat cancer cells [37]. Amar Y *et al.* revealed that Rosmarinus officinalis extracts noticeably exhibit anti-proliferation activity in cancer cells, U937 and CaCo-2, in a concentration- and time dependent manner [38]. Methanolic extract of rosemary inhibited skin cancer initiation in mice [39].

Another study correlates the DMBA inhibition of carcinogenic action and the decrease in breast cancer incidence of *Rosmarinus officinalis* and its ability to increase the activity of glutathione S-transferase (GST) and NAD(P)H-quinone reductase (QR) that participate in the detoxification of xenobiotics in several organs [40, 41]. Supercritical fluid rosemary extract (SFRE) enhances the sensitivity of 5-Flurouracil-resistant cells in both 5-Flurouracil sensitive and resistant tumor cells [42].

Ethanolic extract of *Rosmarinus officinalis* has anti-proliferative activity on human leukemia and breast carcinoma cell lines [43]. Rosemary extract prevents oxidative damage to DNA in CaCo-2 colon cancer cells and hamster lung cells V79 through its anti-oxidant activity and scavenging of oxygen free radicals [44]. Different studies demonstrated that these anticancer activities were exhibited by the phytoconstituents such as rosmarinic acid, carnosic acid, carnosol and ursolic acid. The molecular mechanisms involved in the anticancer activity of rosemary are correlated with different effects such as antioxidant effects, anti angiogenic properties, epigenetic action, immunomodulatory, change of hormone signalling and particular metabolic pathways and overexpression of onco-suppressor genes. In the initial days, the anti-oxidant activities were correlated with its anti-cancer activity (Table **2**).

Table 2. Molecular mechanisms of cytotoxic effects of *Rosmarinus officinalis*.

Type of cancer	Molecular mechanism	Reference
Bladder	Decreases Proliferation	[45]
Breast	Decreases Proliferation Apoptosis Decreases cell transformation Decreases Tumor incidence	[43, 46]
Cervical	Decreases Proliferation	[47]

(Table 2) cont.....

Type of cancer	Molecular mechanism	Reference
Colon	Decreases Proliferation Induces Apoptosis Decreases cell transformation Decreases tumor volume	[48, 49]
Leukemia	Decrease Proliferation	[43, 46]
Liver	Decreases cell viability	[46, 50, 51]
Lung	Decreases Proliferation	[46]
Ovary	Decreases cell viability Apoptosis	[51, 52]
Pancreas	Decreases cell viability Induces Apoptosis Decreases tumor growth	[53, 54]
Prostate	Decreases Proliferation Decreases tumor growth	[46, 26]
Skin	Decrease tumor initiation	[39]
Gastric /oesophagus	Cell cycle arrest	[55]
Hepatic	Reduced apoptosis Capsase stimulation	[56, 57]
Cerebral	Early G2 inhibition; Increased apoptosis;	[58]
Urinary tract	Increased apoptosis	[59]

Carnosic acid (CA), a major polyphenolic diterpene of *Rosmarinus officinalis*, inhibits tumor growth and reduces the aspartate aminotransferase (AST) and alanine aminotransferase (ALT) levels *in vivo* [60]. Carnosic acid was reported to have a cytotoxic effect in human adenocarcinoma AGS cells, Hep G2 hepato cellular carcinoma cells and human lung fibroblasts. Inhibition of growth and stimulation of apoptosis by Carnosic acid in hepatocellular carcinoma HepG2 cells are associated with mitochondrial dysfunction, deactivation of Akt, activation of Caspase-3 and PARP cleavage [61].

Rosmarinic Acid [RA]

In the presence of phytochemicals such as carnosic acid, carnosol and ursolic acid, not only the accumulation of daunorubicin in cell line KB-C2 is increased but also the ATPase activities of P-glycoprotein are stimulated. It is noteworthy to state that carnosic acid increases the sensitivity to vinblastin in KB-C2 cells and thereby reverses multidrug resistance. Carnosol, another important phytochemical that significantly induces autophagy, apoptosis and cell cycle arrest in human osteosarcoma MG-63 through ROS generation [62]. Rosmarinic acid, a caffeic acid analogue of *Rosmarinus officinalis* exerts its anti-cancer activity through different mechanisms.

Rosmarinic acid has a pronounced effect on colon cancer in rats by impairing tumour formation and development, reducing lipid peroxidation by-products and pro-apoptotic protein expression, and increasing the expression of apoptotic proteins [63]. Rosmarinic acid has been reported for its potential inhibitory activity on microtubule affinity regulating kinase (MARK4), which is a drug target for different types of cancer and controls cell division, especially in the early stages [64]. (Anwar *et al.* 2020).

Phytochemistry of *Rosmarinus Officinalis*

Hsiu-Chen Huang *et al.* investigated that urosolic acid, a triterpenoid of rosemary, reduces interleukin-1 beta (IL-1b) or tumour necrosis factor-alpha (TNF-a- -induced C6 glioma cell invasion, and this is correlated with its suppression of activation of NF-kB and downregulation of the MMP-9 protein. It has also been shown to inhibit the interaction between ZIP/p62 and PKC [65].

Different *in-vitro* and *in vivo* studies highlighted the effects of *Rosmarinus officinalis* extracts and phytochemicals in colon cancer. A study revealed that treatment of human colon cancer cells HT-29, HCT116 and SW480 with carnosic acid decreased the survival of these cancer cells. The gene activity of STAT3 in HCT116 cells is blocked by the inhibition of phosphorylation of JAK2 and Src kinases. Production of ROS in these cancer cells is another mechanism involved in the anti-cancer activity of carnosic acid [66].

The phytochemical constituents such as carnosic acid and carnosol modify the protein homeostasis in colon cancer cells by different mechanisms. Carnosic acid enhances the formation of proteins involved in unfolded protein response, mirroring endoplasmic reticulum stress, while carnosol stops the chymotrypsin-like activity of the 20S proteasome [67]. The various molecular mechanisms of rosmarinic acid are represented in the following (Fig. **3**).

A study revealed that rosemary extract shows anti-cancer activity by modifying the cell cycle, especially the G0/G1 phase and the G2/M phase [68]. Dietary carnosol reduced the intestinal tumors' multiplication in a mouse model. Carnosol increased -catenin levels and decreased -catenin phosphorylation at the intestinal enterocyte membrane [69]. On daily administration, an extract of *Rosmarinus officinalis* decreased the growth of colorectal cancer *in vivo* by interrupting RNA post-transcriptional modification, metabolism of amino acids, synthesis of proteins, and inactivation of an oncogene [70].

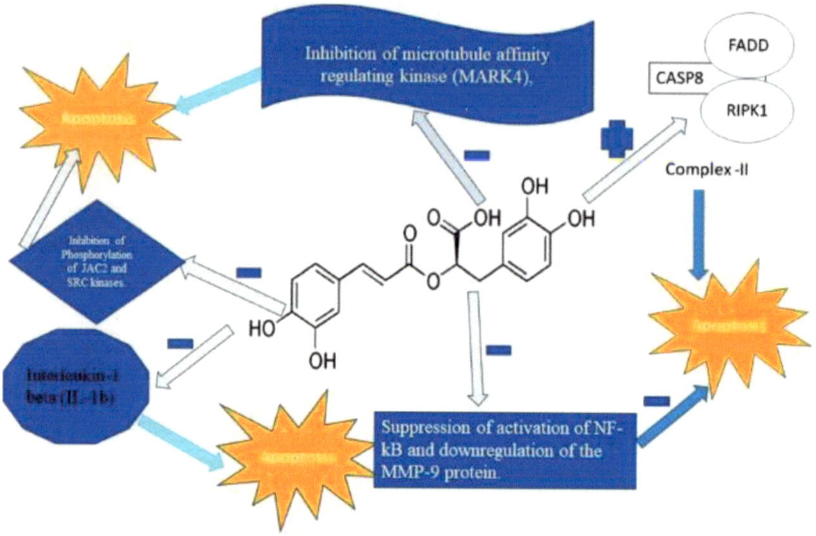

Fig. (3). Molecular mechanisms of Rosmarinic acid in causing cellular apoptosis in cancer cells. Casp8: caspases 8, FADD: Fas associated death domain.

Certain *in vivo* studies have revealed different probable mechanisms, including the reduction of serum miR-15b and other biomarkers of colorectal cancer such as colon cancer-specific antigen-4 and carcinoembryonic antigen, for the anticancer activity of *Rosmarinus officinalis* [71 - 74]. An *in vivo* study using an extract of *Rosmarinus officinalis* in olive oil on HCT116 colon cancer xenografted mice confirmed a reduction in tumour volume in treated animals [75].

An *in vitro* study demonstrated that an extract of *Rosmarinus officinalis* fruit exhibits remarkable cytotoxic activity on gastric cancer cells (AGSs) and KYSE30 cell lines. Cell cycle analysis revealed that Rosmarinus officinalis extract elicits a G2/M cell cycle arrest in gastric cancer cell lines [55]. Sageone, a diterpene obtained from rosemary, induced apoptosis and programmed cell death in SNU-1 human gastric cancer cells. It increased the cytotoxicity of cisplatin in cisplatin-resistant SNU-1 cells. Sageon, when combined with a lower dose of cisplatin, exerts synergistic activity on apoptosis in SNU-1 cells. The combination of sageon and cisplatin was reported to increase the levels of cleaved caspase-3 and caspase-9 [76].

In pancreatic cancer cells and colon cancer cells such as PANC-1, MIA-PaCa-2, SW620, and DLD-1, an increase in the metabolically related gene GCNT3 and a decrease in its potential epigenetic modulator miR-15b are correlated with the anticancer potential of *Rosmarinus officinalis* extract [74]. Rosmarinus officinalis has been extensively reported for its hepatoprotective activity. Ochratoxin- and aflatoxin-induced cell damage, ROS levels, and caspase-3 stimulation have been reduced when HepG2 liver cancer cells are treated with rosmarinic acid [56].

Rosmarinic acid, on the other hand, raises the amount of mRNA for caspase-8, NFBIA, TNFSF9, and Jun while lowering the amount of mRNA for Bcl-2 Lin, C., *et al.*, 2007 [77].Two different studies demonstrated that rosmarinic acid reduces the cell viability of Hep-3B liver tumour cells and increases MRP2 concentrations, Nrf2 nuclear translocation, ARE-luciferin activity, intracellular ATP levels, and efflux of p-glycoprotein [78]. (Wu *et al.* 2016). The essential oil obtained from Rosmarinus officinalis has cytotoxic effects on Bel-7402 cells [51] (Wang *et al.* 2012), and its extract reduces cell viability in a dose-dependent manner with an IC50 of 22.88 g/mL [46].

The effects of *Rosmarinus officinalis* extract on the growth and programmed cell death of human non-small cell lung cancer (NSCLC) cells and its effects on signalling events were studied by Moore *et al.* This study revealed that the rosemary extract inhibited cell growth and decreased the survival of NSCLC adenocarcinoma A549 cells, increased programmed cell death, and significantly decreased total and phosphorylated Akt, p70S6K, and mTOR levels [79].

RA reduces cell proliferation in NCI-H82 and A549 lung tumour cell lines, and this activity was correlated with decreased hCOX2 function (Xu *et al.* 2010). A case study linked rosemary consumption to a lower overall risk of lung tumour development (Fortes *et al.*, 2003). Based on this, different studies were carried out on animal models. Administration of rosmarinic acid to Lewis lung carcinoma (LLC) xenografted mice produced a significant reduction in cancer cells [80]. Cisplatin, in combination with carnosic acid, significantly increased the anti-proliferation effects and apoptosis in LLC xenografts. This synergistic activity is linked to improved CD8+ T cell function and increased IFN-, perforin, granzyme B, and FasL production [81 - 82].

Another study demonstrated that the percentage of myeloid-derived suppressor cells (MDSC) in cancer cells was decreased by the administration of carnosic acid. A study reported that carnosic acid has an anti-proliferative effect on human glioblastoma (GBM) cells. In these cells, carnosic acid enhances early G2 inhibition, increases the expression of p21 WAF, decreases the fraction of cells presenting Ki67, and increases apoptosis. Carnosic acid also increased the degradation of several proteins such as SOX2, retinoblastoma (RB), Cyclin B1, and glial fibrillary acid protein (GFAP), while MYC concentrations were unaltered [83]. (Cortese *et al.* 2016). Another study revealed that carnosic acid induces the production of nerve growth factor (NGF), controlled by the Nrf2 signalling pathway [84, 85].

Carnosic acid increases apoptosis by stimulating caspases and the p38 MAPK in IMR-32 neuroblastoma cells, whereas in SH-SY5Y neuroblastoma cells, CA reduces apoptosis induced by the neurotoxic substance's methylglyoxal and amyloid β, thereby causing cytoprotective action on tumour cells. This cytoprotective activity was interrelated with the improved stimulation of PI3K/Akt signalling, the blocking of cytochrome c release, and the reduction of caspase cascades [86, 87].

Carnosic acid reduces amyloid peptide generation and delivery in U373MG astrocytoma cells and is associated with the stimulation of the -secretase TACE/ADAM17 [88]. Cytotoxic effects and a reduction in the development of cell growth were observed with essential oils obtained from *Rosmarinus officinalis* in various ovarian cancer cell lines [51, 89, 90]. *Rosmarinus officinalis* also showed cytotoxic effects on skin cancer cells.

Carnosol's anti-cancer activity was demonstrated in various cell lines by inhibiting transcription and blocking the diffusion and phosphorylation of specific kinases [65]. In several cell lines, carnosic acid reduced cell viability, adhesion, and diffusion, increased programmed cell death, and caused cell cycle arrest [91, 92].

Topical applications of Carnosol before the administration of 12O-tetradecanoylphorbol-13-acetate (TPA) twice a week significantly decreased the number of papillomas in dimethylbenz(o)anthracene (DMBA)-induced mouse skin cancer. This cytoprotective activity was correlated with its inhibitory action on the TPA-induced stimulation of the ornithine decarboxylase enzyme, an important marker of cancer. Tong *et al.* demonstrated that carnosol absorbs UVB radiation and decreases DNA damage by reducing the UVB-induced reactive ROS and cyclobutane pyrimidine dimers (CPD) production in keratinocytes.

In different studies, it was analysed that rosemary extract prolonged the latency time and reduced the occurrence, size, and load of DMBA and Croton oil-induced mouse skin cancers [93, 94].

Carnosic acid exhibits an inhibitory effect on oral cancer by modifying the expression of different proliferative, apoptotic, inflammatory, and angiogenic components such as c-fos, PCNA, cyclin D1, caspases 3 and 9, Bcl-2, p53, COX-2, NFkB, and VEGF and facilitating the blocking of altered cell growth. Carnosic acid triggered programmed cell death *via* ROS-caused endoplasmic reticular stress and increased the apoptotic markers in human kidney cancer cell lines.

Likewise, rosemary extract produced a noticeable cytotoxic effect on urinary bladder carcinoma cells [59].

The cytotoxic effects of rosemary extract and its phytochemicals on prostate cancer cell types have been widely analyzed. In cancer cell lines 22Rv1 and LNCaP, rosemary extract reduced androgen receptor expression. Different *in vivo* studies revealed that rosemary extract exhibits a 46% reduction in cancer proliferation in xenografted mouse models. Many studies have evidenced the anti-growth properties of carnosol in a time- and dose-dependent manner in prostatic small cell neuroendocrine carcinoma (SCNC) PC3 cells.

Johnson *et al.* studied the effects of carnosol in the cell cycle and demonstrated that carnosol stimulated cell cycle blockade at the G2 phase, increased regulatory proteins such as p21 and p27, reduced cyclin-dependent kinase (cdk) proteins 2 and 6, and cyclin-A, -D1, and -D2. The same study investigated whether carnosol reduces prostate cancer proliferation by blocking the PI3K/Akt and 5′-adenosine monophosphate-activated protein kinase (AMPK) pathways and by reducing the phosphorylation of mTOR, which is a potential therapeutic target [95].

Rosemary extract was reported to interfere with the survival of breast cancer cell lines. Carnosol exerts its anti-cancer activity by interfering with the estrogen receptor (ER) signalling pathway, especially with the ER beta pathway and increased ER/ER ratio. A study found that Carnosol induced ROS-dependent programmed cell death and beciln1-independent autophagy in a triple-negative breast cancer (TNBC) cell line and promoted cell cycle arrest at the G2 phase. In ER-negative human breast cancer cells, carnosol stimulated the expression of genes involved in glutathione synthesis (CYP4F3, GCLC) and transport (SLC7A11). Whereas at high doses it reduced the expression of genes involved in the inhibition of transcription (ID3) and the cell cycle (CDKN2C), carnosol also stimulated the expression of apoptotic genes and certain genes such as AKR1C2, TNXRD1, and HMOX1 involved in anti-oxidant action [96 - 98].

The rosemary extracts and their components have also been reported for their pronounced effects on hematological neoplasms. Rosemary extract demonstrated a reduction in cancer cell growth in the leukemia HL-60, K-562 human cell lines and the murine RAW264.7 cell lines. Rosmarinic acid reduced cancer cell survival, ROS-induced programmed cell death, TNF-α-caused NF-κB activation and ROS production and induced apoptosis in K-562 and U937 leukaemia cell lines [99, 100].

ROSMARINUS OFFICINALIS AS A POTENT ADJUVANT IN CANCER THERAPY

Rosemary and its phytochemical constituents have been shown to reduce chemoresistance and improve chemotherapeutic effects. Table **3** describes the synergic effect of rosemary on chemotherapeutics.

Table 3. Synergic effects of *Rosmarinus officinalis* with anti cancer agents

Anti-cancer drug	Rosemary and its phytoconstituents	Molecular mechanism	Reference
Daunorubicin	Carnosic acid. Carnosol	Accumulation of daunorubicin by increasing the action of ATPase action of P-glycoprotein	[101]
Vinblastine	Carnosic acid Methanolic Extract	Increases the sensitivity to KB-C2 cells in drug-resistant tumors Increases the intracellular accumulation.	[101, 102]
Doxorubicin	Methanolic Extract	Increases the intracellular accumulation.	[102]
5-Fluorouracil	Supercritical fluid rosemary extract (SFRE)	Increases the sensitivity of 5-Fluorouracil by decreasing the TYMS and TK1 enzyme.	[103]
Etoposide	Rosemary Extract	Protects healthy cells from the negative effects of etoposide.	[104]
Cisplatin	Rosemary extract Carnosic acid, Carnosol and Rosmarinic acid.	Synergize with cisplatin in drug-sensitive cells.	[105]
Carmustine and Lomustine	Carnosic acid	Increase cytotoxicity and stimulate cell cycle arrest.	[106]
Tamoxifen	Rosemary extract	Increases the anticancer activity	[107]
Paclitaxel	Rosemary extract	Increases the anticancer activity	[107]
Trastuzumab	Rosemary extract	Increases the anticancer activity	[107]

CONCLUSION

Cancer, is one of the dreadful diseases characterized by uncontrolled cell division and growth and affects millions of people in the world. Recently, anti-cancer drug development has been focused in the search for alternative therapies to lessen the life-threatening side effects and improve patient compliance with the existing chemotherapy. *Rosmarinus officinalis,* one of the culinary herbs, has been reported to possess anti-cancer potentials. Rosemary extract showed anti-cancer activity against different types of cancer including skin cancer, leukaemia, prostate cancer, breast cancer and lung cancer.

Essential oil obtained from *Rosmarinus officinalis* has cytotoxic activity on different cancer cell lines. Different studies have demonstrated the anti-cancer activity of phytochemicals of *Rosmarinus officinalis* such as Rosmarinic acid, carnosic acid, carnosol, ursolic acid and sageone. The anti-cancer activity of *Rosmarinus officinalis* is exhibited by stimulating apoptosis, reducing cell growth, cell cycle arrest, ROS scavenging and reducing the expression of oncogenes. Rosemary extract and its phytoconstituents synergize the anti-cancer activity and sensitivity of chemotherapeutic agents like 5-Flouro uracil, etoposide, paclitaxel, carmustine, lomustine, vinblastine, daunorubicin and cisplatin. Over all *Rosmarinus officinalis* have been shown to have several anti-cancer potentials and more studies are required to analyze its toxic effects on chronic administration.

REFERENCES

[1] Available from: https://www.who.int/news-room/fact-sheets/detail/cancer

[2] Cragg GM, Newman DJ. Natural products: A continuing source of novel drug leads. Biochim Biophys Acta, Gen Subj 2013; 1830(6): 3670-95. [http://dx.doi.org/10.1016/j.bbagen.2013.02.008] [PMID: 23428572]

[3] Sasikumar B. 25 - Rosemary, Food science, Technology and Nutrition, number 227, Handbook of herbs and spices, woodhead publishing, 2012, pages 452-463.

[4] Cuvelier ME, Richard H, Berset C. Antioxidative activity and phenolic composition of pilot-plant and commercial extracts of sage and rosemary. J Am Oil Chem Soc 1996; 73(5): 645-52. [http://dx.doi.org/10.1007/BF02518121]

[5] Ibañez E, Kubátová A, Señoráns FJ, Cavero S, Reglero G, Hawthorne SB. Subcritical water extraction of antioxidant compounds from rosemary plants. J Agric Food Chem 2003; 51(2): 375-82. [http://dx.doi.org/10.1021/jf025878j] [PMID: 12517098]

[6] González-Trujano ME, Peña EI, Martínez AL, *et al.* Evaluation of the antinociceptive effect of Rosmarinus officinalis L. using three different experimental models in rodents. J Ethnopharmacol 2007; 111(3): 476-82. [http://dx.doi.org/10.1016/j.jep.2006.12.011] [PMID: 17223299]

[7] Yamamoto J, Yamada K, Naemura A, Yamashita T, Arai R. Testing various herbs for antithrombotic effect. Nutrition 2005; 21(5): 580-7. [http://dx.doi.org/10.1016/j.nut.2004.09.016] [PMID: 15850964]

[8] Corrêa Dias P, Foglio MA, Possenti A, de Carvalho JE. Antiulcerogenic activity of crude hydroalcoholic extract of Rosmarinus officinalis L. J Ethnopharmacol 2000; 69(1): 57-62. [http://dx.doi.org/10.1016/S0378-8741(99)00133-6] [PMID: 10661884]

[9] Rašković A, Milanović I, Pavlović N, Ćebović T, Vukmirović S, Mikov M. Antioxidant activity of rosemary (Rosmarinus officinalis L.) essential oil and its hepatoprotective potential. BMC Complement Altern Med 2014; 14(1): 225. [http://dx.doi.org/10.1186/1472-6882-14-225] [PMID: 25002023]

[10] Oliviero F, Scanu A, Zamudio-Cuevas Y, Punzi L, Spinella P. Anti-inflammatory effects of polyphenols in arthritis. J Sci Food Agric 2018; 98(5): 1653-9. [http://dx.doi.org/10.1002/jsfa.8664] [PMID: 28886220]

[11] Tagousop CN, Tamokou JD, Ekom SE, Ngnokam D, Voutquenne-Nazabadioko L. Antimicrobial activities of flavonoid glycosides from Graptophyllum grandulosum and their mechanism of

antibacterial action. BMC Complement Altern Med 2018; 18(1): 252.
[http://dx.doi.org/10.1186/s12906-018-2321-7] [PMID: 30219066]

[12] Kim G, Dasagrandhi C, Kang E-H, Eom S-H, Kim Y-M. *In vitro* antibacterial and early stage biofilm inhibitory potential of an edible chitosan and its phenolic conjugates against Pseudomonas aeruginosa and Listeria monocytogenes. Biotech 2018; 8(10): 439.

[13] Ložienė K, Švedienė J, Paškevičius A, Raudonienė V, Sytar O, Kosyan A. Influence of plant origin natural α-pinene with different enantiomeric composition on bacteria, yeasts and fungi. Fitoterapia 2018; 127: 20-4.
[http://dx.doi.org/10.1016/j.fitote.2018.04.013] [PMID: 29689330]

[14] Manoharan RK, Lee JH, Lee J. Antibiofilm and antihyphal activities of cedar leaf essential oil, camphor, and fenchone derivatives against candida albicans. Front Microbiol 2017; 8: 1476.
[http://dx.doi.org/10.3389/fmicb.2017.01476] [PMID: 28824600]

[15] Ramírez J, Gilardoni G, Ramón E, *et al.* Phytochemical Study of the Ecuadorian Species *Lepechinia mutica* (Benth.) Epling and High Antifungal Activity of Carnosol against *Pyricularia oryzae.* Pharmaceuticals (Basel) 2018; 11(2): 33.
[http://dx.doi.org/10.3390/ph11020033] [PMID: 29671794]

[16] Leal Pinto SM, Herrera Sandoval LV, Vargas LY. In vitro susceptibility of *Microsporum* spp. and mammalian cells to *Eugenia caryophyllus* essential oil, eugenol and semisynthetic derivatives. Mycoses 2019; 62(1): 41-50.
[http://dx.doi.org/10.1111/myc.12844] [PMID: 30144163]

[17] Cattaneo L, Cicconi R, Mignogna G, *et al.* Anti-proliferative effect of Rosmarinus officinalis L. extract on human melanoma A375 cells. PLoS One 2015; 10(7): e0132439.
[http://dx.doi.org/10.1371/journal.pone.0132439] [PMID: 26176704]

[18] Sharmila R, Manoharan S. Anti-tumor activity of rosmarinic acid in 7,12-dimethylbenz(a)anthracene (DMBA) induced skin carcinogenesis in Swiss albino mice. Indian J Exp Biol 2012; 50(3): 187-94.
[PMID: 22439433]

[19] Umasankar K, Nambikkairaj B, Backyavathy DM. Effect of topical treatment of rosmarinus officinalis essential oil on wound healing in streptozotocin induced diabetic rats. Nat Environ Pollut Technol 2012; 11: 607-11.

[20] Nejati H, Farahpour MR, Nagadehi MN. Topical Rosemary officinalis essential oil improves wound healing against disseminated Candida albicans infection in rat model. Comp Clin Pathol 2015; 24(6): 1377-83.
[http://dx.doi.org/10.1007/s00580-015-2086-z]

[21] Liu Q, Tang GY, Zhao CN, *et al.* Comparison of antioxidant activities of different grape varieties. Molecules 2018; 23(10): 2432.
[http://dx.doi.org/10.3390/molecules23102432] [PMID: 30249027]

[22] de Lima ME, Ceolin Colpo AZ, Maya-López M, *et al.* Comparing the effects of chlorogenic acid and Ilex paraguariensis extracts on different markers of brain alterations in rats subjected to chronic restraint stress. Neurotox Res 2019; 35(2): 373-86.
[http://dx.doi.org/10.1007/s12640-018-9963-6] [PMID: 30267269]

[23] Liu D, Wang B, Zhu Y, Yan F, Dong W. Carnosic acid regulates cell proliferation and invasion in chronic myeloid leukemia cancer cells *via* suppressing microRNA-708. J BUON 2018; 23(3): 741-6.
[PMID: 30003745]

[24] Ma ZJ, Yan H, Wang YJ, *et al.* Proteomics analysis demonstrating rosmarinic acid suppresses cell growth by blocking the glycolytic pathway in human HepG2 cells. Biomed Pharmacother 2018; 105: 334-49.
[http://dx.doi.org/10.1016/j.biopha.2018.05.129] [PMID: 29864622]

[25] Radziejewska I, Supruniuk K, Nazaruk J, *et al.* Rosmarinic acid influences collagen, MMPs, TIMPs, glycosylation and MUC1 in CRL-1739 gastric cancer cell line. Biomed Pharmacother 2018; 107: 397-407.
[http://dx.doi.org/10.1016/j.biopha.2018.07.123] [PMID: 30099344]

[26] Petiwala SM, Johnson JJ. Diterpenes from rosemary (Rosmarinus officinalis): Defining their potential for anti-cancer activity. Cancer Lett 2015; 367(2): 93-102.
[http://dx.doi.org/10.1016/j.canlet.2015.07.005] [PMID: 26170168]

[27] Lai Y, Li Y, Fu L, *et al.* Combinations of 1,8-cineol and oseltamivir for the treatment of influenza virus A (H3N2) infection in mice. J Med Virol 2017; 89(7): 1158-67.
[http://dx.doi.org/10.1002/jmv.24755] [PMID: 27966790]

[28] Khwaza V, Oyedeji O, Aderibigbe B. Antiviral activities of oleanolic acid and its analogues. Molecules 2018; 23(9): 2300.
[http://dx.doi.org/10.3390/molecules23092300] [PMID: 30205592]

[29] Zhang X-J, Cui H-Y, Yang Y, *et al.* Rosmarinic acid elicits neuroprotection in ischemic stroke *via* Nrf2 and heme oxygenase 1 signaling. Neural Regen Res 2018; 13(12): 2119-28.
[http://dx.doi.org/10.4103/1673-5374.241463] [PMID: 30323140]

[30] Makhathini KB, Mabandla MV, Daniels WMU. Rosmarinic acid reverses the deleterious effects of repetitive stress and tat protein. Behav Brain Res 2018; 353: 203-9.
[http://dx.doi.org/10.1016/j.bbr.2018.07.010] [PMID: 30029998]

[31] Samarghandian S, Borji A, Farkhondeh T. Evaluation of antidiabetic activity of carnosol (phenolic diterpene in Rosemary) in streptozotocin-induced diabetic rats. Cardiovasc Hematol Disord Drug Targets 2017; 17(1): 11-7.
[PMID: 28034282]

[32] Mourya A, Akhtar A, Ahuja S, Sah SP, Kumar A. Synergistic action of ursolic acid and metformin in experimental model of insulin resistance and related behavioral alterations. Eur J Pharmacol 2018; 835: 31-40.
[http://dx.doi.org/10.1016/j.ejphar.2018.07.056] [PMID: 30075220]

[33] Abu-Gharbieh E, Shehab NG, Almasri IM, Bustanji Y. Antihyperuricemic and xanthine oxidase inhibitory activities of *Tribulus arabicus* and its isolated compound, ursolic acid: *In vitro* and *in vivo* investigation and docking simulations. PLoS One 2018; 13(8): e0202572.
[http://dx.doi.org/10.1371/journal.pone.0202572] [PMID: 30114281]

[34] Yao Y, Mao J, Xu S, *et al.* Rosmarinic acid inhibits nicotine–induced C–reactive protein generation by inhibiting NLRP3 inflammasome activation in smooth muscle cells. J Cell Physiol 2019; 234(2): 1758-67.
[http://dx.doi.org/10.1002/jcp.27046] [PMID: 30146678]

[35] Andrade JM, Faustino C, Garcia C, Ladeiras D, Reis CP, Rijo P. *Rosmarinus officinalis* L.: an update review of its phytochemistry and biological activity. Future Sci OA 2018; 4(4): FSO283.
[http://dx.doi.org/10.4155/fsoa-2017-0124] [PMID: 29682318]

[36] Raghavendra NM, Pingili D, Kadasi S, Mettu A, Prasad SVUM. Dual or multi-targeting inhibitors: The next generation anticancer agents. Eur J Med Chem 2018; 143: 1277-300.
[http://dx.doi.org/10.1016/j.ejmech.2017.10.021] [PMID: 29126724]

[37] Elansary HO, Abdelgaleil SAM, Mahmoud EA, Yessoufou K, Elhindi K, El-Hendawy S. Effective antioxidant, antimicrobial and anticancer activities of essential oils of horticultural aromatic crops in northern Egypt. BMC Complement Altern Med 2018; 18(1): 214.
[http://dx.doi.org/10.1186/s12906-018-2262-1] [PMID: 30005652]

[38] Amar Y, Meddah B, Bonacorsi I, *et al.* Phytochemicals, antioxidant and antiproliferative properties of Rosmarinus officinalis L on U937 and CaCo-2 cells. Iran J Pharm Res 2017; 16(1): 315-27.
[PMID: 28496485]

[39] Huang MT, Ho CT, Wang ZY, *et al.* Inhibition of skin tumorigenesis by rosemary and its constituents carnosol and ursolic acid. Cancer Res 1994; 54(3): 701-8. [PMID: 8306331]

[40] Singletary KW. Rosemary extract and carnosol stimulate rat liver glutathione-S-transferase and quinone reductase activities. Cancer Lett 1996; 100(1-2): 139-44. [http://dx.doi.org/10.1016/0304-3835(95)04082-X] [PMID: 8620433]

[41] Singletary K, MacDonald C, Wallig M. Inhibition by rosemary and carnosol of 7,12-dimethylbenz[a]anthracene (DMBA)-induced rat mammary tumorigenesis and *in vivo* DMBA-DNA adduct formation. Cancer Lett 1996; 104(1): 43-8. [http://dx.doi.org/10.1016/0304-3835(96)04227-9] [PMID: 8640744]

[42] González-Vallinas M, Molina S, Vicente G, *et al.* Antitumor effect of 5-fluorouracil is enhanced by rosemary extract in both drug sensitive and resistant colon cancer cells. Pharmacol Res 2013; 72: 61-8. [http://dx.doi.org/10.1016/j.phrs.2013.03.010] [PMID: 23557932]

[43] Cheung S, Tai J. Anti-proliferative and antioxidant properties of rosemary Rosmarinus officinalis. Oncol Rep 2007; 17(6): 1525-31. [http://dx.doi.org/10.3892/or.17.6.1525] [PMID: 17487414]

[44] Slameňová D, Kubošková K, Horváthová E, Robichová S. Rosemary-stimulated reduction of DNA strand breaks and FPG-sensitive sites in mammalian cells treated with H2O2 or visible light-excited Methylene Blue. Cancer Lett 2002; 177(2): 145-53. [http://dx.doi.org/10.1016/S0304-3835(01)00784-4] [PMID: 11825661]

[45] Mothana RAA, Kriegisch S, Harms M, Wende K, Lindequist U. Assessment of selected Yemeni medicinal plants for their *in vitro* antimicrobial, anticancer, and antioxidant activities. Pharm Biol 2011; 49(2): 200-10. [http://dx.doi.org/10.3109/13880209.2010.512295] [PMID: 20942618]

[46] Yesil-Celiktas O, Sevimli C, Bedir E, Vardar-Sukan F. Inhibitory effects of rosemary extracts, carnosic acid and rosmarinic acid on the growth of various human cancer cell lines. Plant Foods Hum Nutr 2010; 65(2): 158-63. [http://dx.doi.org/10.1007/s11130-010-0166-4] [PMID: 20449663]

[47] Berrington D, Lall N. Anticancer activity of certain herbs and spices on the cervical epithelial carcinoma (HeLa) cell line. Evid Based Complement Alternat Med 2012; 2012: 1-11. [http://dx.doi.org/10.1155/2012/564927] [PMID: 22649474]

[48] Valdés A, García-Cañas V, Artemenko KA, Simó C, Bergquist J, Cifuentes A. Nano-liquid chromatography-orbitrap MS-based quantitative proteomics reveals differences between the mechanisms of action of carnosic acid and carnosol in colon cancer cells. Mol Cell Proteomics 2017; 16(1): 8-22. [http://dx.doi.org/10.1074/mcp.M116.061481] [PMID: 27834734]

[49] Ibáñez C, Simó C, García-Cañas V, Gómez-Martínez Á, Ferragut JA, Cifuentes A. CE/LC-MS multiplatform for broad metabolomic analysis of dietary polyphenols effect on colon cancer cells proliferation. Electrophoresis 2012; 33(15): 2328-36. [http://dx.doi.org/10.1002/elps.201200143] [PMID: 22887153]

[50] Peng CH, Su JD, Chyau CC, *et al.* Supercritical fluid extracts of rosemary leaves exhibit potent anti-inflammation and anti-tumor effects. Biosci Biotechnol Biochem 2007; 71(9): 2223-32. [http://dx.doi.org/10.1271/bbb.70199] [PMID: 17827696]

[51] Wang W, Li N, Luo M, Zu Y, Efferth T. Antibacterial activity and anticancer activity of Rosmarinus officinalis L. essential oil compared to that of its main components. Molecules 2012; 17(3): 2704-13. [http://dx.doi.org/10.3390/molecules17032704] [PMID: 22391603]

[52] Tai J, Cheung S, Wu M, Hasman D. Antiproliferation effect of Rosemary (Rosmarinus officinalis) on human ovarian cancer cells *in vitro.* Phytomedicine 2012; 19(5): 436-43.

[http://dx.doi.org/10.1016/j.phymed.2011.12.012] [PMID: 22325591]

[53] González-Vallinas M, Molina S, Vicente G, *et al.* Expression of microRNA-15b and the glycosyltransferase GCNT3 correlates with antitumor efficacy of Rosemary diterpenes in colon and pancreatic cancer. PLoS One 2014; 9(6): e98556.
[http://dx.doi.org/10.1371/journal.pone.0098556] [PMID: 24892299]

[54] Kontogianni VG, Tomic G, Nikolic I, *et al.* Phytochemical profile of Rosmarinus officinalis and Salvia officinalis extracts and correlation to their antioxidant and anti-proliferative activity. Food Chem 2013; 136(1): 120-9.
[http://dx.doi.org/10.1016/j.foodchem.2012.07.091] [PMID: 23017402]

[55] Karimi N, Rashedi J, Mahdavi Poor B, *et al.* Cytotoxic effect of rosemary extract on gastric adenocarcinoma (AGS) and esophageal squamous cell carcinoma (KYSE30) cell lines. Gastroenterol Hepatol Bed Bench 2017; 10(2): 102-7.
[PMID: 28702133]

[56] Renzulli C, Galvano F, Pierdomenico L, Speroni E, Guerra MC. Effects of rosmarinic acid against aflatoxin B1 and ochratoxin-A-induced cell damage in a human hepatoma cell line(Hep G2). J Appl Toxicol 2004; 24(4): 289-96.
[http://dx.doi.org/10.1002/jat.982] [PMID: 15300717]

[57] Lin CS, Kuo CL, Wang JP, Cheng JS, Huang ZW, Chen CF. Growth inhibitory and apoptosis inducing effect of Perilla frutescens extract on human hepatoma HepG2 cells. J Ethnopharmacol 2007; 112(3): 557-67.
[http://dx.doi.org/10.1016/j.jep.2007.05.008] [PMID: 17574356]

[58] Cortese K, Daga A, Monticone M, *et al.* Carnosic acid induces proteasomal degradation of Cyclin B1, RB and SOX2 along with cell growth arrest and apoptosis in GBM cells. Phytomedicine 2016; 23(7): 679-85.
[http://dx.doi.org/10.1016/j.phymed.2016.03.007] [PMID: 27235706]

[59] Min K, Jung KJ, Kwon TK. Carnosic acid induces apoptosis through reactive oxygen species-mediated endoplasmic reticulum stress induction in human renal carcinoma Caki cells. J Cancer Prev 2014; 19(3): 170-8.
[http://dx.doi.org/10.15430/JCP.2014.19.3.170] [PMID: 25337586]

[60] Lin KI, Lin CC, Kuo SM, *et al.* Carnosic acid impedes cell growth and enhances anticancer effects of carmustine and lomustine in melanoma. Biosci Rep 2018; 38(4): BSR20180005.
[http://dx.doi.org/10.1042/BSR20180005] [PMID: 29789400]

[61] Xiang Q, Ma Y, Dong J, Shen R. Carnosic acid induces apoptosis associated with mitochondrial dysfunction and Akt inactivation in HepG2 cells. Int J Food Sci Nutr 2015; 66(1): 76-84.
[http://dx.doi.org/10.3109/09637486.2014.953452] [PMID: 25265205]

[62] Lo YC, Lin YC, Huang YF, *et al.* Carnosol-induced ROS inhibits cell viability of human osteosarcoma by apoptosis and autophagy. Am J Chin Med 2017; 45(8): 1761-72.
[http://dx.doi.org/10.1142/S0192415X17500951] [PMID: 29121803]

[63] Venkatachalam K, Gunasekaran S, Namasivayam N. Biochemical and molecular mechanisms underlying the chemopreventive efficacy of rosmarinic acid in a rat colon cancer. Eur J Pharmacol 2016; 791: 37-50.
[http://dx.doi.org/10.1016/j.ejphar.2016.07.051] [PMID: 27565219]

[64] Anwar S, Shamsi A, Shahbaaz M, *et al.* Rosmarinic acid exhibits anticancer effects *via* MARK4 inhibition. Sci Rep 2020; 10(1): 10300.
[http://dx.doi.org/10.1038/s41598-020-65648-z] [PMID: 32587267]

[65] Huang HC, Huang CY, Lin-Shiau SY, Lin JK. Ursolic acid inhibits IL-1β or TNF-α-induced C6 glioma invasion through suppressing the association ZIP/p62 with PKC-ζ and downregulating the MMP-9 expression. Mol Carcinog 2009; 48(6): 517-31.
[http://dx.doi.org/10.1002/mc.20490] [PMID: 18973186]

[66] Kim DH, Park KW, Chae IG, *et al.* Carnosic acid inhibits STAT3 signaling and induces apoptosis through generation of ROS in human colon cancer HCT116 cells. Mol Carcinog 2016; 55(6): 1096-110.
[http://dx.doi.org/10.1002/mc.22353] [PMID: 26152521]

[67] Valdés A, García-Cañas V, Pérez-Sánchez A, *et al.* Shotgun proteomic analysis to study the decrease of xenograft tumor growth after rosemary extract treatment. J Chromatogr A 2017; 1499: 90-100.
[http://dx.doi.org/10.1016/j.chroma.2017.03.072] [PMID: 28389096]

[68] Pérez-Sánchez A, Barrajón-Catalán E, Ruiz-Torres V, *et al.* Rosemary (Rosmarinus officinalis) extract causes ROS-induced necrotic cell death and inhibits tumor growth *in vivo.* Sci Rep 2019; 9(1): 808.
[http://dx.doi.org/10.1038/s41598-018-37173-7] [PMID: 30692565]

[69] Moran AE, Carothers AM, Weyant MJ, Redston M, Bertagnolli MM. Carnosol inhibits beta-catenin tyrosine phosphorylation and prevents adenoma formation in the C57BL/6J/Min/+ (Min/+) mouse. Cancer Res 2005; 65(3): 1097-104.
[http://dx.doi.org/10.1158/0008-5472.1097.65.3] [PMID: 15705912]

[70] Valdés A, García-Cañas V, Pérez-Sánchez A, *et al.* Shotgun proteomic analysis to study the decrease of xenograft tumor growth after rosemary extract treatment. J Chromatogr A 2017; 1499: 90-100.
[http://dx.doi.org/10.1016/j.chroma.2017.03.072] [PMID: 28389096]

[71] Campo S, Allegra A, D'Ascola A, *et al.* MiRNome expression is deregulated in the peripheral lymphoid compartment of multiple myeloma. Br J Haematol 2014; 165(6): 801-13.
[http://dx.doi.org/10.1111/bjh.12828] [PMID: 24620752]

[72] Allegra A, Alonci A, Campo S, *et al.* Circulating microRNAs: New biomarkers in diagnosis, prognosis and treatment of cancer (Review). Int J Oncol 2012; 41(6): 1897-912.
[http://dx.doi.org/10.3892/ijo.2012.1647] [PMID: 23026890]

[73] Innao V, Allegra A, Pulvirenti N, Allegra AG, Musolino C. Therapeutic potential of antagomiRs in haematological and oncological neoplasms. Eur J Cancer Care (Engl) 2020; 29(2): e13208.
[http://dx.doi.org/10.1111/ecc.13208] [PMID: 31899849]

[74] González-Vallinas M, Reglero G, Ramírez de Molina A. Rosemary (Rosmarinus officinalis L.) extract as a potential complementary agent in anticancer therapy. Nutr Cancer 2015; 67(8): 1223-31.
[http://dx.doi.org/10.1080/01635581.2015.1082110] [PMID: 26452641]

[75] Kim DH, Park KW, Chae IG, *et al.* Carnosic acid inhibits STAT3 signaling and induces apoptosis through generation of ROS in human colon cancer HCT116 cells. Mol Carcinog 2016; 55(6): 1096-110.
[http://dx.doi.org/10.1002/mc.22353] [PMID: 26152521]

[76] Shrestha S, Song YW, Kim H, Lee DS, Cho SK. Sageone, a diterpene from Rosmarinus officinalis, synergizes with cisplatin cytotoxicity in SNU-1 human gastric cancer cells. Phytomedicine 2016; 23(13): 1671-9.
[http://dx.doi.org/10.1016/j.phymed.2016.09.008] [PMID: 27823632]

[77] Lin CS, Kuo CL, Wang JP, Cheng JS, Huang ZW, Chen CF. Growth inhibitory and apoptosis inducing effect of Perilla frutescens extract on human hepatoma HepG2 cells. J Ethnopharmacol 2007; 112(3): 557-67.
[http://dx.doi.org/10.1016/j.jep.2007.05.008] [PMID: 17574356]

[78] Wu J, Zhu Y, Li F, *et al.* Spica prunellae and its marker compound rosmarinic acid induced the expression of efflux transporters through activation of Nrf2-mediated signaling pathway in HepG2 cells. J Ethnopharmacol 2016; 193: 1-11.
[http://dx.doi.org/10.1016/j.jep.2016.07.021] [PMID: 27422165]

[79] Moore J, Megaly M, MacNeil AJ, Klentrou P, Tsiani E. Rosemary extract reduces Akt/mTOR/p70S6K activation and inhibits proliferation and survival of A549 human lung cancer cells. Biomed Pharmacother 2016; 83: 725-32.

[http://dx.doi.org/10.1016/j.biopha.2016.07.043] [PMID: 27470574]

[80] Xu Y, Xu G, Liu L, Xu D, Liu J. Anti-invasion effect of rosmarinic acid *via* the extracellular signal-regulated kinase and oxidation-reduction pathway in Ls174-T cells. J Cell Biochem 2010; 111(2): 370-9.
[http://dx.doi.org/10.1002/jcb.22708] [PMID: 20506543]

[81] Fortes C, Forastiere F, Farchi S, *et al.* The protective effect of the Mediterranean diet on lung cancer. Nutr Cancer 2003; 46(1): 30-7.
[http://dx.doi.org/10.1207/S15327914NC4601_04] [PMID: 12925301]

[82] Liu W, Wu TC, Hong DM, *et al.* Carnosic acid enhances the anti-lung cancer effect of cisplatin by inhibiting myeloid-derived suppressor cells. Chin J Nat Med 2018; 16(12): 907-15.
[http://dx.doi.org/10.1016/S1875-5364(18)30132-8] [PMID: 30595215]

[83] Cortese K, Daga A, Monticone M, *et al.* Carnosic acid induces proteasomal degradation of Cyclin B1, RB and SOX2 along with cell growth arrest and apoptosis in GBM cells. Phytomedicine 2016; 23(7): 679-85.
[http://dx.doi.org/10.1016/j.phymed.2016.03.007] [PMID: 27235706]

[84] Kosaka K, Yokoi T. Carnosic acid, a component of rosemary (Rosmarinus officinalis L.), promotes synthesis of nerve growth factor in T98G human glioblastoma cells. Biol Pharm Bull 2003; 26(11): 1620-2.
[http://dx.doi.org/10.1248/bpb.26.1620] [PMID: 14600414]

[85] Mimura J, Kosaka K, Maruyama A, *et al.* Nrf2 regulates NGF mRNA induction by carnosic acid in T98G glioblastoma cells and normal human astrocytes. J Biochem 2011; 150(2): 209-17.
[http://dx.doi.org/10.1093/jb/mvr065] [PMID: 21596795]

[86] de Oliveira MR, Ferreira GC, Schuck PF, Dal Bosco SM. Role for the PI3K/Akt/Nrf2 signaling pathway in the protective effects of carnosic acid against methylglyoxal-induced neurotoxicity in SH-SY5Y neuroblastoma cells. Chem Biol Interact 2015; 242: 396-406.
[http://dx.doi.org/10.1016/j.cbi.2015.11.003] [PMID: 26577515]

[87] Meng P, Yoshida H, Tanji K, *et al.* Carnosic acid attenuates apoptosis induced by amyloid-β 1–42 or 1–43 in SH-SY5Y human neuroblastoma cells. Neurosci Res 2015; 94: 1-9.
[http://dx.doi.org/10.1016/j.neures.2014.12.003] [PMID: 25510380]

[88] Yoshida H, Meng P, Matsumiya T, *et al.* Carnosic acid suppresses the production of amyloid-β 1-42 and 1-43 by inducing an α-secretase TACE/ADAM17 in U373MG human astrocytoma cells. Neurosci Res 2014; 79: 83-93.
[http://dx.doi.org/10.1016/j.neures.2013.11.004] [PMID: 24295810]

[89] Contini A, Di Bello D, Azzarà A, *et al.* Assessing the cytotoxic/genotoxic activity and estrogenic/antiestrogenic potential of essential oils from seven aromatic plants. Food Chem Toxicol 2020; 138(111205): 111205.
[http://dx.doi.org/10.1016/j.fct.2020.111205] [PMID: 32074490]

[90] Jardak M, Elloumi-Mseddi J, Aifa S, Mnif S. Chemical composition, anti-biofilm activity and potential cytotoxic effect on cancer cells of Rosmarinus officinalis L. essential oil from Tunisia. Lipids Health Dis 2017; 16(1): 190.
[http://dx.doi.org/10.1186/s12944-017-0580-9] [PMID: 28969677]

[91] López-Jiménez A, García-Caballero M, Medina MÁ, Quesada AR. Anti-angiogenic properties of carnosol and carnosic acid, two major dietary compounds from rosemary. Eur J Nutr 2013; 52(1): 85-95.
[http://dx.doi.org/10.1007/s00394-011-0289-x] [PMID: 22173778]

[92] Park S, Song H, Sung MK, Kang YH, Lee K, Park J. Carnosic acid inhibits the epithelial-mesenchymal transition in B16F10 melanoma cells: a possible mechanism for the inhibition of cell migration. Int J Mol Sci 2014; 15(7): 12698-713.
[http://dx.doi.org/10.3390/ijms150712698] [PMID: 25036034]

[93] Sancheti G, Goyal PK. Effect of rosmarinus officinalis in modulating 7,12-dimethylbenz(a)anthracene induced skin tumorigenesis in mice. Phytother Res 2006; 20(11): 981-6. [http://dx.doi.org/10.1002/ptr.1989] [PMID: 16927448]

[94] Laurent C, Chabi B, Fouret G, *et al.* Polyphenols decreased liver NADPH oxidase activity, increased muscle mitochondrial biogenesis and decreased gastrocnemius age-dependent autophagy in aged rats. Free Radic Res 2012; 46(9): 1140-9. [http://dx.doi.org/10.3109/10715762.2012.694428] [PMID: 22607117]

[95] Johnson JJ, Syed DN, Heren CR, Suh Y, Adhami VM, Mukhtar H. Carnosol, a dietary diterpene, displays growth inhibitory effects in human prostate cancer PC3 cells leading to G2-phase cell cycle arrest and targets the 5′-AMP-activated protein kinase (AMPK) pathway. Pharm Res 2008; 25(9): 2125-34. [http://dx.doi.org/10.1007/s11095-008-9552-0] [PMID: 18286356]

[96] Zhao P, Yue-wei LEE D, Ma Z, *et al.* The antioxidant effect of carnosol in bovine aortic endothelial cells is mainly mediated *via* estrogen receptor α pathway. Biol Pharm Bull 2012; 35(11): 1947-55. [http://dx.doi.org/10.1248/bpb.b12-00325] [PMID: 22971524]

[97] Al Dhaheri Y, Attoub S, Ramadan G, *et al.* Carnosol induces ROS-mediated beclin1-independent autophagy and apoptosis in triple negative breast cancer. PLoS One 2014; 9(10): e109630. [http://dx.doi.org/10.1371/journal.pone.0109630] [PMID: 25299698]

[98] Shrivastava A, Kuzontkoski PM, Groopman JE, Prasad A. Cannabidiol induces programmed cell death in breast cancer cells by coordinating the cross-talk between apoptosis and autophagy. Mol Cancer Ther 2011; 10(7): 1161-72. [http://dx.doi.org/10.1158/1535-7163.MCT-10-1100] [PMID: 21566064]

[99] Moon DO, Kim MO, Lee JD, Choi YH, Kim GY. Rosmarinic acid sensitizes cell death through suppression of TNF-α-induced NF-κB activation and ROS generation in human leukemia U937 cells. Cancer Lett 2010; 288(2): 183-91. [http://dx.doi.org/10.1016/j.canlet.2009.06.033] [PMID: 19619938]

[100] Heo SK, Noh EK, Yoon DJ, *et al.* Rosmarinic acid potentiates ATRA-induced macrophage differentiation in acute promyelocytic leukemia NB4 cells. Eur J Pharmacol 2015; 747: 36-44. [http://dx.doi.org/10.1016/j.ejphar.2014.10.064] [PMID: 25481858]

[101] Nabekura T, Yamaki T, Hiroi T, Ueno K, Kitagawa S. Inhibition of anticancer drug efflux transporter P-glycoprotein by rosemary phytochemicals. Pharmacol Res 2010; 61(3): 259-63. [http://dx.doi.org/10.1016/j.phrs.2009.11.010] [PMID: 19944162]

[102] Ciolino HP, Clarke R, Yeh GC, Plouzek CA. Inhibition of P-glycoprotein activity and reversal of multidrug resistance *in vitro* by rosemary extract. Eur J Cancer 1999; 35(10): 1541-5. [http://dx.doi.org/10.1016/S0959-8049(99)00180-X] [PMID: 10673984]

[103] González-Vallinas M, Reglero G, Ramírez de Molina A. Rosemary (*Rosmarinus officinalis L.*) Extract as a Potential Complementary Agent in Anticancer Therapy. Nutr Cancer 2015; 67(8): 1223-31. [http://dx.doi.org/10.1080/01635581.2015.1082110] [PMID: 26452641]

[104] Ozdemir MD, Gokturk D. The effect of Rosmarinus Officinalis and chemotherapeutic etoposide on glioblastoma (U87 MG) cell culture. Turk Neurosurg 2018; 28(6): 853-7. [PMID: 29165747]

[105] Tai J, Cheung S, Wu M, Hasman D. Antiproliferation effect of Rosemary (Rosmarinus officinalis) on human ovarian cancer cells *in vitro*. Phytomedicine 2012; 19(5): 436-43. [http://dx.doi.org/10.1016/j.phymed.2011.12.012] [PMID: 22325591]

[106] Lin KI, Lin CC, Kuo SM, *et al.* Carnosic acid impedes cell growth and enhances anticancer effects of carmustine and lomustine in melanoma. Biosci Rep 2018; 38(4): BSR20180005. [http://dx.doi.org/10.1042/BSR20180005] [PMID: 29789400]

[107] González-Vallinas M, Reglero G, Ramírez de Molina A. Rosemary (*Rosmarinus officinalis L.*) Extract as a Potential Complementary Agent in Anticancer Therapy. Nutr Cancer 2015; 67(8): 1223-31.
[http://dx.doi.org/10.1080/01635581.2015.1082110] [PMID: 26452641]

CHAPTER 13

Cannabis in the Treatment of Various Cancers and its Current Global Scenario

Swati Patil[1,*] and **Mandar Mulik**[1]

[1] *Principal. K.M. Kundnani College of Pharmacy, Mumbai, Maharashtra, India*

Abstract: Cannabis has been used as a drug for centuries, possibly much longer before it was recognised as an illegal substance. The prime psychoactive property is marked on the 9-THC compound. The cannabinoids replicate the action of endocannabinoids by stimulating receptors in the central nervous system and lymphatic system *via* diligent CB1 and CB2, respectively. Cannabinoids, on the other hand, are well known for their dependency, which is less severe than that of other drugs that can be abused. Cannabis' anti-tumor and anti-cancer potential was only discovered at the turn of the twentieth century. Cannabis consumption has been reported to benefit patients with cancer by suppressing nausea, curbing vomiting, elevating appetite, alleviating pain, and pacifying anxiety. Studies envisage that the up-regulation of CB receptors and their associated endogenous ligands correlates with the suppression of tumours. Patients have found cannabis to be effective in reducing side effects and relieving pain when used in conjunction with chemotherapy. Though cannabis prescription is restricted under federal laws in many countries, its lucrative efficacy profile has pushed regulators to reconsider its use in medical causes such as cancer. This chapter is an attempt to emphasise the biological role of cannabis in cancer pathophysiology.

Keywords: Anticancer effect, Cannabis, Cannabinoids, Endocannabinoid , THC.

INTRODUCTION

Cannabis, often referred to as European hemp, is mainly composed of the dried shoots of female plants in blossom condition, specifically Cannabis sativa, Cannabis indica, and Cannabis ruderalis, which are commonly found in India, Pakistan, and Bangladesh. Since 500 BC, Asian traditional medicines have used Cannabis sativa plant extract. Cannabis contains about 300 compounds categorised as cannabinol, cannabidiol, and tetrahydrocannabinol (cannabinoids), consisting of an aromatic portion (C11 or C12), theoretically derivable from six acetate units, and an isoprenoid component [1, 2].

* **Corresponding author Swati Patil:** Principal. K.M. Kundnani College of Pharmacy, Mumbai, Maharashtra, India; E-mail: ss.patil@kmkcp.edu.in

Cannabinoid receptors were discovered much later in humans than in the endocannabinoid system. The theory of non-specific receptor activation for cannabinoids' bioactivity in animals was rejected in the late 1980s when experiments on a rat model characterised specific cannabinoid receptors, CB1 and CB2 [3]. Recent studies suggest that the CB1 receptor is active in the central nervous system (CNS), whereas hematopoietic cells show expression of the CB2 receptor [4]. Endogenous ligands for the CB1 and CB2 receptors, 2-arachidonolyglycerol (2-AG) and N-arachidonoylethanolamine (AEA), have an affinity for groups of G protein-coupled receptors (GPCRs) linked to endocannabinoids and provide relevance of their bioactivity [5, 6].

Recently, the treatment of cancer included cannabinoids after mysterious studies showed the development of CB1 and CB2 receptors in cancer cells, which were responsible for tumour suppression. The hypothesis was confirmed by the characterization of overexpressed CB1 receptors in hepatocellular carcinoma, Hodgkin lymphoma, and epithelial ovarian carcinoma [7 - 11]. Similarly, CB2 has also been found to be overexpressed in HER2+ breast cancers and gliomas [12]. Carchman and co-workers proved the anti-tumor activity of cannabinoids *via* inhibition of DNA synthesis in lung adenocarcinomas, gliomas, breast, pancreas, and prostate lymphomas *in vitro* and *in vivo* models.

The above-reported research has many proposed mechanisms of action, including cell cycle arrest, induction of apoptosis, inhibition of neovascularization, migration, adhesion, invasion, and metastasis. In spite of so many positive findings that support the use of 9-THC-related cannabinoids in cancer research, these compounds are not used clinically because of their psychoactive side effects. The affinity of CBD towards receptors is still questionable [5, 13, 18]. CBD is also reported to interact with other cellular receptors, namely TRPVs, 5-HT1A, GPR55, and PPAR, leading to strong anti-proliferative and pro-apoptotic activities. Besides this, it is also postulated to inhibit the process of metastasis [14 - 17]. The discussion will continue on the anti-tumor activity of CBD, which is linked with the regulation of cell parameters such as ROS, ER stress, and immune modulation, among other probable mechanisms.

Anticancer Effects of Cannabis in the Following Cancers

Glioma

Glioma, or glioblastoma multiforme (GBM), is the most common and hostile type of brain tumour [19]. The GBM remains undetected for up to 5 years, and the rate of survival is reported to be only 4–5% within this period [19]. Most clinical cases are treated with a combined approach of surgery and radiotherapy; however, che-

-motherapy with Temozolomide or Carmustine is necessary to restrict the growth of cancer [20].

Treatment for GBM management is challenging to treat urgent medical needs, hence many scientists' have extended the use of cannabinoids. CBD in combination with other neoplastic drugs showed better cell apoptosis due to the upregulation of TRPV2 receptors, increased *in vitro* inhibition of cell invasion, and decreased *in vivo* angiogenesis, which induce tumour regression [20 - 26]. Ivanov *et al.* establish a link between CBD use, -irradiation, and neoplastic agents in terms of activation of TNF/TNFR1 and TRAIL/TRAIL-R2 for apoptotic pathway fulfillment [27, 28].

Literature suggests that CBD activates apoptotic pathways in glial cells. However, no evidence was found for the role of CBD in glial cell cycle arrest, hence its use as a secondary therapy for patients with high-grade gliomas [29, 30]. The oral administration of CBD along with key players in GBM management such as procarbazine, vincristine, lomustine, *etc.* showed mild adverse effects like rash, nausea, and fatigue, but there were no signs of any lymphopenia, thrombocytopenia, hepatic toxicity, or neurotoxicity [31]. An important study on nine volunteers with grade IV GBM found that a higher dose of CBD (200–400 mg/day) resulted in a prolonged tumour arrest period and no signs of disease progression for three or more years. In conclusion, we must say the results indicate that CBD alone or in combination with routine treatment for GBM shows great promise with relatively mild side effects [25, 27].

Breast Cancer

Breast cancer is the most common type of cancer worldwide. Since 2006, the effects of CBD on breast cancer have been examined, and research in this area has recently expanded [32]. Estrogen receptor (ER)-positive cells (MCF-7, ZR-75-1, and T47D), ER-negative cells (MDA-MB-231, MDA-MB-468, and SK-BR3), and triple-negative breast cancer (TNBC) cells (SUM159, 4T1up, MVT-1, and SCP2) all showed a dose-dependent response to CBD. Very significant results were observed with such a low dose of CBD in MDA-MB-231 after 24 h [26, 33].

As a result, the CBD's IC50 values for the vast majority of cell lines were inadequate. This was a demonstration that CBD's anti-proliferative properties are often responsive to breast cancer cell lines. However, CBD would have no effect on stable breast epithelial cells [34]. The mechanism for the action of CBD on breast cancer progression is limited to apoptosis, autophagy, and cell cycle arrest only. *In vitro* studies of CBD on cell lines such as MDA-MB-231 and MCF-7 showed apoptotic response *via* regulation of caspase-3 and cell cycle arrest at the G1/S phase respectively.

Similarly, the MDA-MB-231cell line envisaged moderate cell arrest by the trigger of CB2 and TRPV1 receptors [15, 35 - 43]. CBD's antiproliferative ability on breast cancer cells has recently been found to be independent of endocannabinoid receptors. CBD has been proven to produce reactive oxygen species (ROS), which hinder cell development and cause death. CBD promotes apoptosis by inhibiting mTOR, AKT, 4EBP1, and cyclin D, while increasing the expression and nuclear localization of PPAR-γ [44 - 47].

Apoptosis levels rose when CBD doses were raised or autophagy was inhibited *via* Beclin-1 translocation and cleavage, according to the researchers [48 - 52]. McAllister *et al.* discovered Id-1 protein downregulation by ER kinase and ROS in CBD-treated MDA-MB-231 and MDA-MB-436 tumours. This reduction in expression was linked to a reduction in tumour invasion and metastases [53].

Lung Cancer

According to epidemiological research conducted by the American Cancer Society, lung malignancy is the second most frequent cancer in both men and women. Small cell lung cancer (SCLC, 13%) and non-small cell lung cancer (NSCLC, 84%) are the two types of lung cancer [54]. In lung cancer cells, CBD treatment increased COX-2-derived products such as prostaglandins E, D, and J. This could be one of the CBD's pro-apoptotic mechanisms, as well as a pathway for endocannabinoid breakdown and PPAR- activation. It was also discovered that treating initial lung carcinoma cells from a patient with brain metastases resulted in COX-2 and PPAR- overexpression. In a lung tumour animal model, PPAR-inhibition by GW9662 consistently abolished CBD's tumor-suppressive effects [41 - 47].

The tissue inhibitor of MMPs (TIMPs) was investigated and shown to be connected to CBD's anti-invasive activity. CBD was discovered to stimulate TIMPs in a time- and concentration-dependent manner. Ramer *et al.* studied the expression of an intercellular molecule, a transmembrane glycoprotein implicated in tumour metastasis, to link CB1, CB2, and TRPV1. TIMP-1 mRNA expression increased as well, but only after intercellular molecule (ICAM-1) mRNA expression increased. The activation of p42/44 MAPK and p38 MAPK was required for the expression of ICAM-1. Both ICAM-1 and TIMP-1 were increased in the *in vivo* model. The use of a neutralising antibody and siRNA to inactivate ICAM-1 resulted in a reduction in TIMP-1 activation as well as CBD's anti-invasive characteristics [52, 55 - 58]. These findings show that MAPKs activate ICAM-1, which in turn enhances TIMP-1 action, preventing tumour invasion [59, 60].

These investigations demonstrate that CBD regulates p38 MAPK *via* CB1, CB2, and TRPV1 receptors, causing ICAM-1 and consequently TIMP-1 to be produced. The increase of ICAM-1 and TIMP-1 inhibits lung cancer invasion. At this time, no clinical trials employing CBD to treat lung cancer patients have been undertaken. As a result, it is impossible to locate published data. The only case study of lung adenocarcinoma self-treated with CBD was an 81-year-old patient. The patient was initially denied chemotherapy and radiation therapy because of his age and the toxicity profile of these therapies when he was diagnosed with several mediastinal masses. The tumour and mediastinal lymph nodes started to regress a year later, according to a computed tomography (CT) scan [61 - 65]. TIMP-1 mRNA expression increased as well; however, this occurred after ICAM-1 mRNA levels increased. The activation of p42/44 MAPK and p38 MAPK was required for ICAM-1 expression. In an *in vivo* A549 model, ICAM-1 and TIMP-1 both controlled CBD's anti-invasive activities [56]. The use of a neutralising antibody to inactivate ICAM-1 ultimately led to an increase in TIMP-1 activity. This was modified when he started consuming 2 percent CBD oil. Slight nausea and a foul taste were among the side effects [57, 60].

Colorectal Cancer

Colorectal cancer (CRC) is the third-leading cause of cancer mortality in both men and women in the United States. Using CRC cell lines as well as proliferative and malignant tissues from CRC patients, researchers suggest that CBD production is substantially enhanced in adenomatous polyps and cancerous colon tissue as well. CB1 and CB2, as well as AEA, 2-AG, and endocannabinoid-metabolizing proteins, including FAAH, are all found in typical human colorectal tissue. Compared to normal colorectal tissues, transformed adenomatous polyps contain higher amounts of 2-AG [66, 67]. CBD can either arrest or enhance the growth of CRC; depending on the stage of the disease, both CBD and inhibitors may be beneficial in the treatment of CRC [68].

CBD has also been studied as an adjuvant to chemotherapy for CRC by a small number of people. The chemotherapy drugs are commonly used to treat CRC. Jeong *et al.* used oxaliplatin and CBD (4 M) to treat oxaliplatin-resistant cell lines. They discovered that CBD increased oxaliplatin-mediated autophagy by decreasing factors in oxaliplatin resistance. Through lowered SOD2 expression, the combination of oxaliplatin and CBD resulted in mitochondrial dysfunction. *In vivo*, these findings were also validated [67 - 70]. The enactment of ER stress-related features, such as Liven, CHOP, and DR5, by CBD and Pathway increased apoptosis. CBD-containing pathways appeared to inhibit tumour growth while increasing the number of apoptotic cells *in vivo*. These findings regarding CBD's synergistic benefits with chemotherapies are quite encouraging and create a strong argument for a future clinical investigation [58, 66 - 69, 71 - 73].

Prostate Cancer

Prostate cancer is the most frequent cancer in males as well as the second leading cause of cancer-related mortality. AR-positive (LNCaP and 22RV1) and AR-negative (LNCaP and 22RV1) prostate cancer cell lines were employed in the experiments (DU-145 and PC-3) [70]. In AR-positive cell lines, CBD has been shown to suppress androgen receptor expression. Depending on the severity, CB1, CB2, or both are upregulated in prostate cancer cells. 22RV1 expresses just CB1, whereas DU-145 expresses only CB2. Despite the fact that CB1 and CB2 are present in both LNCaP and PC-3, PC-3 has substantially higher amounts of these receptors [74]. TRPV1 in DU-145 cells shows the greatest levels of expression. CBD induces anti-proliferative effects and apoptosis-mediated cell death *via* the intrinsic pathway in prostate cancer cells, which may be dependent on CB2, and the transient receptor potential cation-channel receptor (TRPM8) in LNCaP cells. CBD has been shown to inhibit the expression of prostate-specific antigen (PSA), vascular endothelial growth factor (VEGF), and pro-inflammatory cytokines. In LNCaP and PC3 cells, CBD administration caused cell cycle arrest at the G0/G1 transition, whereas in DU-145 cells, it caused cell cycle arrest at the G1/S transition [52, 75 - 77].

Leukemia/Lymphoma

For lymphoma and leukaemia, the EL-4 and Jurkat cell lines are routinely employed. CBD killed these leukaemia and lymphoma cell lines in a dose- and time-dependent manner [3, 78 - 80]. Future considerations must resolve these conflicting outcomes. Regardless, the majority of studies on leukemia and lymphoma confirmed apoptosis in conjunction with other therapy methods such as irradiation, 9-THC, vincristine, and cytarabine [81]. CBD has also been shown in studies to reduce tumour burden and induce apoptosis *in vivo*. CBD therapy also resulted in alterations to cell shape and blebbing of the plasma layer [82]. CBD, like other malignancies, causes ROS in leukaemia and lymphoma. Adding 2.5 mg of CBD to a leukaemia cell line for 24 hours increased ROS levels. CBD's lethal effects were reduced when cells were treated with ROS foragers such as tocopherol and NAC. CBD raised NOX4 and p22phox levels, reduced ROS levels, and prevented CBD-induced cell damage [48 - 51, 83 - 85]. In EL-4 cells, ROS levels were considerably elevated after only two hours of CBD administration, with a concurrent drop in cellular thiols, confirming these findings. CBD inhibited AKT and ribosomal protein S6 phosphorylation, according to the researchers [80]. They also investigated CBD's effects under various nutritional and oxygen circumstances, finding that CBD's anti-proliferative effects were stronger with 1 percent serum than with 5 percent serum, whether alone or in combination with doxorubicin [79]. Olivas-Aguirre *et al.* discovered that even at lower doses of CBD, Jurkat cells proliferated (at 1 μM CBD) and autophagy was enhanced (at 10 μM CBD). The intrinsic apoptotic pathway was triggered at higher doses (30 μM), resulting in cytochrome C release and Ca^{2+} overload inside the mitochondria [4, 86]. AF1q enhanced cell proliferation and decreased ICAM-1 expression in Burkitt lymphoma cell lines, Jiyoye and Mutu I, allowing the cells to become resistant to chemotherapies. The chemo-resistant effect was drastically reduced after 24 hours of CBD administration [13, 14, 87, 88].

CONCLUSION

CBD has been found to have potent anti-cancer effects on cell lines and mice tumour models, as evidenced by the extensive research listed above. CBD, on the other hand, has a softer effect on normal cells in the same tissue or organ. Cell cycle arrest, autophagy, cell death, and combinations of these anti-tumor strategies differ by the tumour type. CBD can also decrease tumour migration, invasion, and neovascularization, suggesting that it affects tumour microenvironment as well. CBDs may have numerous cellular targets and/or various cellular targets in different cancers. CBD appears to work by altering cellular redox homeostasis and producing a significant rise in ROS and ER stress. In order to better understand how CBD treatment disrupts cellular homeostasis in both tumour cells, future studies must elucidate the interplays among different signalling transduction pathways. Clinical studies, which are desperately needed, are the final stage in establishing CBD as an anticancer treatment.

ABBREVIATIONS

5-HT1A-5'-O	(3-Thiotriphosphate) 8-Hydroxy-2-(di-n-propylamino)tetralin
CB	Cannabis
CBD	Cannabidiol (CBD)
CYP	Cytochrome P450
ER	Endoplasmic reticulum
GPR55	G protein-coupled receptor gene- 55
ICAM-1	Intercellular adhesion molecule 1
JNK-AP1	Jun N-terminal kinase
MAPK	-Mitogen activated protein kinase
NOS3	Nitric oxide synthase 3
PPAR	Peroxisome proliferator activated receptor gamma

ROS	Reactive oxygen species
THC	Tetrahydrocannabinol
TRP	Transient receptor potential
TRPV	Transient receptor potential vanilloid
TNFR1	Tumor necrosis factor receptor 1
TRAIL	TNF-related apoptosis-inducing ligand
TZM	Temozolomide
TIMP-1	Tissue Inhibitor of Metalloproteinase 1
TRPV1	Transient receptor potential vanilloid -1

REFERENCES

[1] Macpherson T, Armstrong JA, Criddle DN, Wright KL. Physiological intestinal oxygen modulates the Caco-2 cell model and increases sensitivity to the phytocannabinoid cannabidiol. In Vitro Cell Dev Biol Anim 2014; 50(5): 417-26.
[http://dx.doi.org/10.1007/s11626-013-9719-9] [PMID: 24464350]

[2] Kalenderoglou N, Macpherson T, Wright KL. Cannabidiol Reduces Leukemic Cell Size – But Is It Important? Front Pharmacol 2017; 8: 144.
[http://dx.doi.org/10.3389/fphar.2017.00144] [PMID: 28392768]

[3] Aviello G, Romano B, Borrelli F, *et al.* Chemopreventive effect of the non-psychotropic phytocannabinoid cannabidiol on experimental colon cancer. J Mol Med (Berl) 2012; 90(8): 925-34.
[http://dx.doi.org/10.1007/s00109-011-0856-x] [PMID: 22231745]

[4] Lee W. S.-P.;Liao,M.-H.;Hsu,W.-L.;Wu,H.-Y.;Jan,T.-R.Acomparativestudyoncannabidiol-induced apoptosis in murine thymocytes and EL-4 thymoma cells. Int Immunopharmacol 2008; 8: 732-40.
[http://dx.doi.org/10.1016/j.intimp.2008.01.018] [PMID: 18387516]

[5] Taha T, Meiri D, Talhamy S, Wollner M, Peer A, Bar-Sela G. Cannabis Impacts Tumor Response Rate to Nivolumab in Patients with Advanced Malignancies. Oncologist 2019; 24(4): 549-54.
[http://dx.doi.org/10.1634/theoncologist.2018-0383] [PMID: 30670598]

[6] Togano T, Kim N, Kim N, *et al.* The evaluation of Cannabidiol's effect on the immunotherapy of Burkitt lymphoma. Biochem Biophys Res Commun 2019; 520(1): 225-30.
[http://dx.doi.org/10.1016/j.bbrc.2019.10.001] [PMID: 31587870]

[7] Sakurada R, Odagiri K, Hakamata A, Kamiya C, Wei J, Watanabe H. Calcium Release from Endoplasmic Reticulum Involves Calmodulin-Mediated NADPH Oxidase-Derived Reactive Oxygen Species Production in Endothelial Cells. Int J Mol Sci 2019; 20(7): 1644.
[http://dx.doi.org/10.3390/ijms20071644] [PMID: 30987055]

[8] Simmerman E, Qin X, Yu JC, Baban B. Cannabinoids as a Potential New and Novel Treatment for Melanoma: A Pilot Study in a Murine Model. J Surg Res 2019; 235: 210-5.
[http://dx.doi.org/10.1016/j.jss.2018.08.055] [PMID: 30691796]

[9] Ferro R, Adamska A, Lattanzio R, *et al.* GPR55 signalling promotes proliferation of pancreatic cancer cells and tumour growth in mice, and its inhibition increases effects of gemcitabine. Oncogene 2018; 37(49): 6368-82.
[http://dx.doi.org/10.1038/s41388-018-0390-1] [PMID: 30061636]

[10] Forrester SJ, Kikuchi DS, Hernandes MS, Xu Q, Griendling KK. Reactive Oxygen Species in Metabolic and Inflammatory Signaling. Circ Res 2018; 122(6): 877-902.
[http://dx.doi.org/10.1161/CIRCRESAHA.117.311401] [PMID: 29700084]

[11] Wang YY, Lee KT, Lim MC, Choi JH. TRPV1 Antagonist DWP05195 Induces ER Stress-Dependent Apoptosis through the ROS-p38-CHOP Pathway in Human Ovarian Cancer Cells. Cancers (Basel) 2020; 12(6): 1702.
[http://dx.doi.org/10.3390/cancers12061702] [PMID: 32604833]

[12] Bergamaschi MM, Queiroz RHC, Zuardi AW, Crippa JAS. Safety and side effects of cannabidiol, a Cannabis sativa constituent. Curr Drug Saf 2011; 6(4): 237-49.
[http://dx.doi.org/10.2174/157488611798280924] [PMID: 22129319]

[13] Ståhl A, Johansson K, Mossberg M, Kahn R, Karpman D. Exosomes and microvesicles in normal physiology, pathophysiology, and renal diseases. Pediatr Nephrol 2019; 34(1): 11-30.
[http://dx.doi.org/10.1007/s00467-017-3816-z] [PMID: 29181712]

[14] Lukhele ST, Motadi LR. Cannabidiol rather than Cannabis sativa extracts inhibit cell growth and induce apoptosis in cervical cancer cells. BMC Complement Altern Med 2016; 16(1): 335.
[http://dx.doi.org/10.1186/s12906-016-1280-0] [PMID: 27586579]

[15] Neumann-Raizel H, Shilo A, Lev S, *et al.* 2-APB and CBD-mediated targeting of charged cytotoxic compounds into tumor-like cells suggests the involvement of TRPV2 channels. Front Pharmacol 2019; 10: 1198.
[http://dx.doi.org/10.3389/fphar.2019.01198] [PMID: 31680972]

[16] Jeong S, Jo MJ, Yun HK, *et al.* Cannabidiol promotes apoptosis via regulation of XIAP/Smac in gastric cancer. Cell Death Dis 2019; 10(11): 846.
[http://dx.doi.org/10.1038/s41419-019-2001-7]

[17] Zhang X, Qin Y, Pan Z, *et al.* Cannabidiol Induces Cell Cycle Arrest and Cell Apoptosis in Human Gastric Cancer SGC-7901 Cells. Biomolecules 2019; 9(8): 302.
[http://dx.doi.org/10.3390/biom9080302] [PMID: 31349651]

[18] Blázquez C, Carracedo A, Barrado L, *et al.* Cannabinoid receptors as novel targets for the treatment of melanoma. FASEB J 2006; 20(14): 2633-5.
[http://dx.doi.org/10.1096/fj.06-6638fje] [PMID: 17065222]

[19] Ivanov VN, Wu J, Wang TJC, Hei TK. Inhibition of ATM kinase upregulates levels of cell death induced by cannabidiol and γ-irradiation in human glioblastoma cells. Oncotarget 2019; 10(8): 825-46.
[http://dx.doi.org/10.18632/oncotarget.26582] [PMID: 30783513]

[20] Massi P, Vaccani A, Ceruti S, Colombo A, Abbracchio MP, Parolaro D. Antitumor effects of cannabidiol, a non-psychotropic cannabinoid, on human glioma cell lines. J Pharmacol Exp Ther 2003; 10: 255-67.
[PMID: 14617682]

[21] Vaccani A, Massi P, Colombo A, Rubino T, Parolaro D. Cannabidiol inhibits human glioma cell migration through a cannabinoid receptor-independent mechanism. Br J Pharmacol 2005; 144(8): 1032-6.
[http://dx.doi.org/10.1038/sj.bjp.0706134] [PMID: 15700028]

[22] Ligresti A, Moriello AS, Starowicz K, *et al.* Antitumor activity of plant cannabinoids with emphasis on the effect of cannabidiol on human breast carcinoma. J Pharmacol Exp Ther 2006; 318(3): 1375-87.
[http://dx.doi.org/10.1124/jpet.106.105247] [PMID: 16728591]

[23] Massi P, Valenti M, Vaccani A, *et al.* 5-Lipoxygenase and anandamide hydrolase (FAAH) mediate the antitumor activity of cannabidiol, a non-psychoactive cannabinoid. J Neurochem 2008; 104(4): 1091-100.
[http://dx.doi.org/10.1111/j.1471-4159.2007.05073.x] [PMID: 18028339]

[24] Nabissi M, Morelli MB, Santoni M, Santoni G. Triggering of the TRPV2 channel by cannabidiol sensitizes glioblastoma cells to cytotoxic chemotherapeutic agents. Carcinogenesis 2013; 34(1): 48-57.
[http://dx.doi.org/10.1093/carcin/bgs328] [PMID: 23079154]

[25] Solinas M, Massi P, Cinquina V, *et al.* Cannabidiol, a non-psychoactive cannabinoid compound, inhibits proliferation and invasion in U87-MG and T98G glioma cells through a multitarget effect. PLoS One 2013; 8(10): e76918. [http://dx.doi.org/10.1371/journal.pone.0076918] [PMID: 24204703]

[26] Hernán Pérez de la Ossa D, Lorente M, Gil-Alegre ME, *et al.* Local delivery of cannabinoid-loaded microparticles inhibits tumor growth in a murine xenograft model of glioblastoma multiforme. PLoS One 2013; 8(1): e54795. [http://dx.doi.org/10.1371/journal.pone.0054795] [PMID: 23349970]

[27] Elinav E, Nowarski R, Thaiss CA, Hu B, Jin C, Flavell RA. Inflammation-induced cancer: crosstalk between tumours, immune cells and microorganisms. Nat Rev Cancer 2013; 13(11): 759-71. [http://dx.doi.org/10.1038/nrc3611] [PMID: 24154716]

[28] Marcu JP, Christian RT, Lau D, *et al.* Cannabidiol enhances the inhibitory effects of delta9-tetrahydrocannabinol on human glioblastoma cell proliferation and survival. Mol Cancer Ther 2010; 9(1): 180-9. [http://dx.doi.org/10.1158/1535-7163.MCT-09-0407] [PMID: 20053780]

[29] Mantovani A, Allavena P, Sica A, Balkwill F. Cancer-related inflammation. Nature 2008; 454(7203): 436-44. [http://dx.doi.org/10.1038/nature07205] [PMID: 18650914]

[30] Jacobsson SOP, Rongård E, Stridh M, Tiger G, Fowler CJ. Serum-dependent effects of tamoxifen and cannabinoids upon C6 glioma cell viability. Biochem Pharmacol 2000; 60(12): 1807-13. [http://dx.doi.org/10.1016/S0006-2952(00)00492-5] [PMID: 11108795]

[31] Porta C, Larghi P, Rimoldi M, *et al.* Cellular and molecular pathways linking inflammation and cancer. Immunobiology 2009; 214(9-10): 761-77. [http://dx.doi.org/10.1016/j.imbio.2009.06.014] [PMID: 19616341]

[32] Gill JG, Piskounova E, Morrison SJ. Cancer, Oxidative Stress, and Metastasis. Cold Spring Harb Symp Quant Biol 2016; 81: 163-75. [http://dx.doi.org/10.1101/sqb.2016.81.030791] [PMID: 28082378]

[33] Scott KA, Dennis JL, Dalgleish AG, Liu WM. Inhibiting Heat Shock Proteins Can Potentiate the Cytotoxic Effect of Cannabidiol in Human Glioma Cells. Anticancer Res 2015; 35(11): 5827-37. [PMID: 26504004]

[34] López-Valero I, Saiz-Ladera C, Torres S, *et al.* Targeting Glioma Initiating Cells with A combined therapy of cannabinoids and temozolomide. Biochem Pharmacol 2018; 157: 266-74. [http://dx.doi.org/10.1016/j.bcp.2018.09.007] [PMID: 30195736]

[35] Aparicio-Blanco J, Sebastián V, Benoit JP, Torres-Suárez AI. Lipid nanocapsules decorated and loaded with cannabidiol as targeted prolonged release carriers for glioma therapy: *In vitro* screening of critical parameters. Eur J Pharm Biopharm 2019; 134: 126-37. [http://dx.doi.org/10.1016/j.ejpb.2018.11.020] [PMID: 30472144]

[36] Massi P, Vaccani A, Bianchessi S, Costa B, Macchi P, Parolaro D. The non-psychoactive cannabidiol triggers caspase activation and oxidative stress in human glioma cells. Cell Mol Life Sci 2006; 63(17): 2057-66. [http://dx.doi.org/10.1007/s00018-006-6156-x] [PMID: 16909207]

[37] A Safety Study of Sativex in Combination With Dose-intense Temozolomide in Patients With Recurrent Glioblastoma. ClinicalTrials.gov. 2013.

[38] TN-TC11G (THC+CBD) Combination With Temozolomide and Radiotherapy in Patients With Newly-diagnosed Glioblastoma (GEINOCANN). ClinicalTrials.gov. 2018.

[39] Twelves C, Short S, Wright S. A two-part safety and exploratory efficacy randomized double-blind, placebo-controlled study of a 1:1 ratio of the cannabinoids cannabidiol and delta--tetrahydrocannabinol (CBD:THC) plus dose-intense temozolomide in patients with recurrent

glioblastoma multiforme (GBM). J Clin Oncol 2017; 35(15_suppl): 2046. [http://dx.doi.org/10.1200/JCO.2017.35.15_suppl.2046]

[40] Dall'Stella PB, Docema MFL, Maldaun MVC, Feher O, Lancellotti CLP. Case Report: Clinical Outcome and Image Response of Two Patients With Secondary High-Grade Glioma Treated With Chemoradiation, PCV, and Cannabidiol. Front Oncol 2019; 8: 643. [http://dx.doi.org/10.3389/fonc.2018.00643] [PMID: 30713832]

[41] Likar R, Koestenberger M, Stultschnig M, Nahler G. Concomitant Treatment of Malignant Brain Tumours With CBD – A Case Series and Review of the Literature. Anticancer Res 2019; 39(10): 5797-801. [http://dx.doi.org/10.21873/anticanres.13783] [PMID: 31570484]

[42] Kim Y. American Cancer Society. Cham, Switzerland: Springer Science and Business Media LLC 2019; pp. 1-2.

[43] Sultan AS, Marie MA, Sheweita SA. Novel mechanism of cannabidiol-induced apoptosis in breast cancer cell lines. Breast 2018; 41: 34-41. [http://dx.doi.org/10.1016/j.breast.2018.06.009] [PMID: 30007266]

[44] Ward SJ, McAllister SD, Kawamura R, Murase R, Neelakantan H, Walker EA. Cannabidiol inhibits paclitaxel□induced neuropathic pain through 5□ HT_{1A} receptors without diminishing nervous system function or chemotherapy efficacy. Br J Pharmacol 2014; 171(3): 636-45. [http://dx.doi.org/10.1111/bph.12439] [PMID: 24117398]

[45] McAllister SD, Christian RT, Horowitz MP, Garcia A, Desprez PY. Cannabidiol as a novel inhibitor of Id-1 gene expression in aggressive breast cancer cells. Mol Cancer Ther 2007; 6(11): 2921-7. [http://dx.doi.org/10.1158/1535-7163.MCT-07-0371] [PMID: 18025276]

[46] Shrivastava A, Kuzontkoski PM, Groopman JE, Prasad A. Cannabidiol induces programmed cell death in breast cancer cells by coordinating the cross-talk between apoptosis and autophagy. Mol Cancer Ther 2011; 10(7): 1161-72. [http://dx.doi.org/10.1158/1535-7163.MCT-10-1100] [PMID: 21566064]

[47] Murase R, Kawamura R, Singer E, *et al.* Targeting multiple cannabinoid anti-tumour pathways with a resorcinol derivative leads to inhibition of advanced stages of breast cancer. Br J Pharmacol 2014; 171(19): 4464-77. [http://dx.doi.org/10.1111/bph.12803] [PMID: 24910342]

[48] Kosgodage US, Mould R, Henley AB, *et al.* Cannabidiol (CBD) Is a Novel Inhibitor for Exosome and Microvesicle (EMV) Release in Cancer. Front Pharmacol 2018; 9: 889. [http://dx.doi.org/10.3389/fphar.2018.00889] [PMID: 30150937]

[49] McAllister SD, Murase R, Christian RT, *et al.* Pathways mediating the effects of cannabidiol on the reduction of breast cancer cell proliferation, invasion, and metastasis. Breast Cancer Res Treat 2011; 129(1): 37-47. [http://dx.doi.org/10.1007/s10549-010-1177-4] [PMID: 20859676]

[50] Ramer R, Bublitz K, Freimuth N, *et al.* Cannabidiol inhibits lung cancer cell invasion and metastasis *via* intercellular adhesion molecule□1. FASEB J 2012; 26(4): 1535-48. [http://dx.doi.org/10.1096/fj.11-198184] [PMID: 22198381]

[51] Ramer R, Rohde A, Merkord J, Rohde H, Hinz B. Decrease of plasminogen activator inhibitor-1 may contribute to the anti-invasive action of cannabidiol on human lung cancer cells. Pharm Res 2010; 27(10): 2162-74. [http://dx.doi.org/10.1007/s11095-010-0219-2] [PMID: 20668920]

[52] Lu D, Immadi SS, Wu Z, Kendall DA. Translational potential of allosteric modulators targeting the cannabinoid CB_1 receptor. Acta Pharmacol Sin 2019; 40(3): 324-35. [http://dx.doi.org/10.1038/s41401-018-0164-x] [PMID: 30333554]

[53] Piomelli D. The molecular logic of endocannabinoid signalling. Nat Rev Neurosci 2003; 4(11): 873-84.
[http://dx.doi.org/10.1038/nrn1247] [PMID: 14595399]

[54] Elbaz M, Nasser MW, Ravi J, *et al.* Modulation of the tumor microenvironment and inhibition of EGF/EGFR pathway: Novel anti-tumor mechanisms of Cannabidiol in breast cancer. Mol Oncol 2015; 9(4): 906-19.
[http://dx.doi.org/10.1016/j.molonc.2014.12.010] [PMID: 25660577]

[55] Munro S, Thomas KL, Abu-Shaar M. Molecular characterization of a peripheral receptor for cannabinoids. Nature 1993; 365(6441): 61-5.
[http://dx.doi.org/10.1038/365061a0] [PMID: 7689702]

[56] Howlett AC. The cannabinoid receptors. Prostaglandins Other Lipid Mediat 2002; 68-69: 619-31.
[http://dx.doi.org/10.1016/S0090-6980(02)00060-6] [PMID: 12432948]

[57] Devane WA, Hanuš L, Breuer A, *et al.* Isolation and structure of a brain constituent that binds to the cannabinoid receptor. Science 1992; 258(5090): 1946-9.
[http://dx.doi.org/10.1126/science.1470919] [PMID: 1470919]

[58] Stella N, Schweitzer P, Piomelli D. A second endogenous cannabinoid that modulates long-term potentiation. Nature 1997; 388(6644): 773-8.
[http://dx.doi.org/10.1038/42015] [PMID: 9285589]

[59] Sreevalsan S, Joseph S, Jutooru I, Chadalapaka G, Safe SH. Induction of apoptosis by cannabinoids in prostate and colon cancer cells is phosphatase dependent. Anticancer Res 2011; 31(11): 3799-807.
[PMID: 22110202]

[60] Mechoulam R, Ben-Shabat S, Hanus L, *et al.* Identification of an endogenous 2-monoglyceride, present in canine gut, that binds to cannabinoid receptors. Biochem Pharmacol 1995; 50(1): 83-90.
[http://dx.doi.org/10.1016/0006-2952(95)00109-D] [PMID: 7605349]

[61] Sugiura T, Kishimoto S, Oka S, Gokoh M. Biochemistry, pharmacology and physiology of 2-arachidonoylglycerol, an endogenous cannabinoid receptor ligand. Prog Lipid Res 2006; 45(5): 405-46.
[http://dx.doi.org/10.1016/j.plipres.2006.03.003] [PMID: 16678907]

[62] Chen XP, Yang W, Fan Y, *et al.* Structural determinants in the second intracellular loop of the human cannabinoid CB1 receptor mediate selective coupling to Gs and Gi. Br J Pharmacol 2010; 161(8): 1817-34.
[http://dx.doi.org/10.1111/j.1476-5381.2010.01006.x] [PMID: 20735408]

[63] Lauckner JE, Hille B, Mackie K. The cannabinoid agonist WIN55,212-2 increases intracellular calcium via CB_1 receptor coupling to $G_{q/11}$ G proteins. Proc Natl Acad Sci USA 2005; 102(52): 19144-9.
[http://dx.doi.org/10.1073/pnas.0509588102] [PMID: 16365309]

[64] Roland AB, Ricobaraza A, Carrel D, *et al.* Cannabinoid-induced actomyosin contractility shapes neuronal morphology and growth. eLife 2014; 3: e03159.
[http://dx.doi.org/10.7554/eLife.03159] [PMID: 25225054]

[65] Saroz Y, Kho DT, Glass M, Graham ES, Grimsey NL. Cannabinoid Receptor 2 (CB_2) Signals via G-alpha-s and Induces IL-6 and IL-10 Cytokine Secretion in Human Primary Leukocytes. ACS Pharmacol Transl Sci 2019; 2(6): 414-28.
[http://dx.doi.org/10.1021/acsptsci.9b00049] [PMID: 32259074]

[66] Di Marzo V, Bisogno T, De Petrocellis L. The Biosynthesis, Fate and Pharmacological Properties of Endocannabinoids.Cannabinoids. 2005; pp. 147-85.
[http://dx.doi.org/10.1007/3-540-26573-2_5]

[67] Ryberg E, Larsson N, Sjögren S, *et al.* The orphan receptor GPR55 is a novel cannabinoid receptor. Br J Pharmacol 2007; 152(7): 1092-101.

[http://dx.doi.org/10.1038/sj.bjp.0707460] [PMID: 17876302]

[68] O'Sullivan SE. Cannabinoids go nuclear: evidence for activation of peroxisome proliferator-activated receptors. Br J Pharmacol 2007; 152(5): 576-82. [http://dx.doi.org/10.1038/sj.bjp.0707423] [PMID: 17704824]

[69] Haustrate A, Prevarskaya N, Lehen'kyi V. Role of the TRPV Channels in the Endoplasmic Reticulum Calcium Homeostasis. Cells 2020; 9(2): 317. [http://dx.doi.org/10.3390/cells9020317] [PMID: 32013022]

[70] Sarfaraz S, Adhami VM, Syed DN, Afaq F, Mukhtar H. Cannabinoids for cancer treatment: progress and promise. Cancer Res 2008; 68(2): 339-42. [http://dx.doi.org/10.1158/0008-5472.CAN-07-2785] [PMID: 18199524]

[71] Howlett AC, Barth F, Bonner TI, *et al.* International Union of Pharmacology. XXVII. Classification of cannabinoid receptors. Pharmacol Rev 2002; 54(2): 161-202. [http://dx.doi.org/10.1124/pr.54.2.161] [PMID: 12037135]

[72] Pellati F, Brighenti V, Sperlea J, Marchetti L, Bertelli D, Benvenuti S. New Methods for the Comprehensive Analysis of Bioactive Compounds in Cannabis sativa L. (hemp). Molecules 2018; 23(10): 2639. [http://dx.doi.org/10.3390/molecules23102639] [PMID: 30322208]

[73] Brighenti V, Pellati F, Steinbach M, Maran D, Benvenuti S. Development of a new extraction technique and HPLC method for the analysis of non-psychoactive cannabinoids in fibre-type Cannabis sativa L. (hemp). J Pharm Biomed Anal 2017; 143: 228-36. [http://dx.doi.org/10.1016/j.jpba.2017.05.049] [PMID: 28609672]

[74] Mukhopadhyay B, Schuebel K, Mukhopadhyay P, *et al.* Cannabinoid receptor 1 promotes hepatocellular carcinoma initiation and progression through multiple mechanisms. Hepatology 2015; 61(5): 1615-26. [http://dx.doi.org/10.1002/hep.27686] [PMID: 25580584]

[75] Dumitru CA, Sandalcioglu IE, Karsak M. Cannabinoids in Glioblastoma Therapy: New Applications for Old Drugs. Front Mol Neurosci 2018; 11: 159. [http://dx.doi.org/10.3389/fnmol.2018.00159] [PMID: 29867351]

[76] Jung CK, Kang WK, Park JM, *et al.* Expression of the cannabinoid type I receptor and prognosis following surgery in colorectal cancer. Oncol Lett 2013; 5(3): 870-6. [http://dx.doi.org/10.3892/ol.2012.1081] [PMID: 23426698]

[77] Martínez-Martínez E, Gómez I, Martín P, *et al.* Cannabinoids receptor type 2, CB2, expression correlates with human colon cancer progression and predicts patient survival. Oncoscience 2015; 2(2): 131-41. [http://dx.doi.org/10.18632/oncoscience.119] [PMID: 25859556]

[78] Kim JL, Kim BR, Kim DY, *et al.* Cannabidiol Enhances the Therapeutic Effects of TRAIL by Upregulating DR5 in Colorectal Cancer. Cancers (Basel) 2019; 11(5): 642. [http://dx.doi.org/10.3390/cancers11050642] [PMID: 31075907]

[79] Gallily R, Even-Chen T, Katzavian G, Lehmann D, Dagan A, Mechoulam R. γ-irradiation enhances apoptosis induced by cannabidiol, a non-psychotropic cannabinoid, in cultured HL-60 myeloblastic leukemia cells. Leuk Lymphoma 2003; 44(10): 1767-73. [http://dx.doi.org/10.1080/1042819031000103917] [PMID: 14692532]

[80] McKallip RJ, Jia W, Schlomer J, Warren JW, Nagarkatti PS, Nagarkatti M. Cannabidiol-induced apoptosis in human leukemia cells: A novel role of cannabidiol in the regulation of p22phox and Nox4 expression. Mol Pharmacol 2006; 70(3): 897-908. [http://dx.doi.org/10.1124/mol.106.023937] [PMID: 16754784]

[81] Ramer R, Hinz B. Cannabinoids as Anticancer Drugs. Adv Pharmacol 2017; 80: 397-436. [http://dx.doi.org/10.1016/bs.apha.2017.04.002] [PMID: 28826542]

[82] Bifulco M, Malfitano AM, Pisanti S, Laezza C. Endocannabinoids in endocrine and related tumours. Endocr Relat Cancer 2008; 15(2): 391-408.
[http://dx.doi.org/10.1677/ERC-07-0258] [PMID: 18508995]

[83] Ramer R, Merkord J, Rohde H, Hinz B. Cannabidiol inhibits cancer cell invasion *via* upregulation of tissue inhibitor of matrix metalloproteinases-1. Biochem Pharmacol 2010; 79(7): 955-66.
[http://dx.doi.org/10.1016/j.bcp.2009.11.007] [PMID: 19914218]

[84] Ramer R, Heinemann K, Merkord J, *et al.* COX-2 and PPAR-γ confer cannabidiol-induced apoptosis of human lung cancer cells. Mol Cancer Ther 2013; 12(1): 69-82.
[http://dx.doi.org/10.1158/1535-7163.MCT-12-0335] [PMID: 23220503]

[85] Haustein M, Ramer R, Linnebacher M, Manda K, Hinz B. Cannabinoids increase lung cancer cell lysis by lymphokine-activated killer cells *via* upregulation of ICAM-1. Biochem Pharmacol 2014; 92(2): 312-25.
[http://dx.doi.org/10.1016/j.bcp.2014.07.014] [PMID: 25069049]

[86] Olivas-Aguirre M, Torres-López L, Valle-Reyes JS, Hernández-Cruz A, Pottosin I, Dobrovinskaya O. Cannabidiol directly targets mitochondria and disturbs calcium homeostasis in acute lymphoblastic leukemia. Cell Death Dis 2019; 10(10): 779.
[http://dx.doi.org/10.1038/s41419-019-2024-0] [PMID: 31611561]

[87] De Petrocellis L, Ligresti A, Schiano Moriello A, *et al.* Non-THC cannabinoids inhibit prostate carcinoma growth *in vitro* and *in vivo* : pro-apoptotic effects and underlying mechanisms. Br J Pharmacol 2013; 168(1): 79-102.
[http://dx.doi.org/10.1111/j.1476-5381.2012.02027.x] [PMID: 22594963]

[88] Sharma M, Hudson JB, Adomat H, Guns E, Cox ME. <i>In Vitro</i> Anticancer Activity of Plant-Derived Cannabidiol on Prostate Cancer Cell Lines. Pharmacol Pharm 2014; 5(8): 806-20.
[http://dx.doi.org/10.4236/pp.2014.58091]

CHAPTER 14

Modern Nanotherapeutic Approaches in The Delivery of Phyto Pharmceuticals in Anti Cancer Research

Pavan Kumar Chintamaneni[1,*], Sai Kiran S.S. Pindiprolu[2], Nandhakumar Sathyamoorthy[3], Motamarri Venkata Naga Lalitha Chaitanya[5], Rashmi Saxena Pal[4] and **Malakapogu Ravindra Babu[4]**

[1] *Department of Pharmaceutics, School of Pharmacy, GITAM Deemed to be University, Hyderabad, India*

[2] *Department of Pharmacology, Aditya Pharmacy College, Surampalem, Andhra Pradesh, India*

[3] *Department of Pharmaceutics, Faculty of Pharmacy, Dr. M.G.R. Educational and Research Institute, Chennai, Tamil Nadu, India*

[4] *Department of Pharmacognosy, School of Pharmacy, Lovely professional university, Phagwara, Punjab-144402, India*

[5] *School of Pharmacy, Lovely Professional University Phagwara, 144402 Punjab, India*

Abstract: Cancer has become one of the leading causes of human morbidity and mortality worldwide. A promising approach to tumour prevention is to eliminate cancer cells, preferably with less harm to neighbouring normal cells. Due to the disadvantages associated with current chemotherapy and radiation therapy, there is an increasing interest in developing novel delivery strategies for these natural products. Many phytochemicals show promise in cancer prevention and treatment due to their biocompatibility, low cytotoxicity, low resistance, and dynamic physiochemical properties that discriminate normal cells in the treatment of various cancer types. However, their low aqueous solubility, poor stability, unfavourable bioavailability, and low target specificity make their administration at therapeutic doses unrealistic. Recently developed nanotechnology has transformed drug delivery concepts and paved the way for the development of phytochemical-loaded nanoparticles for cancer prevention and treatment. Polymeric nanoparticles, lipid nanoparticles, carbon-based nanoparticles, and cell-derived nanoparticles can increase the stability and solubility of phytochemicals and also help in overcoming the disadvantages associated with conventional chemotherapy and phytochemicals. In the current chapter, we have men-

* **Corresponding author Pavan Kumar Chintamaneni:** Department of Pharmaceutics, School of Pharmacy, GITAM Deemed to be University, Hyderabad, India;
E-mail: pchintam@gitam.edu

Motamarri Venkata Naga Lalitha Chaitanya, Galvina Pereira, & Heyam Saad Ali (Eds.)

tioned the importance of nanotechnology in the delivery of phytochemicals and also added a note on the significance of delivery with current chemotherapeutics, including present challenges and future perspectives.

Keywords: Cancer, Chemotherapy, Cell cycle, Co-delivery, Checkpoints, Carbon nanoparticles, Drug delivery, Exosomes, Lipid nanoparticles, Nanoparticles, Phyto- chemicals, Phytomedicine, Polymeric nanoparticles.

INTRODUCTION

Cancer is one of the leading causes of death across the world. In 2018 alone, there were around 18.1 and 9.5 million new cancer cases and cancer-related mortalities, respectively. It is anticipated that there would be 29.5 and 16.4 million new cancer cases and cancer-related mortalities, respectively, by 2040. Cancer incidence is often higher in countries with a higher life expectancy and standard of living. According to statistics from 2015–2017, cancer would be diagnosed in approximately 39.5 percent of men and women at some point in their lives. In 2020, a projected number of 16,850 children and adolescents aged 0 to 19 would be diagnosed with different types of cancer, with 1,730 dying from cancers.

In 2018, the expected national cancer care expenses in the United States were $150.8 billion, and the costs are likely to climb in the coming years with the progression of age. As a result, enhancing overall survival and maintaining the quality of life are always necessary in order to reduce the worldwide burden of cancer. Future work will focus on improving current treatment options through dosing regimen optimization and the creation of successful chemotherapeutic combos.

Cancer Biology and Cell Cycle Checkpoints

The cell undergoes different phases for the evolution of new cells, which is generally called the "cell cycle." The cell cycle was divided into different phases and events. G1 phase, S phase, G2 phase, and M phase are the different phases undergone by the cell, which will give rise to two daughter cells, and again that cell will undergo the cell cycle process, and the process continues. In the cell cycle process at the G1 phase, the cell prepares to divide and then moves to the S phase, where the DNA and genetic material are copied by the cell, and then to the G2 phase, where the genetic material is organised by the cell, and finally to the M phase, where the cell undergoes mitosis, where the genetic material is divided, and two daughter cells are formed [1]. External and intracellular factors will influence and control the cell cycle progression by interfering with the cyclin/CDK task, resulting in a cell cycle pause, which is also known as a "checkpoint." In this case, the cells are given time to repair the damaged DNA, and various levels of growth factors are obtained to transfer the genetic material to the next phase. If severe damage has occurred to the DNA, it will start the

apoptotic signalling cascades to stop the damaged DNA from inhibiting its replication and further passage to the next phase of the cell cycle [2] (Fig. **1**).

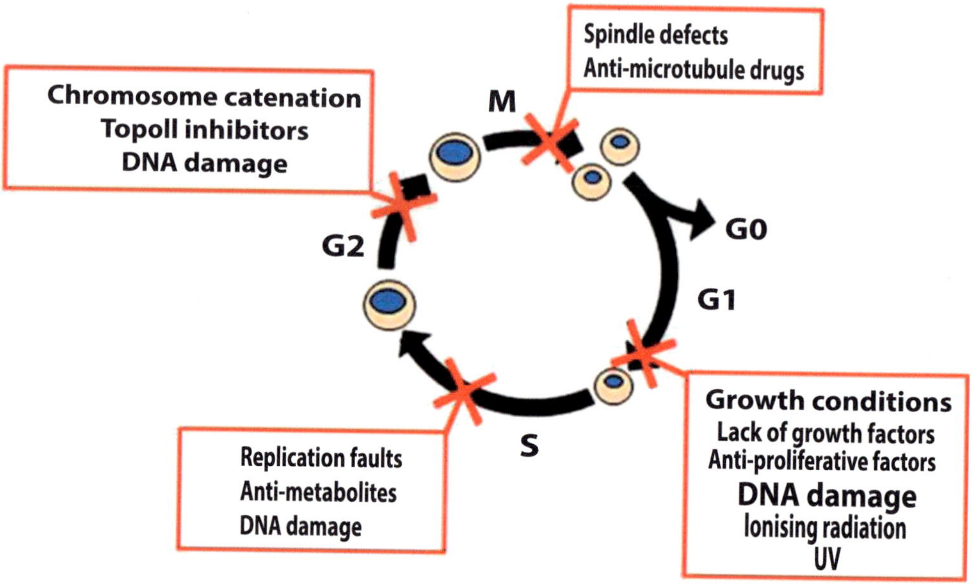

Fig. (1). Cell cycle Check points, reproduced from Gabrielli B, Brooks K, Pavey S. Defective cell cycle checkpoints as targets for anti-cancer therapies. Frontiers in pharmacology. 2012 Feb 2;3:9, under the terms of the Creative Commons Attribution Non Commercial License

During cell cycle, four major checkpoints have been identified: the restriction check point (G0/G1), the G1 check point, the G2 check point, and the mitosis-associated spindle-associated check point (SAC). The G0/G1 checkpoint is present in the G1 phase, which is controlled by the Rb/E2F signalling pathway. The E2F transcription factors were released from the Rb, which activates the genes and initiates the replication of DNA, which then enters the S phase. If the upstream regulators of Rb and the inactivating mutations present in RB1 are overexpressed, the degradation of this check point occurs, and early activation DNA occurs. Delayed DNA replication during the G1 checkpoint results in DNA damage.

This can be controlled by the p53, p21, and MDM2 pathways. The G2 checkpoints are of two types: the G2 checkpoint of DNA damage and the G2 checkpoint of decantation. The G2 checkpoint of DNA damage will delay the mitosis initiation that leads to DNA damage by seizing the inactive cyclin B1/cdk1 present in the cytoplasm that prevents entry into the mitosis, the decantation, and DNA damage. G2 check points are controlled by the ATM/Chk2/p53 pathway. The spindle assembly checkpoints are present in the mitotic phase, which leads to a delay in anaphase until the chromosomes show bipolar attachment to the mitotic spindle. This checkpoint was controlled by APC/C, BudR1, and Mad2 [1, 3].

To process the DNA damage repair prior to DNA replication and mitosis, the DNA damage response requires the integration of cell cycle regulation *via* checkpoint signalling. The importance of these checkpoint pathways, in response to DNA damage (both endogenous and exogenous) justifies the use of checkpoint inhibitors to enhance the efficiency of cancer chemo and radiotherapies. Chemo and radiation are significant inducers of the DNA damage response pathways, inducing various forms of DNA damage and activating checkpoints in varied degrees, and blocking these checkpoints might improve the cytotoxic efficacy of many anticancer medications. Targeting the S and G2 checkpoints of cell cycle appeared advantageous in cancer therapy, as the mutation on the p53 gene leads to loss of G1 control point in cancer cells and this makes them rely on S and G2 checkpoints in preventing DNA damage and cell death. Normal cells, on the other hand, rely on a functional G1 checkpoint [4].

Current Therapeutic Approaches and Associated Challenges

The most extensive and effective modes of management of cancer today are chemotherapy and radiotherapy. However, these current treatment methods suffer from several adverse effects like hepatotoxicity, cardiotoxicity, nephrotoxicity, neurotoxicity, and gastrointestinal toxicities. They also have other side effects like fatigue, reduced immunity, infections, loss of appetite, constipation, anemia, *etc.* due to off-target actions [5, 6]. As a result, these negative effects frequently decrease cancer patients' quality of life and may lead to therapy withdrawal. Hence, it is critical to establish appropriate alternate treatment methods that can counter chemotherapy- and radiotherapy-related side effects [7].

Need of Phytochemicals

The principal drawbacks of chemotherapy are cancer relapse, drug resistance, and off-target side effects, which consequently decrease the patient's quality of life.

This restricts the use of anticancer medications. To address the inadequacies of the present therapy, researchers are still looking for novel potential molecules with anticancer activity with improved efficacy and reduced side effects. Phytochemicals are structurally varied and consist of scaffolds that are particularly designed to bind to and down-regulate the functions of a wide variety of key proteins. These phytochemical molecules have more chiral centres and a greater spectrum of ring structures in comparison to synthetic pharmaceuticals. This structural complexity is responsible for increasing target selective activity, reducing the non-specific binding and thereby, reducing the unfavourable effects [8].

Plants have historically been used to cure a number of diseases, including cancer. Plants, animals, marine species, and microorganisms all contribute to anti-cancer drugs, making nature an interesting source of new therapeutic entities [9]. Natural goods, such as crude extracts, bioactive component-enriched fractions, pure chemicals produced from herbs, and herbal formulations, have been shown to prevent and treat cancer [10]. Some natural compounds have been shown in clinical trials and preclinical studies to minimise chemotherapy- and radiotherapy-induced toxicities [6]. Natural anticancer medications include taxanes, vinca alkaloids and their analogues, camptothecin and its derivatives, anthracyclines, podophyllotoxin, *etc.* Natural products or their derivatives derived from tiny molecules or macromolecules found in nature account for half of all anti-cancer medications licensed worldwide. Plant phytochemicals and derivatives are promising alternatives for increasing therapeutic efficacy and decreasing unwanted effects in cancer patients. Several of these phytochemicals are physiologically active compounds that exist naturally and have anticancer action [11, 12]. Several of these phytochemicals are physiologically active compounds that exist naturally and have an anticancer action. From common sources, a diverse spectrum of phytochemicals has been identified and described, including, vegetables like broccoli and onion; fruits like grapes and apple; spices line pepper, turmeric and nutmeg; brews like red wine, oolong tea and green tea. All the natural sources are rich in antioxidants.

These antioxidants aid in the prevention and treatment of cancer and other disorders by protecting cells from damage caused by extremely reactive oxygen molecules known as "free radicals." Quercetin, quercitrin, and kaempferol are common flavonoids found in roughly 70% of all plants [13].

Here we have listed out some examples of phytochemicals that can effectively inhibit cancer cell growth.

- *Cordyceps cicadae* is a type of fungus which belongs to the family of

Cordycipitaceac that was used in the Chinese medicine. The alcoholic extracts from the cordyceps cicadae are used to treat gastric cancer by targeting the SGC-7901 cell lines of cancer. It has been shown to inhibit the proliferation of SGC-7901 which increases the cellular stress and cell cycle inhibition of S phase [14].

- *Allium sativum* belongs to the *Amaryllidaceae*. The allicin is the extract from the *Allium sativum* that is used to inhibit the SGC-7901 cell lines of cancer and G2/M phase cycle arrest [15].
- Camptothecin (CPT), obtained from the stem wood of a Chinese tree, *Camptotheca acuminata* inhibits topoisomerase I and promotes apoptosis in human leukaemia cell lines, PLB-985 [16].
- Plumbago Zeylanica shows anti-cancer activity by showing effects on different cancer cell lines like MKN-28, AGS, SGC-7901 [17].
- *Saussera lappa* acts on cancer cell lines AGS, BGC-823. The action on AGS results in the G2 phase arrest of the cell cycle [14].
- Euphorbia lunulata acts on the cancer cell lines like MCF-7 and NCI-H460 which inhibits the cell cycle at the G2/M phase and cell apoptosis is observed [18].
- Croton regelianus Mull. Arg has shown anti-activity on brain cancer cell lines HL-60 and SF-295 [19].
- The root extract of the Sanguinaria Canadensis called Sanguinarine acts as anti-cancer drug on MDA-231 breast cancer cells [20].
- Piperine extracted from the Piper nigrum has shown anti-cancer activity on 4T1 breast cancer cells [21].

Challenges in Delivery of Phytopharmaceuticals

A majority of anticancer medications currently in clinical use suffer from a lot of limitations. These limitations include limited water solubility, the inability to be delivered orally, poor specificity, and a very short biological half-life. The treatment regimen associated with this short biological half-life is associated with the development of systemic toxicities and multiple drug resistance (MDR). which is mostly caused by the overexpression of proteins from the ATP-binding cassette (ABC) transporter superfamily. These MDR proteins, particularly P-glycoprotein (Pgp), are responsible for energy-dependent drug efflux, resulting in less chemotherapeutic agent present in cancer cells [22]. It has also fuelled increased research activity toward the development of novel analogues of existing nature-derived treatments and the search for novel compounds from natural sources, furthering the use of nanotechnology to improve the safety and efficacy of these drugs. Cancer diagnosis and therapy could be transformed by nanotechnology. Tumor angiogenesis is poorly controlled, and a tumour is often accompanied by a faulty, leaky vascular architecture. Because the faulty lymphatic system drains the interstitial fluid within a tumor, submicron-sized particles can easily extravasate into and be retained at the tumour site. This phenomenon is termed the "enhanced permeation and retention" (EPR) effect.

The EPR effect, in turn, will benefit nanoparticle systems that use passive targeting to localise at the tumour site. Active targeting techniques work by combining chemotherapeutic nanocarriers with compounds that bind to overexpressed antigens or receptors on target cells. However, because of the recent breakthroughs in surface-engineering technology, the biodistribution profile of nanocarriers can be fine-tuned by altering their surface physicochemical qualities to target the tissues of interest. This increases the amount of medicine that reaches the targeted tumour sites while minimising systemic pharmacological effects [22 - 24]. Nanotechnologically modified drugs and drug delivery systems are becoming increasingly frequent in cancer treatment, with several already being used in clinical trials with promising results. As a result, it can be used to improve cancer diagnosis, medicine delivery into tumour cells, and molecularly targeted cancer therapy, all of which improve the therapeutic management of cancer patients. The majority of existing nanotechnology-based chemotherapy solutions include the repackaging of traditional anticancer medicines into various nanometer-sized delivery vehicles. Thus, nanotechnology has provided a platform for improving phytochemical delivery by employing novel concepts and carriers that conventional technologies were unable to achieve [25].

Nanotechnology in the Delivery of Phytopharmaceuticals in Cancer Therapy

Polymeric Nanoparticles

A polymer is synthesised using many organic compounds, which can then be combined to form a nanoparticle with hydrophilic and hydrophobic regions. As a result, polymeric nanoparticles protect pharmaceuticals from degradation while also increasing their solubility and bioavailability. Polymeric nanoparticles were created using a variety of biodegradable polymers, such as PLA, PLGA, *etc.*, along with surfactants or stabilizers. The polymeric nanoparticles range in size from 10 to 1000 nm. Polymeric nanoparticle characteristics such as size, charge, structure, and release kinetics can be adjusted during synthesis by selecting the suitable polymer length and solvent. Furthermore, the alteration can be performed on functional groups located on the polymeric nanoparticles' exterior [26].

Nikita Sharma *et al.* investigated the beneficial effects of diosgenin (DS)-loaded poly-glycerol malate co-dodecanedioate (PGMD) nanoparticles for improved anticancer efficacy. The authors employed the nanoprecipitation method for preparing DS-loaded PGMD nanoparticles (7:3 and 6:4 variants) and optimised them with the Box-Behnken design. The independent variables were the concentrations of each PGMD, diosgenin, and PF-68. Particle size and polydispersity index (PDI) are the dependent variables used for optimising the formulation. The particle sizes were 133.6 nm and 121.4 nm for PGMD 7:3 and PGMD 6:4 nanoparticles, respectively, with an entrapment efficiency range of 77–83%. The IC50 in A549 lung cancer cells after 48 hours was found to be 27.14 M, 15.15 M, and 13.91 M for DS, PGMD 7:3, and PGMD 6:4, respectively [27].

Jian-dong Yuan *et al.*, prepared curcumin (Cur) and doxorubicin (Dox) nanoparticles (CURDOX-NPs) using monomethoxy (polyethylene glycol)-b-P (D,L-lactic-co-glycolic acid)-b-P (L-glutamic acid) polymers for simultaneous targeting of cancer and cancer stem cells (CSCs). CURDOX-NPs (107.5 nm) have a zeta potential of−13.7 mV and entrapment efficiencies (EE) of 80.30% and 96.2%, for Cur and Dox, respectively. There is a significant drug release at tumour pH (5.0) compared to the physiological pH (7.4). CURDOX-NPs exhibited significant cytotoxicity *in vitro* against CSC-enriched MCF-7/ADR mammospheres. Further, CURDOX-NPs also showed significant CSC-enriched tumour regression in the xenograft mouse model. The combined delivery of Cur and Dox was proven to be a potentially useful therapeutic strategy for refractory breast cancer [28].

In another study by, Jinming Zhang *et al.*, co-delivery of pro-apoptotic agent (Dox) and anti-angiogenic agent (Cur) ((D+C)/NPs)) was carried out for synergistic tumor regression in hepatocellular carcinoma (HCC). (D+C)/NPs resulted in enhanced cellular uptake in SMMC 7721 cells and human umbilical vein endothelial cells (HUVECs) compared to their free forms and improved their cytotoxic effects in SMMC 7721 cells. Besides, (D+C)/NPs also exhibited stronger anti-angiogenic effects as evident from inhibition of VEGF mediated HUVEC proliferation, migration, invasion, and tube formation. Betulinic acid (BA) is an anti-angiogenic phytochemical with cytotoxic effects on breast cancers including triple negative breast cancer (TNBC).

However, the off-target effects, low solubility, and low bioavailability of BA are its limitations for its applications as an anticancer agent. It was recently reported that lactoferrin (Lf) attached to BA nanoformulation (Lf-BAnp) improved the anticancer activity of BA in TNBC (MDA-MB-231) and laryngeal (HEp-2) cancer cells. The association of LF and BA was evident from SDS-PAGE and FT-IR. Lf-Banp (147.7 nm) has a zeta potential of -28.51 mV and a 75.38% EE, followed a non-fickian drug release pattern, inhibiting the cell cycle in the sub-G1 population, and possessed greater cytotoxic effects with intracellular uptake within 30 min. Lf-Banp design, therefore, has a propensity for therapeutic application in TNBC. Pigallocatechin-3-gallate (EGCG) is another phytochemical from green tea with a broad spectrum of cytotoxicity [29].

Julekha Kazi *et al.*, developed a folate receptor (FR) targeted polymeric drug delivery system of EGCG for the treatment of breast cancer (FP-EGCG-NPs). The preclinical efficacy of FP-EGCG-NPs was evaluated in MDA-MB-231 and MCF-7 cells. The FA peptide conjugated, FP-EGCG-NPs formulation has greater cytotoxicity and intracellular uptake than the unconjugated NPs with a longer half-life. Furthermore, when compared to naive EGCG, the FP-EGCG-NPs formulation has a higher plasma concentration and a much higher mitochondrial depolarization impact. In scintigraphy imaging research, FP-EGCG-NPs were radiolabeled with technetium-99m and their selectivity towards MDA-MB-231 tumours in nude mice was studied. The preclinical examination indicated that FP-EGCG-NPs had better tumour regression than the naive medication and unconjugated nanoformulation [30].

Lipid Nanoparticles

Amphiphilic lipid molecules can assemble into a specific configuration of one or more concentric bilayer structures when distributed in a polar solvent such as water; these concentric bilayer structures are called vesicles. Vesicular systems provide a good answer to a variety of pharmacological issues with drugs, such as insolubility, short half-life, and toxicity. Drugs that are insoluble can be made soluble by entrapping them in vesicular networks. Furthermore, these vesicular systems shield and delay drug metabolism from xenobiotic metabolising enzymes, allowing for extended drug release throughout the body. Another key benefit of the lipid-based vesicular system is that it protects body tissues from direct contact with harmful medications, which are then selectively ingested by body cells. Hydrophilic and hydrophobic medicines can both entrap lipid-based vesicular systems. In general, hydrophobic medications are confined within the vesicular system's internal compartment, whereas hydrophobic drugs are coupled with the vesicular system's lipid membrane layer *via* hydrophobic interactions. Surfactant molecules, in addition to lipids, were utilised to create the vesicular nanostructures. The physiochemical properties of vesicular systems are determined by the size, elasticity, surface charge, and membrane lamellarity. These physiochemical and colloidal variables can affect the vesicular system's shape, stability, entrapment effectiveness, and drug-delivery capability. To boost bilayer plasticity and defend against aggregation, the lipid bilayer can be merged with cholesterol and other charged compounds [26, 31].

Satveer Jagwani *et al.*, developed Resveratrol (RS) loaded cationic liposomes (RLs) for specific delivery of RS to hepatocellular carcinoma (HepG2) cells. The optimized RLs (145.78 nm) were spherical with a ZP of 38.03 mV and EE of 78.14%. *In vitro* efficacy studies revealed greater cellular uptake and cytotoxicity of RLs compared to naïve RS. Further, the *in vivo* efficacy of RL was evaluated in N-nitrosodiethylamine (NDEA) induced hepatic cancer (HCC) in rats. RL possesses significant anticancer activity compared to free RS in HCC tumor-bearing rats. Further, RL also reversed the HCC-induced alterations in hepatic enzymes (alanine transaminase, alkaline phosphatase, aspartate transaminase, total bilirubin levels, γ-glutamyl trans-lpeptidase, and α-fetoprotein) compared to disease group and free RS treated groups. The findings of this study were also supported by histopathological analysis, and demonstrated NDEA-induced detrimental effects on rat livers and the protective effects of RL. A Pharmacokinetic evaluation demonstrated increased localization of RL in cancerous liver tissues with 3.2- and 2.2-fold increases in AUC and Cmax, respectively, when compared to the free RS group. In another study [32]. Chinnaiyan Senthil Kumar *et al.* fabricated chitosan-coated-trans-resveratrol (RSV) and ferulic acid (FER) loaded SLNs surface modified with folic acid (FA) (C-RSV-FER-FA-SLNs). C-RSV-FER-FA-SLNs exhibited better stability under acidic conditions for tumour targeted drug delivery applications. Further, the optimised C-RSV-FER-FA-SLNs possess greater cytotoxicity in colon cancer (HT-29) cells. C-RSV-FER-FA-SLNs effectively increased the cytotoxicity of HT29 cells compared to free RSV-FER and serve as a promising candidate for novel nanodrug formulations in cancer therapy [33]. Vahab Ghalehkhondabi *et al.*, reported the improved anticancer effects of silibinin (SLB)-loaded folic acid (FA)-conjugated Pluronic F127 folate targeted nanomicelles (SLB-F127-FA) for the treatment of liver cancer. FA was conjugated.

In a recent study [34], Boshra Amiri *et al.* used a thin film hydration technique to create a PEGylated Niosomal Formulation (Pn-VB) to improve the anticancer effects of vinblastine (VB) by increasing cellular bioavailability. Pn-VB (234.3 nm) exhibited greater regression of tumours in murine lung cancer (TC-1) cells and tumor-bearing C57BL/6 mice compared to free VB. Furthermore, when compared to the free drug, Pn-VB increased survivability in tumor-bearing mice [35].

Walid S. Kamoun *et al.* explored the synergistic effects of novel EphA2-targeted liposomal docetaxel (EphA2-ILs-DTXp) and anti-PD-1. The combination of EphA2-ILs-DTXp with anti-PD-1 effectively prevented the tumour relapse in the EMT-6 tumour model. EphA2-ILs-DTXp resulted in an increased AUC of docetaxel by 15 times, from 52.1 to 785 ng/mL/h. A dose reduction study of EphA2-ILs-DTXp showed a dose-response relationship between both tumour growth inhibition and the CD8/Treg ratio [36].

Carbon Nanoparticles

Neha Singh *et al.*, fabricated single-walled carbon nanotubes (SWCNTs) of Curcumin (Cur) surface modified with alginate (ALG) and chitosan (CHI). Surface modification renders a high %EE and targeting efficacy of SWCNTs. *In vitro* release studies revealed the pH-dependent release of Cur from SWCNTs. In human lung adenocarcinoma (A549) cells, Cur-loaded SWCNTs exhibited greater cytotoxicity than free Cur, by induction of apoptosis (37).

In another study, Zhong Tian *et al.* prepared polyethyleneimine (PEI), folic acid, and functionalized multiwalled carbon nanotubes (f-MWNTs) for enhanced Paclitaxel (PTX) drug delivery *via* noncovalent - stacking interactions. f-MWNTs resulted in enhanced cytotoxicity with high stability and safety. Further f-MWNTs resulted in improved cellular internalisation of PTX [38].

Rossella Arrigo ***et al.*** reported that, for quercetin (Q), CNTs have been formulated and used in the preparation of ultra-high molecular weight polyethylene (UHMWPE) nanocomposites for enhanced antioxidant activity. The rheological behaviour reveals the remarkable stabilising action, due to the strong physical interaction between Q and CNTs. In particular, the presence of Q molecules causes the formation of CNT structural defects, remarkably amplifying the intrinsic CNT radical scavenging activity [39].

Chuanjin Wang ***et al.*** **prepared** multiwalled carbon nanotubes encapsulated with ORI (MWCNTs-ORI) for enhancing the antitumor potency and reducing the cytotoxicity of ORI. The EE of ORI is 82.6% (w/w). There was improved tumour regression of ORI with nanoformulations both *in vitro* and *in vivo* in tumour-bearing mice [40].

Julia M. Tan, ***et al.*****,** prepared carboxylic acid-functionalized single-walled carbon nanotubes (f-SWCNTs) of BA. The binding of BA onto the surface of f-SWCNTs was confirmed by FTIR and Raman spectroscopies. Powder XRD analysis showed that the structure of the conjugate was unaffected by the loading of BA. f-SWCNTs significantly enhanced the cytotoxicity in A549 than HepG2 cell line and proved to be an efficient drug carrier to conjugate drugs for anticancer applications [41].

Exosomes

Javier Donoso-Quezada ***et al.*** showed that exosomes encapsulated with saponins and flavonoids obtained from Phaseolus vulgaris L. have enhanced anticancer activity. The authors demonstrated co-loading of three different phytochemicals in one step for intracellular delivery into tumour cells. The efficacy studies revealed greater cytotoxic effects of exosomes compared to other formulation components. In this study, the authors demonstrated exosomes as a promising delivery system for tumour-targeted delivery of nutraceuticals [42].

Huan Liu *et al.*, developed triptolide-loaded exosomes delivery system (TP-Exos), to improve the anticancer efficiency of triptolide, by improving the bioavailability and reducing side effects such as hepatotoxicity, and nephrotoxicity. Further, the tumor targeting efficiency and toxicity of exosomes was measured by monitoring the tumor volume of mice, and TUNNEL assay, in ovarian cancer models. The results revealed that, TP-Exos showed high encapsulation efficiency, and significant uptake by SKOV3 cells *in vitro* as well as tumor site *in vivo*.

The cytotoxic and apoptotic effects of TP-Exos showed greater tumour growth inhibition and cell proliferation, when compared to free TP. However, the TP-Exos showed toxic effects on the liver and spleen. As a result, clinical translation of these TP-Exos necessitates addressing liver and spleen damage [43].

Co delivery of Phytochemical and Chemotherapeutic Agent/Genetic Material

Drug combinations are frequently used to treat serious diseases such as AIDS and cancer. The major goal is to achieve a reduction in dose and toxicity, a synergistic therapeutic impact, and to reduce or postpone drug resistance induction. Synergistic interactions are important in phytomedicine, which explain why extremely low doses of active components in herbal formulations are effective. Traditional medicine is predicated on the idea that a whole or partially purified plant extract outperforms a single isolated ingredient. Synergism also contributes to toxicity reduction and resistance minimization. Though vinblastine is efficient on its own, it is increasingly being studied in combination with other anticancer medications, primarily for the treatment of recurrent or advanced cancers resistant to conventional chemotherapy. The advent of clinical treatment resistance has highlighted the significance of looking for new chemotherapeutic drugs as well as better combinations of existing agents. Synergy is often regarded as having more than additive therapeutic effects when compared to the efficacy of each drug alone. Combination therapies have recently been studied, with the theory being that targeting two independent pathways will result in increased cytotoxicity, whether additive or synergistic. Several researchers have attempted to boost the performance of well-known anti-cancer drugs such as vinblastine and paclitaxel by combining them with cisplatin, etoposide, and doxorubicin (Table **1** and **2**).

Table 1. Phytochemicals in combination with other anticancer drugs in clinical practice which showed synergistic activity

Plant secondary metabolite	Synergy with anti-cancer agents	Experimental models & Outcomes	References
Apigenin	Tamoxifen Fulvestrant	Improved sensitivity of Tamoxifen and fulvestrant MCF7 human breast cancer cells.	[44]
Berberine	Cisplatin	Ovarian cancer cell line VCAR3, enhanced more ovarian cancer cell death by inducing apoptosis and necroptosis.	[45]
	Doxorubicin	Murine melanoma B16F10 cells, showed inhibition of cancer cell proliferation and increase in apoptotic cell death.	[46]
Curcumin	Cisplatin, Doxorubicin	Human and rat glioblastoma cell lines, improved the sensitivity of glioma cells to chemotherapeutic agents.	[47]
	Oxaliplatin/cisplatin	Human ovarian carcinoma cell lines (2008 and C13), curcumin was also able to increase sensitivity of resistant ovarian cancer cells to cisplatin/oxaliplatin.	[48]
	SiRNA	Mouse melanoma cells (B16F10), greater depth penetration and tumor regression.	[49]
	SiRNA	Human bladder cancer cell line, decreased proliferation and increased apoptosis of bladder cancer cells.	[50]
Genistein	Cisplatin	Human pancreatic carcinoma cell line (BxPC-3), murine xenograft model of BxPC-3 cells, improved NF-κB binding and inactivation.	[51]
	Camptothecin	Human cervical cancer cell line (HeLa), human ovarian carcinoma line [OAW-42), increased cytotoxicity, damage to DNA and greater inhibited cell-cycle progression.	[52]
(-)-epigallocatechin 3-gallate (EGCG)	Cisplatin	Human ovarian cancer cell lines (SKOV3, CAOV3, and C200), increased cisplatin potency by three to six-fold.	[53]
	Doxorubicin	Murine xenografts of human carcinoma DOX-resistant cells (KB-A-1), improved the sensitivity of the cells.	[54]
Eupatin	Mitoxantrone	NCI-H460 human lung non-small-cell carcinoma cells, improved sensitivity of resistant cells to mitoxantrone.	[55]
Indirubin	Arylidene derivative	Human non□small cell lung carcinoma cells, improved apoptotic cell death	[56]

(Table 1) cont.....

Plant secondary metabolite	Synergy with anti-cancer agents	Experimental models & Outcomes	References
	Vinblastine	HeLa cells, synergistically enhanced the anti-mitotic and anti-proliferative activity of vinblastine.	[57]
Kaempferol	Vinblastine	Cervical carcinoma cell lines (KB-V1, KB---1), inhibition of P glycoprotein and improved chemo sensitization.	[58]
Luteolin	Doxorubicin	4T1 and MCF-7 cells, improved cell proliferation with adjunct action.	[59]
Quercetin	Cisplatin	Human laryngeal carcinoma cell line (Hep-2), improved activity by mitochondrial-mediated apoptosis.	[60]
Resveratrol	Doxorubicin	Human acute myeloid leukemia cell lines (ML-2/DX30, AML-2/DX100, and AML-2/DX300), helps in overcoming doxorubicin resistance, or in sensitizing doxorubicin-resistant AML cells to anti-leukemic agents.	[61]
Silybin	Cisplatin	Human prostate carcinoma cell line DU145, improved efficiency and increased apoptosis.	[62]

Table 2. Marketed Nanophyto pharmaceuticals for anticancer therapy

Product (Trade name)	Manufactured by	Approved year	Application in cancer
Pegylated liposomal doxorubicin	Intas Pharmaceuticals Ltd.	1999	Kaposi' sarcoma, ovary, breast
Liposomal cytarabine (Depocyt)	Pacira BioSciences, Inc	1999	Lymphomatous meningitis
Liposomal mifamurtide (Mepact)	Takeda UK Ltd.	2009	Osteosarcoma
NAB-paclitaxel (Abeaxane)	Celgene corporation	2012	Breast, lung, pancreas
Liposomal vincristine (Marqibo)	Spectrum Pharmaceuticals Ltd.	2012	Adult acute lymphoblastic leukemia
Irinotecan (NaI-IRI)	Merrimack Pharmaceuticals, Inc	2015	Awaiting new drug application
Liposomal daunorubicin: Cytrabine (Vyxeos)	Jazz Pharmaceuticals plc	2017	Kaposi' sarcoma
Liposomal doxorubicin (PEGADRIA 50)	Intas Pharmaceuticals Ltd.	2018	Breast Cancer

Conclusion and Future Perspectives

Over the last decade, advances in nanobiotechnology and nanomaterial science have aided in imaging diagnostics and tailored cancer therapy by developing efficient drug delivery systems. A variety of nano drug delivery systems incorporating traditional anticancer medications or phytochemicals have been developed to improve increased permeability and retention (EPR) in cancer. To gain a deeper understanding of the physicochemical properties of nanoparticles, such as their form, size, charge, surface chemistry, and toxicity, creative nanoencapsulation designs and the creation of efficient anticancer phytochemicals are necessary. Many natural substances have been proven to be effective in cultured cells and animals while being low in toxicity, such as anacardic acid, betulinic acid, curcumin, EGCG, ferulic acid, gambogic acid, ginsenosides, kaempferol, lycopene, and resveratrol. However, due to poor solubility, stability, rapid clearance by RES phagocytosis, drug distribution, degradation, and resistance, many phytochemicals have not exhibited significant anticancer activity in people. Phytochemical-encapsulated NPs, on the other hand, have been shown to boost antitumor effects in a range of cancers by blocking several pathways and reducing drug resistance.

However, for a specific molecular target, the distinction between nano-phytochemicals and free phytochemicals or NPs alone should be examined further by analysing the synergistic or additive effects of NPs and free phytochemicals. Furthermore, the repeatability and reliability of NP-phytochemical encapsulations, as well as their potential toxicity and the best routes of administration (oral, intravenous, transdermal), must be guaranteed. Furthermore, because some phytochemicals can cause negative side effects despite being less toxic than synthetic anticancer drugs, their pharmacodynamic and pharmacokinetic properties should be studied in a variety of preclinical and randomised clinical trials.

Furthermore, more research is required to understand the detailed molecular mechanism of nanodrugs within the tumour environment for active drug delivery, to lengthen the circulation period, and to examine RES evasion, sensitive drug release, and tailored co-delivery of diverse chemicals. Finally, in addition to overcoming the obstacles, an appropriate strategy for reducing manufacturing costs and scaling up the production of anticancer phytochemical candidates should be developed to ensure their success in the pharmaceutical market.

REFERENCES

[1] Gabrielli B, Brooks K, Pavey S. Defective cell cycle checkpoints as targets for anti-cancer therapies. Front Pharmacol 2012; 3: 9.
[http://dx.doi.org/10.3389/fphar.2012.00009] [PMID: 22347187]

[2] Andersson E. The control of the cell cycle with particular emphasis on the G1/S transition. 2014.

[3] Barnum KJ, O'Connell MJ. Cell cycle regulation by checkpoints Cell cycle control. Springer 2014; pp. 29-40.

[4] Kastan MB, Bartek J. Cell-cycle checkpoints and cancer. Nature 2004; 432(7015): 316-23. [http://dx.doi.org/10.1038/nature03097] [PMID: 15549093]

[5] Charles L, Levy OG. Highlights of Recent Findings on Quality-of-Life Management for Patients With Cancer and Their Survivors. 2016.

[6] Zhang QY, Wang FX, Jia KK, Kong LD. Natural product interventions for chemotherapy and radiotherapy-induced side effects. Front Pharmacol 2018; 9: 1253. [http://dx.doi.org/10.3389/fphar.2018.01253] [PMID: 30459615]

[7] Turcotte LM, Liu Q, Yasui Y, *et al.* Temporal trends in treatment and subsequent neoplasm risk among 5-year survivors of childhood cancer, 1970-2015. JAMA 2017; 317(8): 814-24. [http://dx.doi.org/10.1001/jama.2017.0693] [PMID: 28245323]

[8] Mansoori B, Mohammadi A, Davudian S, Shirjang S, Baradaran B. The different mechanisms of cancer drug resistance: a brief review. Adv Pharm Bull 2017; 7(3): 339-48. [http://dx.doi.org/10.15171/apb.2017.041] [PMID: 29071215]

[9] Cragg GM, Pezzuto JM. Natural products as a vital source for the discovery of cancer chemotherapeutic and chemopreventive agents. Med Princ Pract 2016; 25(Suppl 2) (Suppl. 2): 41-59. [http://dx.doi.org/10.1159/000443404] [PMID: 26679767]

[10] Sanders K, Moran Z, Shi Z, Paul R, Greenlee H, Eds. Natural products for cancer prevention: clinical update 2016. Seminars in oncology nursing 2016; 32(3): 215-40.

[11] Greenwell M, Rahman PK. Medicinal plants: their use in anticancer treatment. Int J Pharm Sci Res 2015; 6(10): 4103-12. [PMID: 26594645]

[12] Khan T, Gurav P. PhytoNanotechnology: Enhancing delivery of plant based anti-cancer drugs. Front Pharmacol 2018; 8: 1002. [http://dx.doi.org/10.3389/fphar.2017.01002] [PMID: 29479316]

[13] Doughari JH. Phytochemicals: extraction methods, basic structures and mode of action as potential chemotherapeutic agents Phytochemicals - A Global Perspective of Their Role in Nutrition and Health. Rijeka, Croatia: INTECH Open Access 2012.

[14] Nakonieczna S, Grabarska A, Kukula-Koch W. The Potential Anticancer Activity of Phytoconstituents against Gastric Cancer—A Review on *in vitro, in vivo*, and Clinical Studies. Int J Mol Sci 2020; 21(21): 8307. [http://dx.doi.org/10.3390/ijms21218307] [PMID: 33167519]

[15] Forma A, Chilimoniuk Z, Januszewski J, Sitarz R. The Potential Application of Allium Extracts in the Treatment of Gastrointestinal Cancers. Gastroenterol Insights 2021; 12(2): 136-46. [http://dx.doi.org/10.3390/gastroent12020012]

[16] Pal A, Sengupta S, Kundu R. Tiliacora racemosa leaves induce oxidative stress mediated DNA damage leading to G2/M phase arrest and apoptosis in cervical cancer cells SiHa. J Ethnopharmacol 2021; 269: 113686. [http://dx.doi.org/10.1016/j.jep.2020.113686] [PMID: 33309918]

[17] Li J, Shen L, Lu F, *et al.* Plumbagin inhibits cell growth and potentiates apoptosis in human gastric cancer cells *in vitro* through the NF-κB signaling pathway. Acta Pharmacol Sin 2012; 33(2): 242-9. [http://dx.doi.org/10.1038/aps.2011.152] [PMID: 22231395]

[18] Fu Z, Han X, Du J, *et al.* Euphorbia lunulata extract acts on multidrug resistant gastric cancer cells to inhibit cell proliferation, migration and invasion, arrest cell cycle progression, and induce apoptosis. J Ethnopharmacol 2018; 212: 8-17.

[http://dx.doi.org/10.1016/j.jep.2017.08.014] [PMID: 28811220]

[19] Bezerra DP, Filho JDBM, Alves APNN, *et al.* Antitumor activity of the essential oil from the leaves of Croton regelianus and its component ascaridole. Chem Biodivers 2009; 6(8): 1224-31. [http://dx.doi.org/10.1002/cbdv.200800253] [PMID: 19697341]

[20] Croaker A, King G, Pyne J, Anoopkumar-Dukie S, Liu L. Sanguinaria canadensis: traditional medicine, phytochemical composition, biological activities and current uses. Int J Mol Sci 2016; 17(9): 1414. [http://dx.doi.org/10.3390/ijms17091414] [PMID: 27618894]

[21] de Almeida GC, Oliveira LFS, Predes D, *et al.* Piperine suppresses the Wnt/β-catenin pathway and has anti-cancer effects on colorectal cancer cells. Sci Rep 2020; 10(1): 11681. [http://dx.doi.org/10.1038/s41598-020-68574-2] [PMID: 32669593]

[22] Fakhar ud Din , Aman W, Ullah I. Effective use of nanocarriers as drug delivery systems for the treatment of selected tumors. International Journal of Nanomedicine 2017.

[23] Yao Y, Zhou Y, Liu L, *et al.* Nanoparticle-based drug delivery in cancer therapy and its role in overcoming drug resistance. Front Mol Biosci 2020; 7: 193. [http://dx.doi.org/10.3389/fmolb.2020.00193] [PMID: 32974385]

[24] Jeevanandam J, Barhoum A, Chan YS, Dufresne A, Danquah MK. Review on nanoparticles and nanostructured materials: history, sources, toxicity and regulations. Beilstein J Nanotechnol 2018; 9(1): 1050-74. [http://dx.doi.org/10.3762/bjnano.9.98] [PMID: 29719757]

[25] Jin C, Wang K, Oppong-Gyebi A, Hu J. Application of nanotechnology in cancer diagnosis and therapy-a mini-review. Int J Med Sci 2020; 17(18): 2964-73. [http://dx.doi.org/10.7150/ijms.49801] [PMID: 33173417]

[26] Sajid M, Cameotra SS, Khan MSA, Ahmad I. Nanoparticle-based delivery of phytomedicines: challenges and opportunities New Look to phytomedicine. Elsevier 2019; pp. 597-623. [http://dx.doi.org/10.1016/B978-0-12-814619-4.00024-0]

[27] Sharma N, Singhal M, Kumari RM, *et al.* Diosgenin Loaded Polymeric Nanoparticles with Potential Anticancer Efficacy. Biomolecules 2020; 10(12): 1679. [http://dx.doi.org/10.3390/biom10121679] [PMID: 33339083]

[28] Yuan J-D. pH-sensitive polymeric nanoparticles of mPEG-PLGA-PGlu with hybrid core for simultaneous encapsulation of curcumin and doxorubicin to kill the heterogeneous tumour cells in breast cancer. Artificial cells, nanomedicine, and biotechnology 2018; 46(supl 1): 302-13.

[29] Zhang J, Li J, Shi Z, *et al.* pH-sensitive polymeric nanoparticles for co-delivery of doxorubicin and curcumin to treat cancer *via* enhanced pro-apoptotic and anti-angiogenic activities. Acta Biomater 2017; 58: 349-64. [http://dx.doi.org/10.1016/j.actbio.2017.04.029] [PMID: 28455219]

[30] Das M, Sahoo SK. Folate decorated dual drug loaded nanoparticle: role of curcumin in enhancing therapeutic potential of nutlin-3a by reversing multidrug resistance. PLoS One 2012; 7(3): e32920. [http://dx.doi.org/10.1371/journal.pone.0032920] [PMID: 22470431]

[31] Jain S, Jain V, Mahajan S. Lipid based vesicular drug delivery systems. Advances in Pharmaceutics 2014. [http://dx.doi.org/10.1155/2014/574673]

[32] Jagwani S, Jalalpure S, Dhamecha D, Jadhav K, Bohara R. Pharmacokinetic and pharmacodynamic evaluation of resveratrol loaded cationic liposomes for targeting hepatocellular carcinoma. ACS Biomater Sci Eng 2020; 6(9): 4969-84. [http://dx.doi.org/10.1021/acsbiomaterials.0c00429] [PMID: 33455290]

[33] Senthil Kumar C, Thangam R, Mary SA, Kannan PR, Arun G, Madhan B. Targeted delivery and apoptosis induction of trans-resveratrol-ferulic acid loaded chitosan coated folic acid conjugate solid

lipid nanoparticles in colon cancer cells. Carbohydr Polym 2020; 231: 115682. [http://dx.doi.org/10.1016/j.carbpol.2019.115682] [PMID: 31888816]

[34] Ghalehkhondabi V, Soleymani M, Fazlali A. Folate-targeted nanomicelles containing silibinin as an active drug delivery system for liver cancer therapy. J Drug Deliv Sci Technol 2021; 61: 102157. [http://dx.doi.org/10.1016/j.jddst.2020.102157]

[35] Amiri B, Ahmadvand H, Farhadi A, Najmafshar A, Chiani M, Norouzian D. Delivery of vinblastine-containing niosomes results in potent *in vitro* / *in vivo* cytotoxicity on tumor cells. Drug Dev Ind Pharm 2018; 44(8): 1371-6. [http://dx.doi.org/10.1080/03639045.2018.1451880] [PMID: 29532687]

[36] Kamoun WS, Dugast AS, Suchy JJ, *et al.* Synergy between EphA2-ILs-DTXp, a novel EphA2-targeted nanoliposomal taxane, and PD-1 inhibitors in preclinical tumor models. Mol Cancer Ther 2020; 19(1): 270-81. [http://dx.doi.org/10.1158/1535-7163.MCT-19-0414] [PMID: 31597714]

[37] Singh N, Sachdev A, Gopinath P. Polysaccharide functionalized single walled carbon nanotubes as nanocarriers for delivery of curcumin in lung cancer cells. J Nanosci Nanotechnol 2018; 18(3): 1534-41. [http://dx.doi.org/10.1166/jnn.2018.14222] [PMID: 29448627]

[38] Tian Z, Shi Y, Yin M, Shen H, Jia N. Functionalized multiwalled carbon nanotubes-anticancer drug carriers: synthesis, targeting ability and antitumor activity. Nano Biomed Eng 2011; 3(3) [http://dx.doi.org/10.5101/nbe.v3i3.p157-162]

[39] Arrigo R, Dintcheva NT, Guenzi M, Gambarotti C. Nano-hybrids based on quercetin and carbon nanotubes with excellent anti-oxidant activity. Mater Lett 2016; 180: 7-10. [http://dx.doi.org/10.1016/j.matlet.2016.05.096]

[40] Wang C, Li W. Preparation, characterization, and *in vitro* and *vivo* antitumor activity of oridonin-conjugated multiwalled carbon nanotubes functionalized with carboxylic group. Journal of Nanomaterials 2016; 2016

[41] Tan JM, Karthivashan G, Arulselvan P, Fakurazi S, Hussein MZ. Sustained release and cytotoxicity evaluation of carbon nanotube-mediated drug delivery system for betulinic acid. Journal of Nanomaterials 2014; 2014 [http://dx.doi.org/10.1155/2014/862148]

[42] Donoso-Quezada J, Guajardo-Flores D, González-Valdez J. Enhanced exosome-mediated delivery of black bean phytochemicals (Phaseolus vulgaris L.) for cancer treatment applications. Biomed Pharmacother 2020; 131: 110771. [http://dx.doi.org/10.1016/j.biopha.2020.110771] [PMID: 33152932]

[43] Liu H, Shen M, Zhao D, Ru D, Duan Y, Ding C, *et al.* The effect of triptolide-loaded exosomes on the proliferation and apoptosis of human ovarian cancer SKOV3 cells. BioMed research international 2019; 2019 [http://dx.doi.org/10.1155/2019/2595801]

[44] Long X, Fan M, Bigsby RM, Nephew KP. Apigenin inhibits antiestrogen-resistant breast cancer cell growth through estrogen receptor-α-dependent and estrogen receptor-α-independent mechanisms. Mol Cancer Ther 2008; 7(7): 2096-108. [http://dx.doi.org/10.1158/1535-7163.MCT-07-2350] [PMID: 18645020]

[45] Liu L, Fan J, Ai G, *et al.* Berberine in combination with cisplatin induces necroptosis and apoptosis in ovarian cancer cells. Biol Res 2019; 52(1): 37. [http://dx.doi.org/10.1186/s40659-019-0243-6] [PMID: 31319879]

[46] Mittal A, Tabasum S, Singh RP. Berberine in combination with doxorubicin suppresses growth of murine melanoma B16F10 cells in culture and xenograft. Phytomedicine 2014; 21(3): 340-7. [http://dx.doi.org/10.1016/j.phymed.2013.09.002] [PMID: 24176840]

[47] Dhandapani KM, Mahesh VB, Brann DW. Curcumin suppresses growth and chemoresistance of human glioblastoma cells via AP-1 and NFκB transcription factors. J Neurochem 2007; 102(2): 522-38.
[http://dx.doi.org/10.1111/j.1471-4159.2007.04633.x] [PMID: 17596214]

[48] Montopoli M, Ragazzi E, Froldi G, Caparrotta L. Cell-cycle inhibition and apoptosis induced by curcumin and cisplatin or oxaliplatin in human ovarian carcinoma cells. Cell Prolif 2009; 42(2): 195-206.
[http://dx.doi.org/10.1111/j.1365-2184.2009.00585.x] [PMID: 19236381]

[49] Jose A, Labala S, Ninave KM, Gade SK, Venuganti VVK. Effective skin cancer treatment by topical co-delivery of curcumin and STAT3 siRNA using cationic liposomes. AAPS PharmSciTech 2018; 19(1): 166-75.
[http://dx.doi.org/10.1208/s12249-017-0833-y] [PMID: 28639178]

[50] Xing ZH, Wei JH, Cheang TY, *et al.* Bifunctional pH-sensitive Zn(ii)–curcumin nanoparticles/siRNA effectively inhibit growth of human bladder cancer cells *in vitro* and *in vivo.* J Mater Chem B Mater Biol Med 2014; 2(18): 2714-24.
[http://dx.doi.org/10.1039/c3tb21625j] [PMID: 32261437]

[51] Sharma V, Hupp C, Tepe J. Enhancement of chemotherapeutic efficacy by small molecule inhibition of NF-kappaB and checkpoint kinases. Curr Med Chem 2007; 14(10): 1061-74.
[http://dx.doi.org/10.2174/092986707780362844] [PMID: 17456020]

[52] Papazisis KT, Kalemi TG, Zambouli D, *et al.* Synergistic effects of protein tyrosine kinase inhibitor genistein with camptothecins against three cell lines *in vitro.* Cancer Lett 2006; 233(2): 255-64.
[http://dx.doi.org/10.1016/j.canlet.2005.03.022] [PMID: 15893418]

[53] Chan MM, Soprano KJ, Weinstein K, Fong D. Epigallocatechin-3-gallate delivers hydrogen peroxide to induce death of ovarian cancer cells and enhances their cisplatin susceptibility. J Cell Physiol 2006; 207(2): 389-96.
[http://dx.doi.org/10.1002/jcp.20569] [PMID: 16402374]

[54] Zhang Q, Wei D, Liu J. *In vivo* reversal of doxorubicin resistance by (−)-epigallocatechin gallate in a solid human carcinoma xenograft. Cancer Lett 2004; 208(2): 179-86.
[http://dx.doi.org/10.1016/j.canlet.2004.01.033] [PMID: 15142676]

[55] Henrich CJ, Bokesch HR, Dean M, *et al.* A high-throughput cell-based assay for inhibitors of ABCG2 activity. SLAS Discov 2006; 11(2): 176-83.
[http://dx.doi.org/10.1177/1087057105284576] [PMID: 16490770]

[56] Rajagopalan P, Dera A, Abdalsamad MRC, C Chandramoorthy H. Rational combinations of indirubin and arylidene derivatives exhibit synergism in human non-small cell lung carcinoma cells. J Food Biochem 2019; 43(7): e12861.
[http://dx.doi.org/10.1111/jfbc.12861] [PMID: 31353710]

[57] Mohan L, Raghav D, Ashraf SM, Sebastian J, Rathinasamy K. Indirubin, a bis-indole alkaloid binds to tubulin and exhibits antimitotic activity against HeLa cells in synergism with vinblastine. Biomed Pharmacother 2018; 105: 506-17.
[http://dx.doi.org/10.1016/j.biopha.2018.05.127] [PMID: 29883946]

[58] Limtrakul P, Khantamat O, Pintha K. Inhibition of P-glycoprotein function and expression by kaempferol and quercetin. J Chemother 2005; 17(1): 86-95.
[http://dx.doi.org/10.1179/joc.2005.17.1.86] [PMID: 15828450]

[59] Du GJ, Song ZH, Lin HH, Han X, Zhang S, Yang Y. Luteolin as a glycolysis inhibitor offers superior efficacy and lesser toxicity of doxorubicin in breast cancer cells. Biochem Biophys Res Commun 2008; 372(3): 497-502.
[http://dx.doi.org/10.1016/j.bbrc.2008.05.080] [PMID: 18503759]

[60] Kuhar M, Imran S, Singh N. Curcumin and quercetin combined with cisplatin to induce apoptosis in human laryngeal carcinoma Hep-2 cells through the mitochondrial pathway. J Cancer Mol 2007; 3(4): 121-8.

[61] Kweon SH, Song JH, Kim TS. Resveratrol-mediated reversal of doxorubicin resistance in acute myeloid leukemia cells *via* downregulation of MRP1 expression. Biochem Biophys Res Commun 2010; 395(1): 104-10.
[http://dx.doi.org/10.1016/j.bbrc.2010.03.147] [PMID: 20350534]

[62] Dhanalakshmi S, Agarwal P, Glode LM, Agarwal R. Silibinin sensitizes human prostate carcinoma DU145 cells to cisplatin- and carboplatin-induced growth inhibition and apoptotic death. Int J Cancer 2003; 106(5): 699-705.
[http://dx.doi.org/10.1002/ijc.11299] [PMID: 12866029]

SUBJECT INDEX

A

B

C

D

E

F

G

H

I

K

L

M

N

X

Made in the USA
Las Vegas, NV
03 November 2026

57422016R00193